Atlas of Urologic Endoscopic Surgery

Atlas of Urologic Endoscopic Surgery

Hans J. Reuter

Translated by
Roland J. Kohen
Matthias A. Reuter

Foreword by Victor A. Politano

1982

W. B. Saunders Company
Philadelphia London Toronto Mexico City Rio de Janeiro Sydney

Georg Thieme Verlag Stuttgart

Prof. Hans J. Reuter, M.D.
Urologic Hospital
Humboldtstr. 16
D-7000 Stuttgart 1
West Germany

Roland J. Kohen, M.D., F.A.C.S.
Mount Sinai Hospital
Miami Beach, Florida/U.S.A.

Matthias A. Reuter, M.D.
University of Tuebingen
West Germany

W. B. Saunders Company: West Washington Square
Philadelphia, PA 19105

1 St. Anne's Road
Eastbourne, East Sussex BN21 3UN, England

1 Goldthorne Avenue
Toronto, Ontario M8Z 5T9, Canada

Apartado 26370 – Cedro 512
Mexico 4, D.F., Mexico

Rua Coronel Cabrita, 8
Sao Cristovao Caixa Postal 21176
Rio de Janeiro, Brazil

9 Waltham Street
Artarmon, N.S.W. 2064, Australia

Original German edition *Atlas der urologischen Endoskopie, Vol. 1*

Authorized English edition copublished 1982 by W. B. Saunders Company, Philadelphia, and Georg Thieme Verlag, Stuttgart.

ISBN 3-13-601901-6 (Thieme)
ISBN 0-7216-7567-0 (Saunders)
LC catalog card No. 81-52134

Atlas of Urologic Endoscopic Surgery ISBN 0-7216-7567-0

Dedicated to the urologists and endoscopists, who are my models and to whom I am personally indebted:

Max Hösel
Vincent Vermooten
John L. Emmet
Rubin H. Flocks
Roger W. Barnes
Luis Cifuentes Delatte
Einar Ljunggren
Roberto Rocha Brito
Martin Stolze

on the occasion of the 20th anniversary of the Urologische Klinik Professor Dr. Reuter, Stuttgart, Germany.

Foreword

Transurethral surgery blossomed with the development and subsequent improvement of endoscopic instruments. Better lens systems that afford greater visibility; fiberoptic light sources; improved working elements; electrosurgical units with rapid, clean cutting currents and precise pinpoint coagulation—all contributed to this success story.

Fiberoptic teaching attachments have improved and simplified the teaching of endoscopy and transurethral surgery. Blood replacement, antibiotics, monitoring of electrolytes and fluids and improved anesthesia have made transurethral surgery safe and practical.

In spite of these many scientific and technical advancements, good endoscopic surgery requires a clear understanding of the anatomy and landmarks of the bladder, bladder neck, prostatic urethra and membranous urethra. This new *Atlas of Urologic Endoscopic Surgery* by Doctor H.J. Reuter is a precise, clear and beautifully illustrated book that will help teach and orient the student of endoscopic surgery. The already experienced endoscopist will be improved by the many fine points of technique presented. The author's original concepts of low pressure continuous flow during endoscopic surgery are well illustrated and described.

The chapters devoted to cryosurgery of the prostate and bladder tumors reveal the tremendous expertise gained in this field and may well represent the largest experience in the world. Detailed descriptions with illustrations and color photographs are most explicit.

A statistical review of the large experience in both transurethral surgery and cryosurgery is presented. The mortality rate for transurethral prostatic surgery has been reduced to 0.3 per cent. Complications and their frequency of occurrence are reviewed.

The beautiful color photographs of surgery in progress truly bring transurethral surgery to life. Both as a teaching aid and as a reference guide, this Atlas should become a part of the armamentarium of all physicians interested in endoscopic surgery.

VICTOR A. POLITANO, M.D.

Preface

The purpose of this atlas is to explain and illustrate "low pressure transurethral resection" with continuous aspiration of irrigant via the suprapubic trocar or the return flow-resectoscope. This procedure was developed at our hospital and is performed as total transurethral prostatectomy for adenoma and as total or radical resection of prostatic cancer and of bladder tumors.

The atlas is also intended to demonstrate the advantages of "low pressure TUR" over the conventional method (high pressure TUR) and to evaluate our material statistically. During low pressure TUR the tissues of the prostatic capsule and the bladder neck can be identified clearly because hemorrhage is minimal. Irrigant absorption and the TUR syndrome are thus prevented, so that there is a low rate of complications and mortality. The operating time is almost unlimited. The new technique increases the ability of a skilled resectionist and facilitates teaching, since the interruption for bladder evacuation is superfluous and coagulation is easier.

Another purpose is to acquaint the reader with the new technique of endoscopic cryosurgery. This new method avoids the disadvantages of the blind technique. In addition, the ice ball can be measured exactly and thus controlled intravesically and subvesically. Furthermore, we have developed a central freezing technique with a trocar cryoprobe (trocar cryosurgery). For the first time, long-term results of these methods are presented. Trocar TUR and cryosurgery have caused a significant decrease in the total mortality and complications from our prostatic operations.

Open surgery of the lower urinary tract, prostate and bladder tumors can be significantly but not totally replaced by operative endoscopy. Often both methods complement each other, as, for instance, radical TUR, cryosurgery and lymphadenectomy for treatment of cancer. The preference for open surgery in the treatment of certain kinds of prostatic and bladder carcinomas, for example, is not jeopardized. In these cases endoscopy is also important as a diagnostic tool and useful as a therapeutic method for recurrent tumors. This applies also to irradiation, chemotherapy and immunotherapy. In addition, we demonstrate regional lymphatics by radionuclide scintigraphy and utilize operative angiography therapeutically.

It is necessary for me to pay my respects to men like Edwin Beer, Maximilian Stern, Joseph F. McCarthy, Roger W. Barnes, Reed M. Nesbit, Reinhold Wappler and Maurice J. Gonder. These urologists, following in the footsteps of Max Nitze, Josef Leiter and Georg Wolf, laid the foundation for transurethral operations. The perfection of TUR and more recently cryosurgery would not have been possible without the meticulous and often misunderstood early work of these men. In particular, George O. Baumrucker described the mistakes and dangers of TUR in an inimitable way.

The instrument makers also contributed to TUR. Personally I am obliged to Annemarie and Richard Wolf, who have continued the great Berlin tradition of instrument making. They developed the excellent modern resectoscope used by my teacher Max Hösel, who introduced TUR successfully into Germany in the 1940s. In 1968 our first continuous-flow urethroscope was constructed with an irrigating chamber (R. Wolf). The first continuous-flow resectoscope was presented in 1973 during the third international symposium, and was later equipped with a channel for measuring bladder pressure after M.A. Reuter (1975). Subsequently, the continuous-flow urethrotome was developed. In 1979, in his dissertation at the University of Freiburg, M. A. Reuter explained the principles of irrigation during TUR.

I wish to thank Doctor Günther Hauff from the Georg Thieme Verlag, Stuttgart, Germany, for the generous format of this book.

Stuttgart, Autumn 1979 H. J. Reuter

Contents

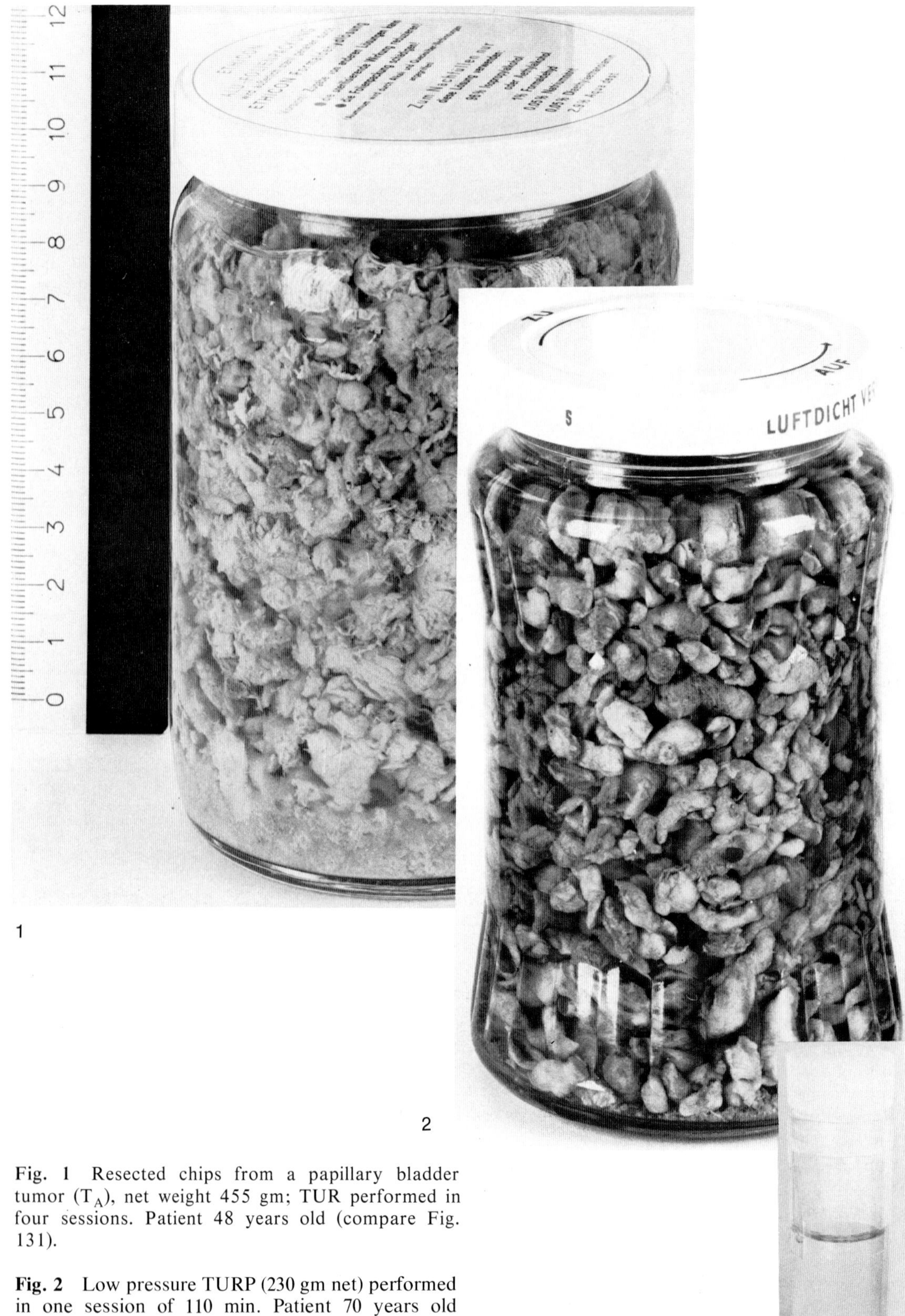

Fig. 1 Resected chips from a papillary bladder tumor (T_A), net weight 455 gm; TUR performed in four sessions. Patient 48 years old (compare Fig. 131).

Fig. 2 Low pressure TURP (230 gm net) performed in one session of 110 min. Patient 70 years old (compare Figs. 55–56).

Fig. 3 TUR of a sclerotic sphincter: 78 chips resected in 30 minutes in a 5-year-old boy (compare Fig. 70).

Transurethral Resection — TUR

"All that can be obtained by suprapubic, retropubic, or the conservative way of perineal prostatectomy can be obtained by TUR as well" (R. H. Flocks 1969).

The new technique of transurethral prostatectomy (TURP with physiologic low pressure irrigation and continuous aspiration of irrigant) reduces postoperative complications and mortality significantly when compared to conventional transurethral resection (TUR) and open prostatectomy.

The new technique of endoscopic cryosurgery of adenoma (in the poor risk patient) and of carcinoma of the prostate is an optimal complement to TUR; it reduces mortality of prostatic operations to a minimum hitherto unreached.

INTRODUCTION

The technique of transurethral prostatectomy (TURP) can be acquired by every urologist with average talent, but in reality the number of perfect resectionists is very small. Sometimes partial TUR, which is not up to standards, is performed in place of TURP, especially of larger adenomas over 30 gm (Fig. 2).

The reasons are the following: TUR requires a more perfect technique than do other operations. The skills needed to perform open surgical prostatectomy can be achieved after a few dozen operations. TURP, however, requires the training of several hundred operations if tumors larger than 50 gm are to be resected without difficulty. For a TURP of 100 gm, 1 or, better, 2 gm of adenomatous tissue should be resected per minute, including time needed for coagulation.

Physiologic low pressure irrigation with continuous aspiration of irrigant (see p. 25) facilitates TURP so that the resection speed of the surgeon is doubled within a short time of training. This stretches the indications for TURP to include the patient with higher operative risk. Who wants to perform open surgical prostatectomy, for instance, on a 75-year-old patient with cerebral sclerosis, diabetes or cardiac insufficiency? Particularly when one considers that these patients often have, because of their age, very large prostatic adenomas.

The student does not always know the theoretic and technical basis of TUR. Furthermore, he lacks exact knowledge of the structure of the different layers of prostatic tissue (see p. 40). It is the task of this atlas to help remedy this situation. The technique of TUR cannot be learned by passive watching. The teacher has to use the teaching attachment and the student the resectoscope. He should operate on several cases with small adenomas (up to 20 gm) and larger adenomas (from 30 to 50 gm) each week to perfect his TUR technique.

For many reasons TURP cannot be the routine procedure for every adenoma. Partial TUR is doubtless not an adequate alternative to open surgical prostatectomy. Here, endoscopic cryosurgery is closing the gap.

Postoperative mortality can be decreased definitively when the three techniques of prostatic operations are performed as follows:

(1) TURP as a routine operation for about 85 per cent of prostatic adenomas and radical TUR for selected prostatic carcinomas in stages T_1 to T_3.

(2) Endoscopic cryosurgery for poor-risk patients with prostatic adenoma (about 10 per cent) and with selected cases of prostatic carcinoma stages T_2 to T_4 (an exception is the young patient with prostatic carcinoma in stage T_1).

(3) Open surgical prostatectomy for patients below 70 years of age without operating risk (risk degree 0; see p. 6) with a large adenoma (80 gm or more). Radical open prostatectomy is used for patients with prostatic carcinoma in stage T_2; here, however, radical TUR and cryosurgery and implantation of radioactive iodine (Whitmore) are indicated as well.

Why are endoscopic procedures preferred over open surgical operations? Good TURP with continuous low pressure irrigation under conduction anesthesia spares the patient the risks of open surgery and its pains as well as the dangers general anesthesia holds for the geriatric heart and brain. Besides that, effective costs of endoscopic surgery are significantly lower for patient and hospital than those of open surgery (care, anesthesia, surgical assistance, transfusion).

Postoperative mortality of TURP is 0.3 per cent in our hospital (1000 cases in 6 years) and 1.2 per cent as a mean of several authors. This success has not been matched by any open surgical method, where postoperative mortality is still between 3 and 4 per cent (collective statistics of several authors, Table 8, p. 234).

Patients over 70 years of age should not be operated on by open surgery. The choice of the appropriate operative procedure is facilitated by the classification of operating risk (see p. 6).

Definition of TUR

TUR (*t*rans*u*rethral *r*esection) is too universal a term for use in this discussion. The term "TURP" is often used incorrectly for partial TUR. A precise definition is therefore necessary (Fig. 4).

(1) *Pseudo-TUR.* Here only a small part of the adenoma is resected (0 to 30 per cent, mostly less than 10 gm), with a few cuts into the bladder neck (barrier), into the median lobe in the form of a channel, or TUR of the median lobe alone. Rectal findings are the same as before TUR. No excavation of the prostatic mass is demonstrated by cystography. The pseudo-TUR is inadequate in any case.

(2) *Partial TUR.* Only 30 to 90 per cent of the adenoma is resected.

(a) *Palliative resection.* TUR of a maximum of 50 per cent is performed, most often forming a crater in the proximal third of the prostatic mass at the bladder neck. The result is not good. Most of the patients have to be resected again one to five years later. This has given TUR a bad reputation.

(b) *Subtotal TUR.* Up to 90 per cent of the adenoma is resected. A cone is resected off the fossa: its tip lying within the apex and its base within the bladder neck. The apex, the most difficult part of TUR, is not resected totally. Long-term results of this TUR are mostly good. A significantly smaller prostate is found by rectal palpation after subtotal TUR. The prostatic fossa is not completed as demonstrated on the cystogram (see Fig. 57). Endoscopically, rough adenomatous residuals are verified at the apex, especially on the anterior part between 9 and 3 o'clock (see Fig. 108).

(3) *TURP (total TUR: transurethral prostatectomy).* Approximately 100 per cent of the adenoma is resected, as in open surgical prostatectomy. In addition, parts of the trigone, bladder neck and prostatic capsule (e.g., inflammatory infiltration) are resected. The internal and external sphincter both form a completely round opening; the prostatic fossa has the shape of a hollow sphere (Figs. 4, 107). On rectal palpation the capsule is felt only as a flat plate; a prominent adenoma is not palpable. A regular tongue-shaped excavation is seen on the cystogram below the bladder (Fig. 7). Endoscopically, a prostatic urethra with smooth walls and no adenomatous residuals is seen (Fig. 91). TURP is the only adequate alternative to open surgical prostatectomy.

(4) *(Sub-)radical TUR.* The prostatic carcinoma, the coincident adenoma and the prostatic capsule are resected totally. The carcinomatous infiltration is resected into the healthy periprostatic tissue. Radical TUR requires special indications involving the age of the patient, operative risk and the stage of the carcinoma. Often, larger parts of the capsule remain after incorrect radical TURP. Lymphadenectomy and vesiculectomy eventually must be performed as well.

By rectal palpation only the wall of the rectum over the hard bone of the symphysis is felt. The typically firm consistency of the prostatic capsule cannot be palpated. On the cystogram, the prostatic fossa is unusually large, and not infrequently is misshapen on one side (fat deposits; Fig. 61). Endoscopically, extraprostatic tissues, e.g., muscle of the levator ani and longitudinal muscle of the rectum, are seen (Fig. 95). Radical TUR has relatively good results; its rate of causing incontinence is low (about 2 per cent).

(5) *Diagnostic TUR.* A certain part of the prostate is resected — for cxample, a suspicious carcinomatous node. It is advisable to resect a simultaneously existing adenoma totally. Diagnostic TUR is also performed in prostatic abscess, tuberculosis, bilharziasis, leiomyoma, prostatic stone and diverticulum.

Finally, it should be mentioned that the results of TUR can be confirmed by transurethral and transrectal ultrasonic scanning (Watanabe, H. et al.; Gammelgard, J.).

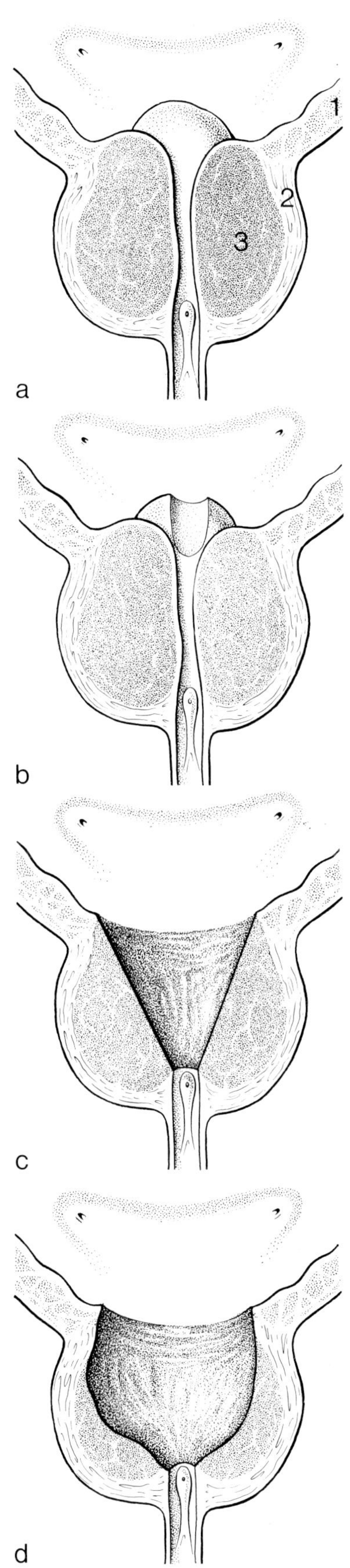

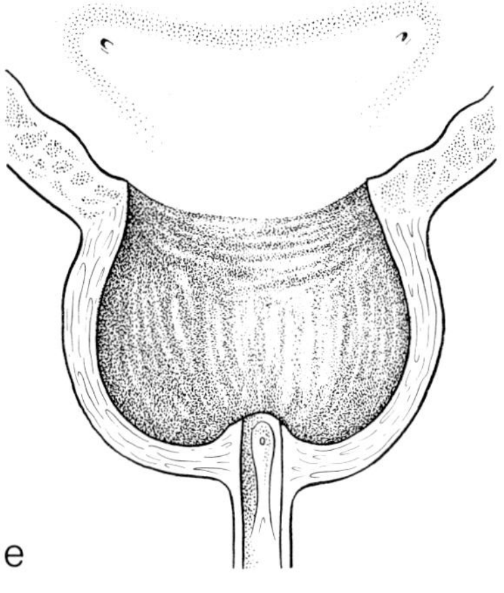

Fig. 4, a–e Value of endoscopic prostatic operations (longitudinal sections through the prostatic fossa comparable to x-ray cystograms).

(a) Subvesical prostatic adenoma: 1 = bladder wall; 2 = capsule; 3 = adenoma (compare Figs. 55, a, 64, a, 67, a); (b) Pseudo-TUR: groove in the middle lobe (not verifiable by cystogram); (c) Partial TUR: funnel reaching down to the verumontanum (compare Fig. 5); (d) Subtotal TUR: adenomatous remainders at the apex (compare Fig. 58, a); (e) (total TUR) TURP; hollow sphere without adenomatous remnants, result equivalent to open surgical prostatectomy (compare Fig. 62, b).

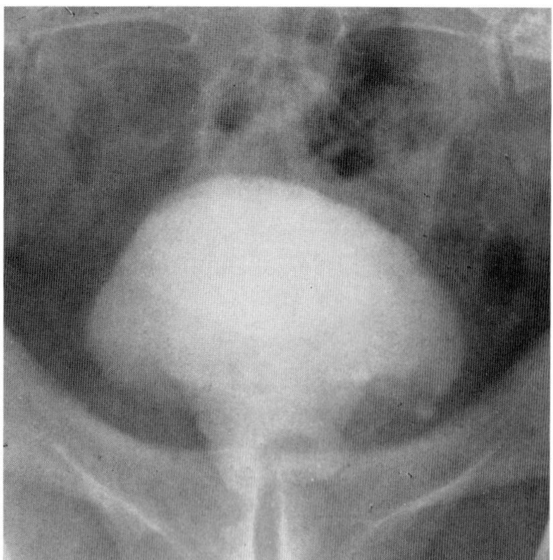

Fig. 5 Partial TUR of a large adenoma (about 80 gm) in a poor-risk patient.

The postoperative cystogram (13 × 18 cm) shows a crater-shaped prostatic fossa (4 × 2 cm) below a mushroom bladder shadow four days after TUR (60 gm net in 50 min). The bladder neck has an irregular outline, especially at the left, suggesting adenomatous remnants of the lateral lobes. The crater is not completely cut below; here, adenomatous tissue remained at the apex. TUR was performed only partially in this 83-year-old patient because of high risk (group III) and short life expectancy. Voiding leaves no residual urine; good permanent result.

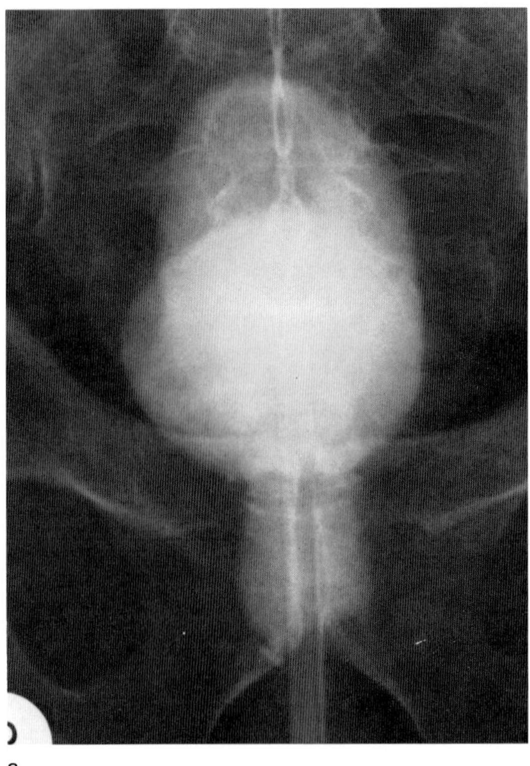

a

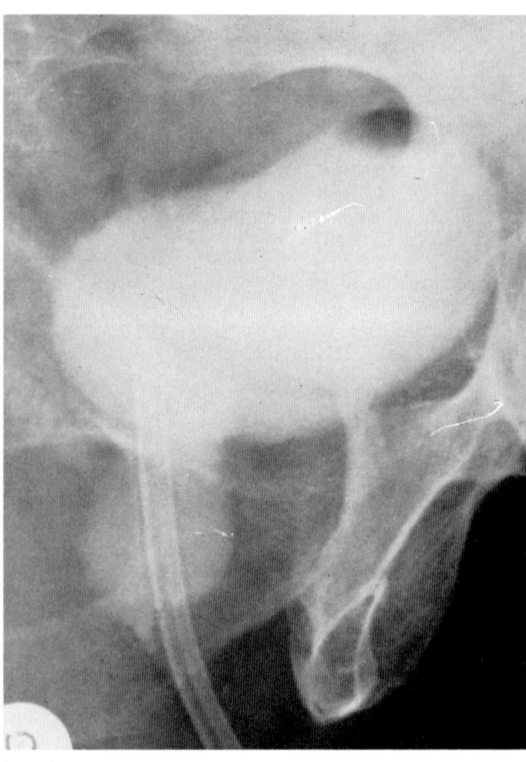

b

Fig. 6, a–b Subtotal TURP with small adenomatous remnants at the apex.

In this 60-year-old patient, an adenoma of 60 gm net was resected in 55 min. Low pressure irrigation with continuous trocar aspiration was used.

(a) The bladder is well contracted. It shows a double contour on the AP film (13 × 18 cm) caused by a hood (see Fig. 6, b) on top of the bladder. The internal sphincter delineates the pear-shaped prostatic fossa (3.5 × 2.5 cm) well from the bladder. An adenomatous remnant at the left apex is verified as a convexity of the fossa (column of the lateral "lobe").

(b) The oblique lateral exposure (13 × 18 cm) demonstrates the typical pear shape of the fossa (3.5 × 3 cm). Adenoma remained ventrally at the apex (12 o'clock). It fits into a small groove that seems to be cut into the right (Fig. 6, a) and lateral part of the external sphincter. The patient is not incontinent. The tip of the catheter lies within the bladder (5-cc balloon deflated).

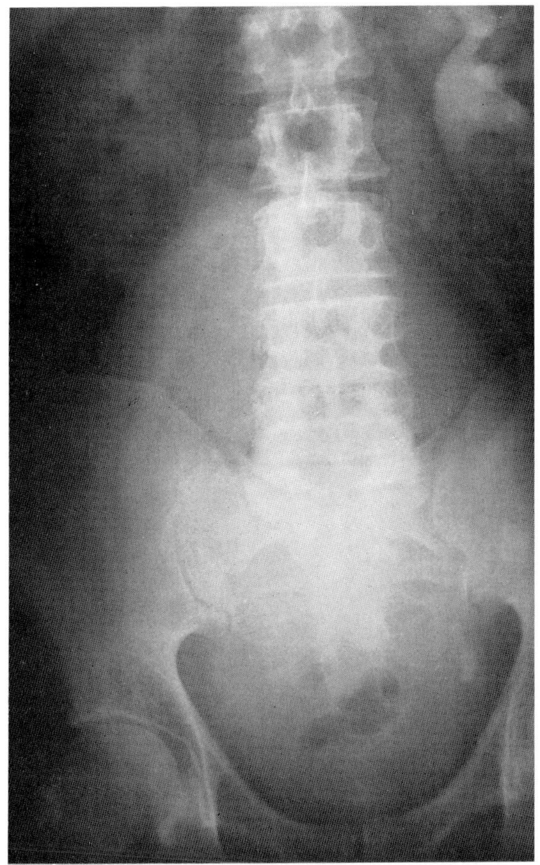

a

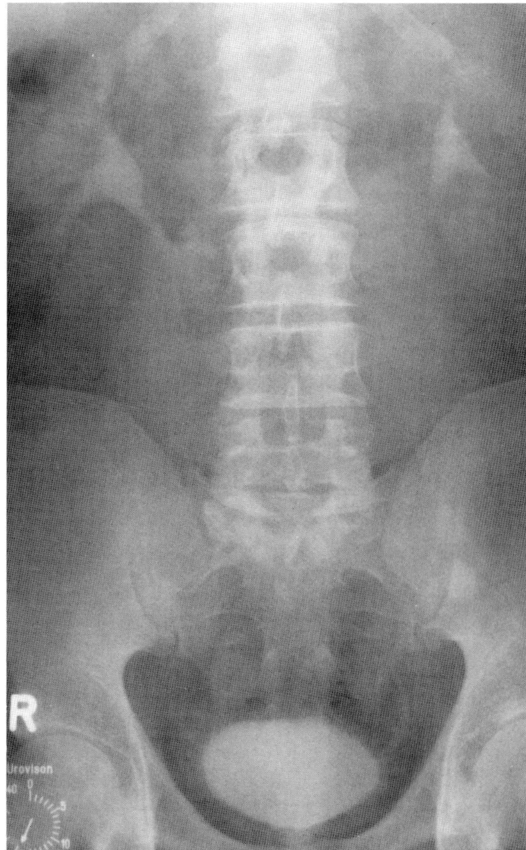

c

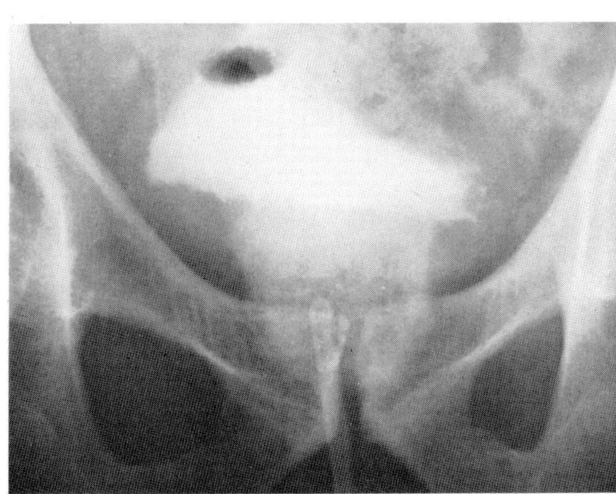

b

Fig. 7, a–c TURP of a large subvesical prostatic adenoma in an extremely atonic bladder.

(a) IV urogram before the operation (35 × 40 cm film). Two hours after injection of contrast medium, an overlarge bladder (2.2-liter content) and significantly congested kidneys were seen. This 58-year-old patient was referred for evaluation of an abdominal tumor. No urologic complaints; micturition reported to be without disturbance. Two-month preoperative preparation with a permanent catheter was necessary.

(b) Cystogram (13 × 18 cm) with 50 cc of contrast medium after TURP of 85 gm net adenomatous tissue. The bladder lies slack over the broad horizontal bladder neck; below hangs a regular tongue-shaped fossa 5 × 6 cm in diameter. The catheter (20 Fr., 5-cc balloon, three-way) is seen at the apex.

(c) IV urography four years after TURP (35 × 40 cm film). Apart from a small forebladder at the bladder neck, the urinary tract is completely normal.

A New Concept of Prostatic Surgery

Thanks to low-pressure TUR and endoscopic cryosurgery, the total mortality of prostatic operations over the past ten years was reduced to less than 1 per cent (Table 10). As shown below, the indications for the different procedures are determined by the risk-degree of the patient:

(1) *TUR.* Patients with risk-degree 0 to II (III in the exceptional case) = 74 per cent of our prostatic operations (mortality 0.36 per cent).

(2) *Cryosurgery.* High-risk patients with prostatic adenoma (risk-degree II to IV) are mainly treated with cold, as are about 50 per cent of prostatic carcinoma patients = 26 per cent of our cases (mortality 1.8 per cent). This unusually high percentage represents our referred patient population.

(3) *Open Surgical Prostatectomy.* Open surgery is restricted to a few patients less than 70 years old (for mortality, see Table 8) with risk degree 0 and an overly large adenoma (over 100 gm).

TUR is performed as a rule as transurethral prostatectomy (TURP) or for prostatic cancer as (sub)radical TUR. Aseptic, physiologic conditions are maintained with a closed continuous irrigation system (low-pressure TUR). Intervals of irrigation and traumatization of the bladder and prostatic fossa are avoided by continuous aspiration of irrigant from the nearly empty and thus inactivated bladder (trocar TUR or backflow resectoscope). Conduction anesthesia (peridural) is preferred over general anesthesia.

Trocar TUR prevents the TUR syndrome. Arterial and venous hemorrhages are significantly reduced, since the blood pressure does not rise, as usually occurs in high-pressure irrigation (owing to irrigant absorption) and since the filled bladder does not obstruct venous drainage of the prostate. Catheter compression (balloon with 30 to 50 cc) is applied only in extreme bleeding of venous sinuses (in less than 1 per cent; see p. 62; compare Fig. 48). Blood transfusion is rarely necessary (Table 6, p. 233).

Postoperatively, continuous suprapubic low pressure irrigation is applied to the bladder and prostatic fossa. (A small tube or a 12 Fr Foley catheter is introduced suprapubically through the trocar after TUR and a 18 Fr Foley catheter with a 5-cc balloon transurethrally; the irrigant bag is suspended only about 20 cm over the patient.) Electronic catheter control prevents complications due to obstruction of the irrigating system (chills, fever). Antibiotics are not routinely applied (hospitalism). They are replaced by instillation and suprapubic continuous irrigation with solutions of 10 per cent iodine (povidone–iodine: for instillation, 1:50; for irrigation, 1:200 dilution).

Strict hygiene of the nursing staff is enforced (sterile gloves, repeated disinfection of the patient's hands, etc.; see Statistics. p. 231).

Classification of Operative Risk

Guidelines for the rating of risk of prostatic operations (Schlegel).

0. Patient in Normal Condition

Age up to 70 years; several minimal deviations from normal:

(a) Blood pressure: up to 160/100 mm Hg (if untreated essential hypertonia is the only abnormal finding, a blood pressure of up to 200/110 mm Hg is tolerated).

(b) Uncomplicated diabetes, well managed by diet.

(c) Chronic urinary infection but normal renal function established by intravenous pyelogram and renal function scintigraphy; serum urea and creatinine within normal limits; normal creatinine clearance: the specific gravity of urine after concentration test over 1.015; residual urine but no chronic alterations of the bladder (diverticula, stones and atony).

I. Patients with Moderate Operative Risk

Several defects related to general condition and age; no need for intensified therapeutic effort. Renal function is not reduced significantly.

II. Patient with Mean Operative Risk

Significant chronic diseases or residuals needing constant medical care — e.g., diabetes, hypertension and long-standing angina pectoris requiring medication; condition following one or two mild myocardial infarctions; pulmonary emphysema with a vital capacity of 2500 to 3000 cc; moderate bronchial asthma; cardiac insufficiency well stabilized by prolonged glycoside therapy; compensated liver insufficiency; condition after major surgery requiring continuous replacement therapy. Age over 80 years; progressive cerebral sclerosis; compensated renal insufficiency.

Obvious but not extreme alterations of the intravenous pyelogram and renal function scintigram. Significant changes of blood electrolytes with deviation of blood pH; creatinine clearance not below 80 per cent.

III. High Risk Patient

Life expectancy less than five years; decompensated diseases requiring constant therapy, e.g., diabetes dependent on administered insulin; cardiac insufficiency difficult to compensate; significant changes of the ECG after myocardial infarction; grave cardiac arrhythmia; excessive hypertension not responsive to antihypertensive agents; severe bronchial asthma; paraplegias following cerebrovascular accident; considerable cerebral sclerosis; age over 90 years; poor general condition; isosthenuria, serum urea up to 90 mg/dl, creatinine clearance below 50 per cent; considerable changes in renal function on scintigram.

IV. Poor Risk Patient

Life expectancy less than one year; several of the defects described under III coexistent. Examples of these conditions include uremia; serious cerebral diseases; peripheral paralysis; cachexia; marasmus; leukemia; terminal prostatic carcinoma or other malignant disease.

Commentary

When estimating the operative risk for a patient, his age, general condition, other diseases and history must be considered. Significant residuals from previous operations will exclude his classification as a normal patient, Group 0. Transitions from one group to another are frequent. The various operative procedures (open surgical, transurethral prostatectomy, cryosurgery) place different strains on the patient. The classification of operative risk, therefore, is intended to help select the correct operative procedure that will correspond to the risk-degree of the patient. Using this system consistently, it is possible to lower total postoperative mortality. We have been able to reduce the postoperative mortality of prostatic operations to 0.7 per cent (Table 10, p. 234).

Teaching of TUR

The large adenoma (30 to 50 gm) is more appropriate for teaching purposes than the smaller lesion. Student errors, e.g., undermining of the lateral lobes, do not lead as quickly to serious complications (perforation, damage to the sphincter, etc.). TUR of the small adenoma is more difficult than TURP of large tumors.

(1) Preliminary instruction may use an animal model (cow's udder) or a cadaver. However, only the technique can be taught, since the typical movements of living tissue and associated hemorrhage are lacking.

(2) Next, the student may practice management of the instrument in a patient at the start and termination of TUR (introduction of the resectoscope, rectal control, irrigation, endoscopy including suprapubic trocar cystoscopy, evacuation of the bladder, sphincter test, catheter).

(3) The structure of the tissue can be studied with the teaching attachment and on films and photographs.

(4) Finally, active participation begins (first cuts, coagulation). By looking through the teaching attachment, the instructor can correct cutting technique. First, the trainee has to learn how to resect the channel for irrigation off the median lobe down to the verumontanum. Only then can he view the whole prostatic urethra and learn to avoid from the beginning a typical pseudo-TUR at the bladder neck. The adenoma is to be thought of as a sphere. Its mass can be totally resected only if all cuts are begun behind the center of the sphere and then brought down to the apex, i.e., the verumontanum (Fig. 8).

The knob on the sheath of the resectoscope is a good teaching aid. It is set at the apex by rectal palpation (see p. 45). Here it lies within the center of rotation of the resectoscope during cutting. Each cut is controlled by rectal palpation. Thus a one-handed resectoscope is essential.

The next step is preparation of the internal sphincter between the 3 and 9 o'clock positions (TUR of the median lobe; then a correct first cut into the lateral lobes). The most difficult part of TUR is at the end of the procedure: preparation of the apex and external sphincter (Figs. 101–103).

Resection of residuals in a follow-up procedure is the best way to learn TUR. All mistakes are promptly seen in the secondarily inflamed indurated tissue, and are easily corrected.

Today, teaching is facilitated by effective new methods: fiberoptics (teaching attachment); low pressure irrigation with continuous aspiration including suprapubic cystoscopy through the trocar sheath; the control knob on the sheath of the resectoscope and the rectal shield. Control of TUR is also possible by TV monitor and magnetic tape.

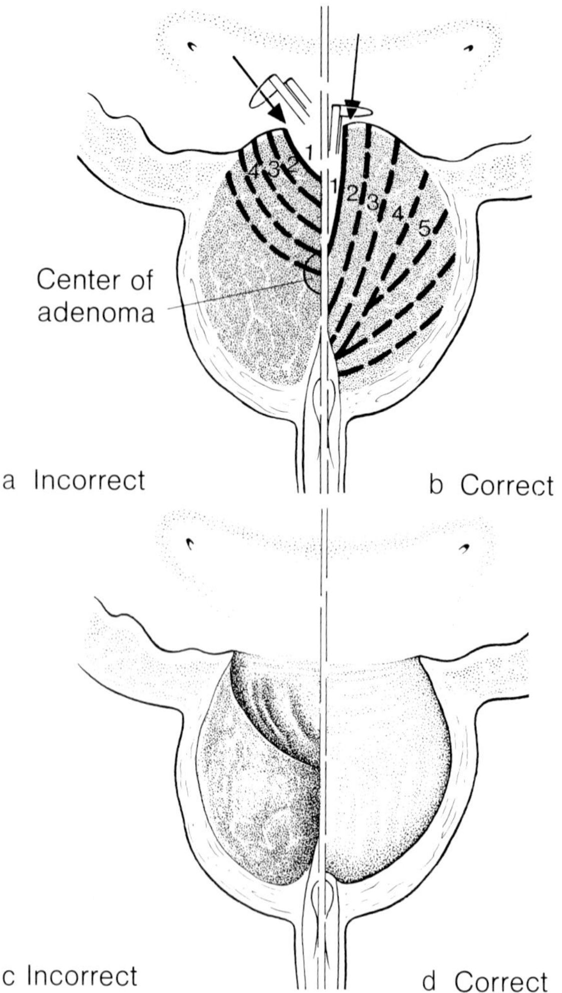

Fig. 8, a–d Guiding the cut during TURP in relation to the mass, particularly the center of the adenoma (frontal section).

(a) The left half of the picture represents schematically a widely used but incorrect cutting technique. The resectoscope is positioned at an angle, and the cutting loop is scarcely extended. Short oblique cuts result; these do not reach beyond the center of the adenoma. The distal mass, including the apex, is not resected here.

(b) The right half of the picture shows correct cutting, the resectoscope positioned axially. The first cuts are already carried distally over the center. In the beginning, the loop is hooked blindly onto the bladder neck until the fibers of the internal sphincter are visible (in this example, from the fourth cut on).

(c) The incorrect technique results in partial resection of the adenoma (partial TUR).

(d) Correct total resection of the adenoma by TURP.

Summary

TUR is useful only if performed totally (TURP). Only years of daily training and secondary resection of every partial TUR will lead to technical mastery of TURP. There is no specialist in TUR who has not experienced perforation, uncoagulable hemorrhage, water intoxication, patient incontinence and other complications.

With continuous low pressure irrigation, efficiency of TUR increases as the rate of complications (hemorrhage, water intoxication) decreases. As an average, 50 gm to a maximum of 150 gm of adenomatous tissue can be resected in one hour, including time spent on coagulation.

Cryosurgery is a possible alternative to partial TUR (e.g., when the operator is not adequately trained in TUR and especially in the poor risk patient and in prostatic cancer).

Open prostatectomy is seldom performed by an experienced resectionist (less than 1 per cent in our hospital) although it is without doubt preferable (especially in risk degree 0) to partial TUR or cryosurgery.

Technical Basics of TUR

The High Frequency Generator

The quality of the cutting and coagulating current is more important in TUR than the most perfect resectoscope (Fig. 9). Careful selection and maintenance of the high frequency generator are essential.

The generator produces two different currents: (1) Tube current for cutting (sinus); (2) Spark-gap current for coagulation (sawtooth).

The cutting current allows smooth cutting without affecting deep tissues, causing no primary necroses of tissue but also no coagulation.

The coagulating current destroys the tissue until it chars, causing necroses several millimeters deep. It therefore is not suited for cutting. These currents can today be simulated electronically.

Bleeding vessels should be coagulated promptly to avoid creating extended areas of necrosis, which can cause dangerous hemorrhage 10 to 30 days postoperatively, when they separate from intact tissue. For this reason, any blind coagulation is to be avoided. Continuous aspiration of irrigant from the bladder will facilitate endoscopic visualization of the bleeder (see Low Pressure Irrigation, p. 25). TUR also may be performed with mixed current; however, we advise use of the two distinct currents during TURP. A mixed current doubles the risk of damage to the prostatic capsule, causing increased rates of bladder neck stricture. Furthermore, the surface of the cut becomes rough, and differentiation of the tissues is made more difficult. Combined currents are less harmful in partial TUR because adenomatous tissue is not as sensitive as the prostatic capsule.

Hazards of the High Frequency Generator

(1) The general hazards of any electrical equipment (defective switches, incomplete grounding, loose connections, incorrect cable layout).

(2) Wrong connection or defective grounding due to confusion of cables and/or defects within the resectoscope. Burning of the patient or surgeon can be the consequence. Connections and switches within cables should be checked or exchanged once a year.

(3) Defects in the foot-switch or the high frequency unit. A dangerous situation develops when the current is not cut off by removing the foot from the switch. The loop of the resectoscope may continue to cut unnoticed. We know of two cases of intraperitoneal perforation that resulted from such a failure. This danger can be avoided only by combining the current with an audible signal. Thus, for example, when examining the bladder for papillomas, the cutting loop must be retracted within the sheath.

(4) Deep coagulation — e.g., of tumors of the bladder roof and anterior wall — is an obsolete technique that can lead to necrosis and traversing peritonitis. We have never experienced these complications after resection of the bladder wall or after covered perforation.

(5) A defective cutting loop can produce a short-circuit in the resectoscope or dangerous, uncontrollable cutting.

(6) The surgeon can burn his fingers when touching the cutting loop for cleaning or shaping if the footswitch has inadvertently been pressed.

(7) The lines between unit and resectoscope must be secured with elastic to prevent uncontrolled tearing of the tissues if the instrument is moved accidentally.

(8) Deadly accidents have been reported as a consequence of attempting to regulate the spark gap while the current is on. An open spark brings danger of explosion. (Do not use disinfectant sprays: the spray gas may explode!) Today, only tube-generators are allowed.

The Resectoscope

The resectoscope is stored as a set together with all the other instruments necessary for TUR and kept sterile in a steel box. The cover of the box is removed before starting TUR, and the envelope of the set (plastic or cotton) is opened. Thus, all the instruments are untouched and ready to use (Fig. 9).

The optical system of a resectoscope resembles a urethroscope: the urethra and bladder are seen from beneath (unlike suprapubic trocar cystoscopy, where they are seen from above; Fig. 10). For operative cystoscopy, an optical system with a 90° to 110° angle of view is introduced into the resectoscope sheath. This facilitates detection of small papillomas, diverticula, stones etc.

Cutting guidance. Because the adenoma is more or less spherical, the ideal cutting loop has the form of a semi-circle. Rotation of the loop around its long axis would be the ideal way of cutting (Fig. 11).

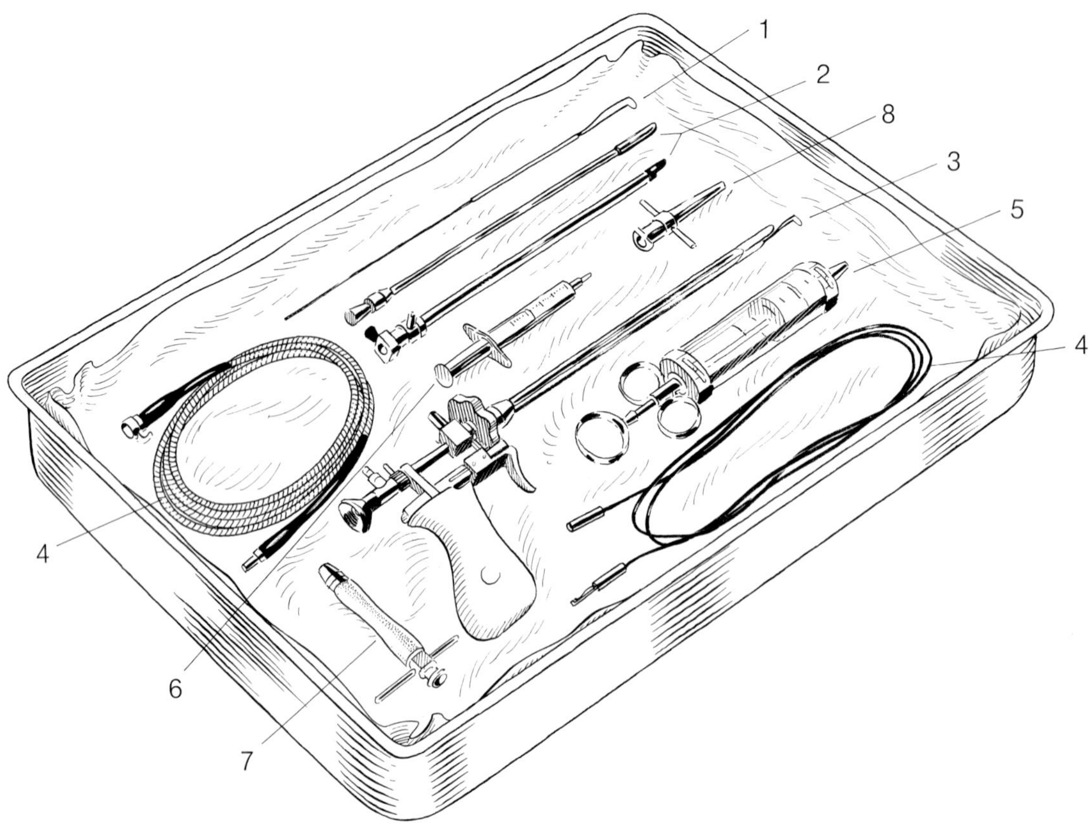

Fig. 9 Complete set of instruments for TUR in a steel container ready for use.

1 = cutting loop (spare part); 2 = sheath and obturator; 3 = electrotome with cutting loop and optical system; 4 = cables (for light and current); 5 = syringe for aspiration (100 cc); 6 = 5-cc syringe with lubricant containing 10 per cent povidone-iodine; 7 = connecting piece between syringe and sheath; 8 = connecting piece for syringe and catheter.

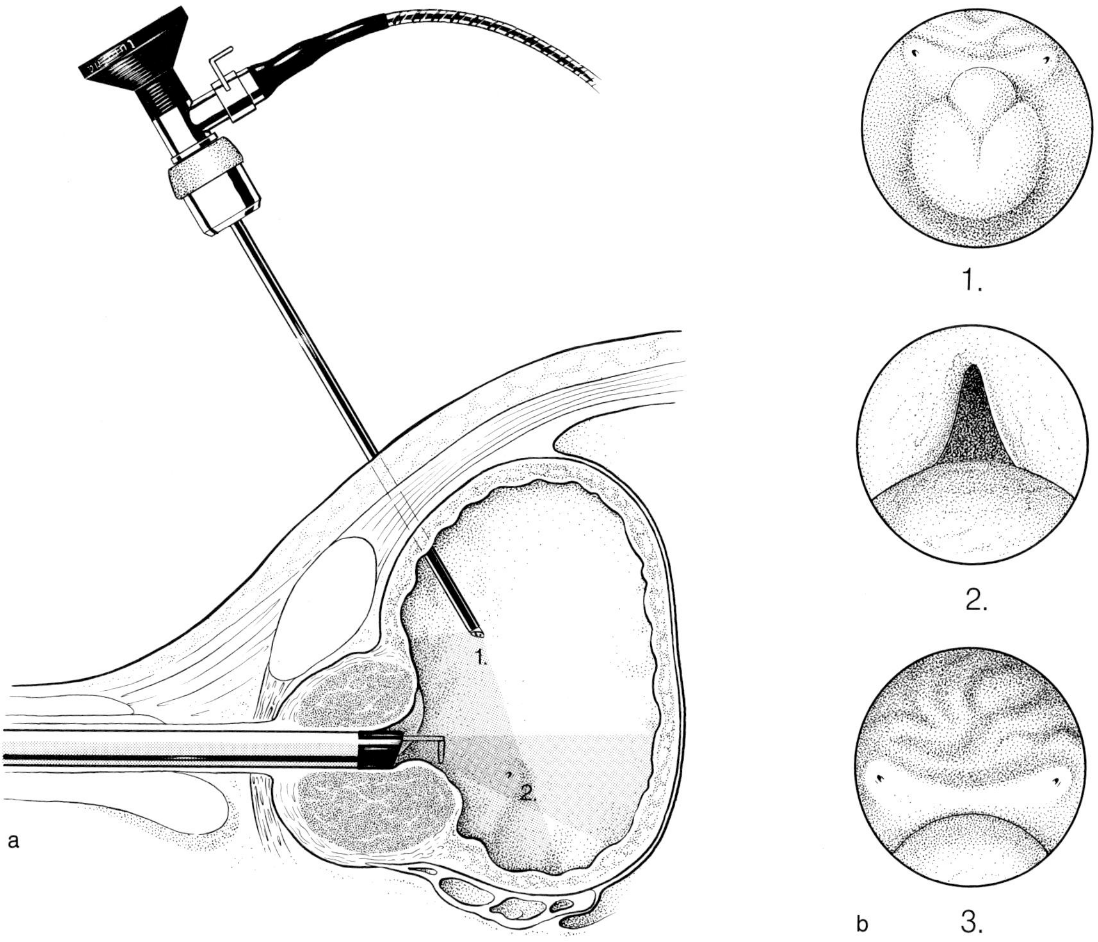

Fig. 10, a–b Bladder neck with prostatic adenoma.

(a) Sagittal section. Comparison of the width of the view (a_1) with the trocar cystoscope (b_1) and the view (a_2) with the resectoscope, urethroscope (b_2) and cystoscope (b_3).

(b) Endoscopic views: 1 = Trocar cystoscopy through the suprapubic aspiration trocar. An optical system like that used for cystoscopy (110° view) is introduced into the trocar sheath (bladder neck; see Fig. 83). 2 = Urethroscopy (160° view): prostatic urethra (see Fig. 85). 3 = Cystoscopy (110° view): trigone (see Figs. 135, 149, c).

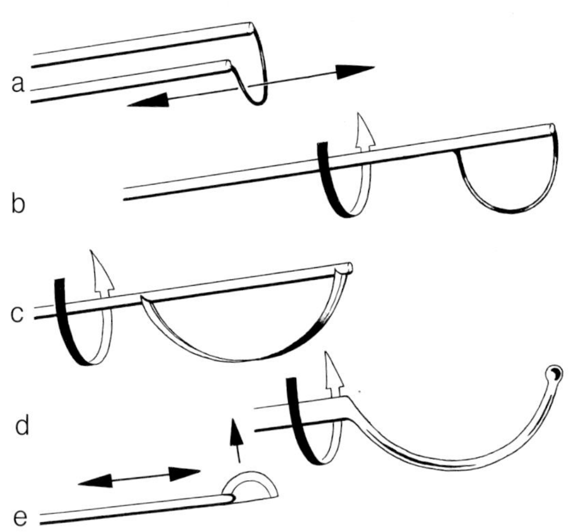

Fig. 11, a–e Possible means of guiding transurethral cutting. The warm cutting loop in the usual resectoscope (a and b); cold cutting with the spherical knife and bougie (c and d) and the urethrotome (e).

(a) Conventional axial cutting guidance (Stern-McCarthy); (b) optimal circular cutting guidance (instrument still on trial); (c) circular cutting guidance with the cold knife (razor blade); (d) blunt, blind luxation with the curved bougie (comparable to the finger in open prostatectomy); (e) axial cutting with the urethrotome.

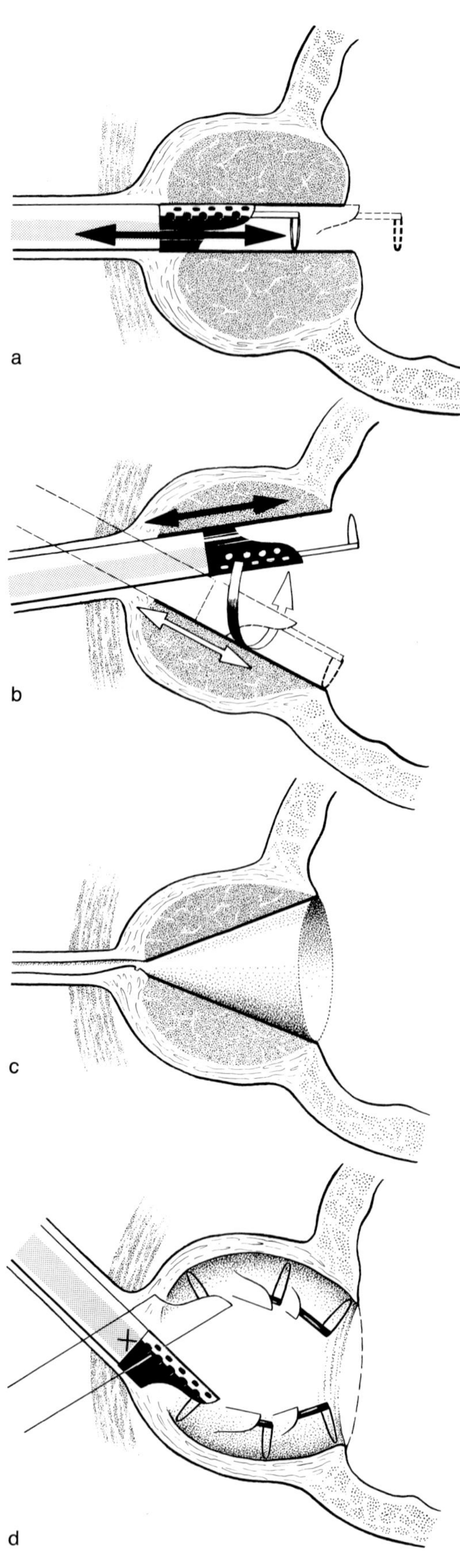

The construction of the modern resectoscope makes possible the cutting of a hollow sphere out of the prostatic urethra by means of a series of complex movements (Fig. 12):

(1) The cutting loop can only be moved back and forth in the axis of the sheath.

(2) Cutting in other planes requires coordinated movement of the cutting loop and the sheath, with the center of rotation in the urogenital diaphragm (apex, external sphincter, verumontanum), resulting in the formation of a crater.

(3) The optimal shape of a hollow sphere in the prostatic fossa can be achieved by two techniques: (a) coordinated movement of the cutting loop and the sheath; (b) lifting and stretching the prostatic capsule into an even plane by introducing the index finger into the rectum.

(4) Other movements include protrusion and retraction of the resectoscope during cutting. The form and volume of the elastic prostatic fossa can be altered by changing the dynamic pressure of the irrigation.

(5) The optical system can provide only a two-dimensional view. The third dimension is determined in part by rectal palpation. The cutting loop acts only as a fine tweezer to check the inside of the fossa. Its movements can be felt by the finger in the rectum. The thickness and quality of the tissue (capsule, adenoma) between the two can be judged with astonishing precision: the consistency helps the operator to differentiate the following tissues: adenoma; capsule; seminal vesicles; carcinomatous infiltration; inflammatory infiltration; abscess; prostatic stones and bone (symphysis in radical TUR). The external sphincter is felt as a fine bulge around the sheath; the internal sphincter and the trigone are felt as a plate.

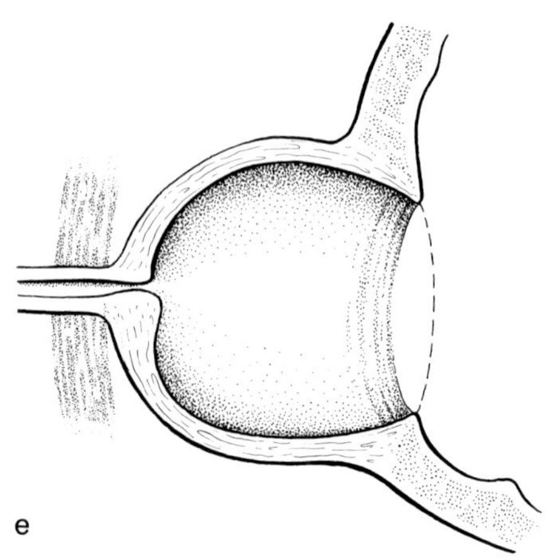

◀
Fig. 12, a–e Variations in movement of the cutting loop and (return-flow-) resectoscope (compare Fig. 41, sagittal section).

(a) Axial movement of resectoscope and loop.

(b) Angulation of the resectoscope at the urogenital diaphragm results in a crater (c); (d) coordinated movement of cutting loop and resectoscope sheath results in a hollow sphere (e).

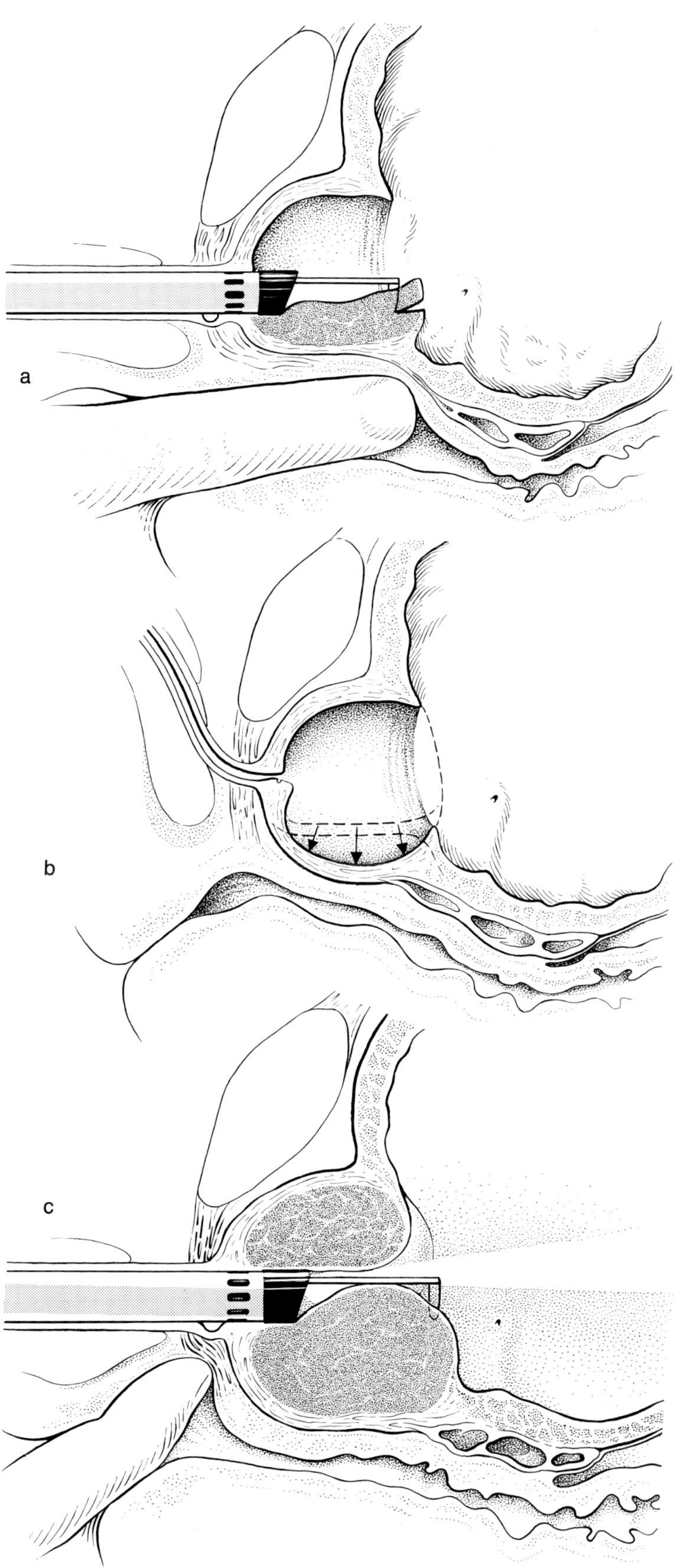

Fig. 13, a–c (a) Adjustment of the cutting surface by lifting the finger inserted in the rectum. The simple axial cutting movement is more efficient and removes the tissue faster and more easily than the combined concave movement with an angulated sheath. ▶

(b) The plane becomes a concave surface (capsule) after removing the finger from the rectum.

(c) Control knob at the apex for blind orientation. The view is restricted by the adenoma.

In complicated situations the spatial relation between operating field and instrument is felt more exactly and reliably than it is seen through the optics. Here the control knob of the sheath is a great help. It is set at the apex by rectal palpation.

The one-handed resectoscope with pistol grip and revolving electrode facilitates TUR of large adenomas (50 to 300 gm), where the operating time is one hour or longer (Fig. 2). Without doubt the surgeon will prefer the resectoscope with which he was trained. Subsequent changes of instrument seem difficult. Today, the two-handed resectoscope of Stern-McCarthy (1926–1931) is still used by some.

The one-handed resectoscope is based on a construction by Nesbit (1939). The pistol grip was introduced in 1946 by Baumrucker; the rotating sheath in 1947 by Scott. M. Hösel united the two principles of construction in the instruments of R. Wolf, which are the ones we operate with today (Figs. 9, 14, 76).

(1) *The Sheath of the Resectoscope.* For the last 25 years we have used almost exclusively a 28 Fr. sheath in adults. The 24 Fr. sheath has been used only rarely. The newer resectoscopes (except for the continuous flow instruments) have a diameter of 26 Fr. with the same size cutting loop.

Statistical investigation of our cases did not reveal any relationship between diameter of sheath used and the rate of incidence of postoperative strictures. Here, the skill of the surgeon seems to be the main factor: trauma during introduction of the sheath; small cuts with high intensity current; a thick catheter for postoperative care (over 20 Fr.); perforation of the capsule; high pressure irrigation with trauma to tissue, etc. As recommended in the first edition of this book in 1963, we apply a lubricant containing 50 per cent cortisone (more recently povidone-iodine has been added) as a prophylactic measure against strictures of the distal urethra. The shape of the obturator is of some importance for proper introduction of the sheath through the urethra into the bladder. We prefer the hinged obturator (after Timberlake), which imitates the effect of a Mercier catheter.

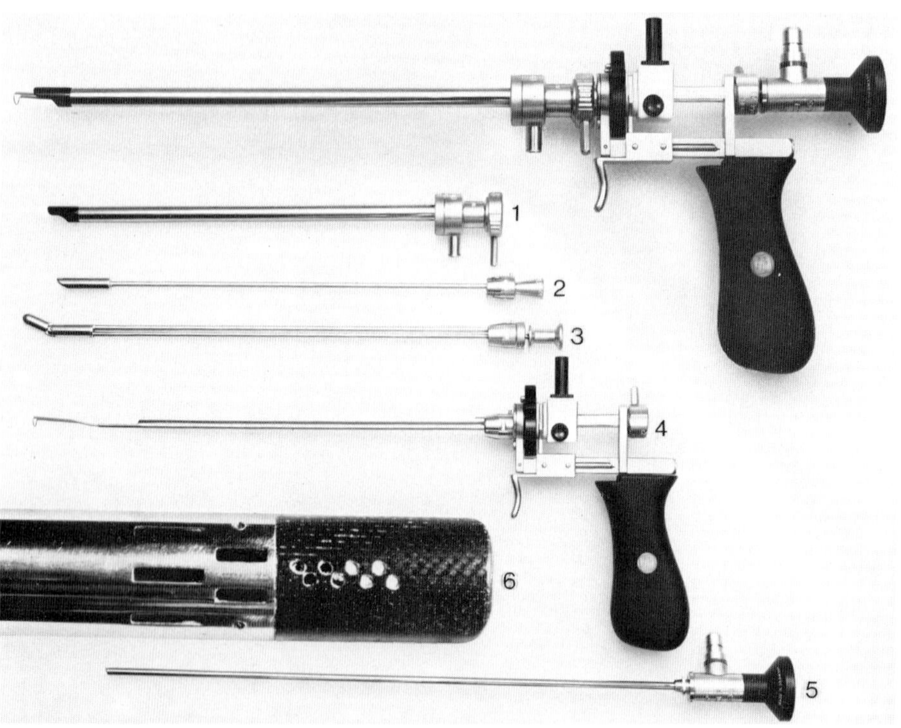

Fig. 14 Resection instrument with pistol grip and revolving electrode (after Hösel, modernized by Reuter).

1 = sheath with revolving collar (outflow), also with return-flow sheath (compare Figs. 15, 81, 87); 2 and 3 = obturator; 4 = electrotome with revolving collar; 5 = optical system (160° vision); 6 = beak of the return-flow sheath.

Fig. 14a **Resectoscope** with simultaneous irrigation and suction (K. Storz)

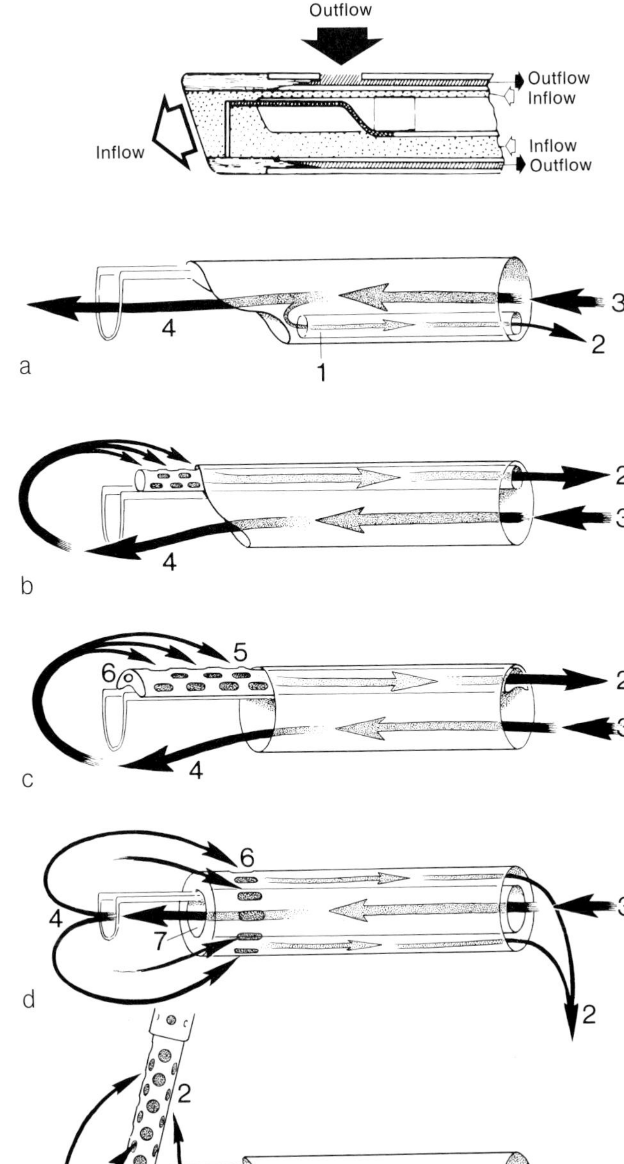

Fig. 15, a–e Development of the return-flow resectoscope since 1968.

(a) Precursor of the return-flow sheath (Iglesias, A.U.A. meeting, New York, 1973). The thin return-flow tube (1) returns only clear irrigant (2 = wrong direction of flow); 3 = inflow; 4 = outflow.

(b) Correct direction of flow in return-flow irrigation by Reuter (following discussion and correction with Iglesias of (a) in Newark, May 1973). This correction was based on many years of experience with low pressure irrigation and on the following instruments: 1. the return-flow urethroscope constructed in 1968 and demonstrated by us in 1969 at the I. Int. Symposium in Stuttgart (R. Wolf; see urethrotome, Fig. 54); 2. the suprapubic trocar (see Fig. 27). The passive outflow (1) and siphon effect later used with the trocar (Madsen; passive suction by gravity) are not sufficient to empty the bladder through the return-flow sheath. Only active suction (c and e) with a water jet or an electric suction pump guarantees function of the system during TUR (compare Figs. 26, 43).

(c) Return-flow resectoscope (Reuter). The return-flow pipe (5) protects the bladder wall from being cut by the loop during TUR (see Fig. 124). The measuring channel (6) is used for bladder pressure measurement (after M. A. Reuter).

(d) Corrected return-flow resectoscope after Iglesias, built by Storz (correction of b). This instrument was tried and presented first in Stuttgart (Reuter, July 1973, III. Int. Symposium). Disadvantages of the return-flow resectoscope include: The openings for aspiration are blocked during TURP (unlike c) by the wall of the urethra and/or the prostatic fossa; the bladder wall can be accidentally sucked onto the tip of the sheath (6) and damaged during TUR. The double sheath reduces the effective lumen (7). For cleaning the return-flow openings of the sheath (6), the entire instrument must be retracted from the urethra and reintroduced. The inflow is stronger than the outflow. Therefore, the bladder often is filled unintentionally (see Fig. 22). In high pressure irrigation (irrigating reservoir higher than 60 cm), an unphysiologic high pressure is established in the bladder and prostatic fossa without warning (see Figs. 21, 24, 29, b).

(e) Suprapubic trocar. The conditions of flow are well balanced, i.e., inflow and outflow are equivalent in trocar irrigation (compare Fig. 29, b). The cutting loop is one third larger than in the resectoscope (d) and has an accordingly higher efficiency. An optical system can be introduced for endoscopic control of TUR through the trocar (1) (trocar cystoscopy; see Fig. 87); (2) the bladder can be evacuated retrograde after TUR (McDonald); (3) a plastic tube for postoperative suprapubic irrigation (with povidone-iodine 1%) can be introduced (compare Fig. 48, e).

(2) The Electrotome. These instruments vary greatly in technical features. The only important differences are the diameter and length of the path of the cutting loop, which determine the efficiency of the cut. The larger the cut and the faster the TUR the less stress is placed on the tissue by the electric current.

The wire of the electrode should not be too thick; otherwise, the current becomes too intense. For bladder papillomas, for example, we use a thinner wire. We coagulate only by placing the cutting loop on the bleeder.

(3) The Optical System. The quality of the optical system often is overemphasized. In fact, this has not been improved substantially in the last 20 years. The optical system helps mainly in positioning the instrument between the internal sphincter and the colliculus seminalis and in differentiation of tissues. The cut itself cannot be seen. Modern optics with external light sources tend to be too bright and to alter the colors of the tissue. Differentiation is more difficult (see Fig. 91). Orientation is faster by rectal palpation than by relying on the optical system. Stereo-TUR is achieved with a double optical system.

Testing of the Cutting and Coagulating Efficiency of the High Frequency Generator

(1) *Cutting*

(a) The current is too weak when the cutting loop meets marked resistance; the cut surface produced is too rough. The loop bends, and the cut tissue remains fixed at its base, resembling floating polyps.

(b) There is too much current if the cutting loop meets no resistance, as if it were cutting butter or air.

(c) With the correct amount of current the loop cuts with low resistance and produces a smooth surface.

(2) *Coagulation*

(a) When the current is too low, the vessels continue to bleed or bleed again shortly after coagulation.

(b) When there is too much current the cutting loop is covered by a tough, black coagulum that insulates the wire.

(c) The correct current stops a spouting artery at once. Black coagulum forms only after several seconds of coagulation. Coagulated tissue retracts only minimally.

Fig. 16 ERBOTOM T 400.

Electrosurgical equipment for transurethral resections. This well-tried unit is equipped with a powerful transistor generator that tolerates the rapid sequences of cutting and coagulation needed during low pressure and trocar TUR. Intensity and quality of the HF currents for cutting and coagulation can be adjusted independently (ERBE, Elektromedizin, Tübingen).

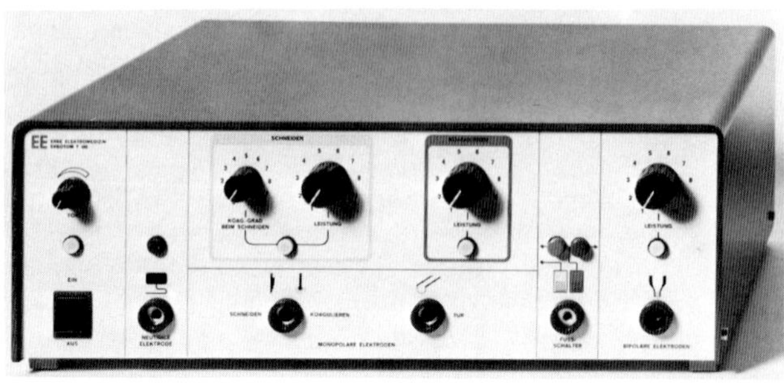

THE OPERATION (TUR)

Preparation of the Patient

The patient is prepared as for regular surgery. The biologic rhythm of the older patient is disturbed as little as possible. His habits of eating and drinking are observed, and alcohol and medications are given as usual. The preparatory measures performed before major surgical procedures — exaggerated laxative doses and sedation — are not given. The evening before the operation the patient should drink one half to one liter of fluid and should eat a light meal. This is especially important in alcoholic or diabetic patients and in those with cerebrovascular disease and/or renal insufficiency. We recommend oral administration of electrolyte solutions (Modifast; Clinifeed). These diets may be taken six to eight hours before the operation and on the first postoperative day – at first in addition to and later as a replacement for intravenous infusions.

Psychologic preparation is important. We tell the patient about his disease, the operating method and its risks, the vasotomy and about the postoperative phase with the indwelling catheter. Often the best information can be provided by having the patient read a book, such as *Medical Advice for Prostatic Patients*, Reuter, Thieme, 1979.

The enlightened patient has a certain amount of choice concerning the operating procedure and the anesthesia — if there is a choice. He therefore bears a small but psychologically important part of the responsibility. Contact with other surgical patients is desirable. Psychologic preparation raises the patient's confidence in the doctor, which is necessary for a good operative result.

Anesthesia

The risk of TUR is reduced significantly when the patient is able to cooperate passively during the operation by communicating his general condition, pains in the bladder or abdomen, feelings of nausea and so on. These symptoms indicate imminent complications that may go unrecognized with general anesthesia: e.g., overdistention of the bladder, perforation and water intoxication. If necessary, diazepam (5 to 10 mg), pethidine (0.5 to 1 ml) or an intravenous anesthetic can be administered during TUR.

Conduction anesthesia (Fig. 17) is preferred for TUR. Serious complications of peridural anesthesia are rare. The spinal ascent of anesthetic (procaine) leading to respiratory paraly-

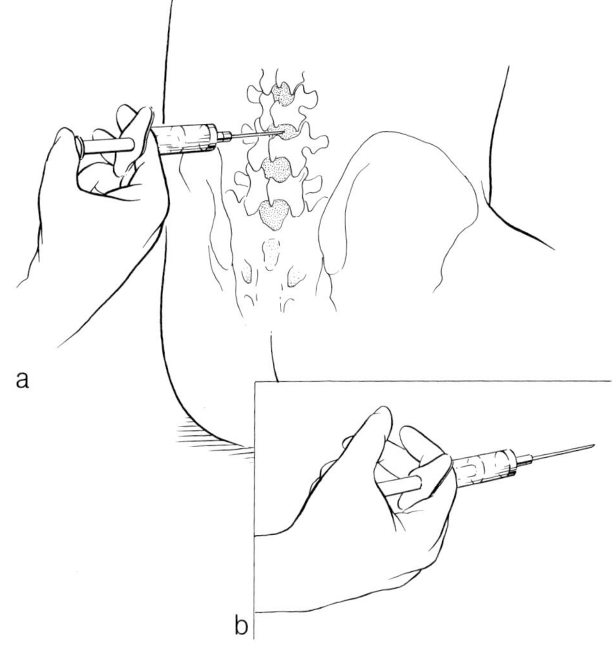

Fig. 17, a–b Conduction anesthesia (epi- and peridural anesthesia).

(a) The anesthetic usually is injected between the third and fourth lumbar vertebrae (eventually between L_4 and L_5 or L_5 and the sacrum). This is preferred to general anesthesia because:

1. Passive cooperation of the patient avoids complications.
2. The risks of general anesthesia in the elderly are avoided (cerebral, pulmonary and cardiac risks). Technical and personnel costs of regional anesthesia are lower.
3. Postoperative care is easier; postoperative recovery is quicker and does not require narcotics and analgesics.

If epidural anesthesia is to be successful, two technical points must be observed:

1. The piston of the syringe has to be loose and move easily; i.e., it should not spoil the effect of "falling in."
2. The piston of the syringe must be under firm manual pressure while feeling the way in so that the effect of falling into the peridural space becomes evident.

(b) We prefer to hold the syringe between the index and middle fingers and the ball of the thumb, pressing the piston forcefully.

sis has not occurred in our hospital for the last 15 years. Hypotonic circulatory collapse seldom occurs during or after injection of the anesthetic. It is treated with usual vasopressors. The possibility of an accidental myocardial infarction or cerebrovascular accident must always be considered. Psychogenic causes of collapse can be eliminated by conversation with the patient during the manipulation. Listening to music through earphones has proved to be relaxing for the patient during the operation (Matuschek).

Anesthesia is achieved with 20 ml of 2 per cent carticaine with 0.006 mg epinephrine. Epinephrine prolongs the anesthetic effect. Rarely, peridural anesthesia becomes lumbar anesthesia; this is recognized when the legs quickly become paralytic. Accidental lumbar anesthesia should be prevented, because lumbar anesthesia requires only one third as much of the tetracaine derivative. The great psychologic advantage of peridural anesthesia is that active motion of feet and legs is not eliminated completely. A few hours after the operation, the patient can get out of bed.

Infusion and Blood Transfusion

Physiologic low pressure irrigation is the most important and most nearly perfected measure against water intoxication. Infusion therapy is supplementary, and is begun before peridural conduction anesthesia. We infuse one liter of hypertonic electrolyte solution per hour during TUR. A diuretic (furosemide) is administered to patients with renal insufficiency. A diuretic (mannitol) added to the irrigant has no effect, since intravenous absorption is insignificant during continuous low pressure irrigation. With conventional high pressure irrigation (reservoir 60 to 120 cm above the bladder), 20 to 50 ml of a 10 per cent sodium chloride solution is added to one liter of intravenous infusion in case of increased venous bleeding or water intoxication. This prevents hyponatremia. A blood transfusion rarely is required when the new technique of TUR is used (low pressure irrigation, efficient coagulation). (See Table 9, p. 234.)

Prophylaxis of the TUR Syndrome

(Numbers (2), (4) and (5) are used mainly in high pressure irrigation.)

(1) Low pressure irrigation (see p. 25).

(2) Drug-induced diuresis.

(3) Hypertonic infusion of electrolytes (1 to 2 L).

(4) Ten per cent sodium chloride solution IV (20 to 50 cc).

(5) Blood transfusion because of vigorous bleeding and extended TUR.

(6) Patient positioned with the chest raised (Fowler's position), causing augmentation of the pelvic venous pressure. By using low pressure irrigation, the supine position may be possible.

Positioning of the Patient

One's perspective of the operating field in the prostatic fossa can be adjusted by changing the patient's position by vertical and rotational movements of the operating table (Figs. 18 and 19).

(a) Vertical raising and lowering of the operating table causes passive changes in the angle of view and the distance to the fossa. The center of rotation of the resectoscope lies within the urogenital diaphragm (external sphincter).

(b) Rotation of the patient around the transverse axis of the table below the pelvis causes even greater passive changes in the angle of view and the distance. Both passive movements, vertical and rotational, often are combined to obtain a good viewing angle. Active movement of the resectoscope can be used to adjust the angle to its optimal position.

(1) Position at the Beginning of TUR. The patient lies supine with his chest raised (Fowler's position). The operating table is lifted almost to the level of the surgeon's head so that he can hold the resectoscope horizontally.

(2) Positioning During TUR of the Posterior Fossa at 6 o'Clock. The operating table is lowered and its headpiece is raised. The resectoscope thus is passively angled downward.

(3) Positioning During TUR of the Anterior Fossa at 12 o'Clock. The operating table is lifted and its headpiece lowered (maximum about 30 degrees). Thus the resectoscope tip looks upward. This position also facilitates resection of an overhanging (undermined) lateral lobe. Frequent change of the patient's position facilitates the TUR and especially the coagulation of a heavy bleeder. Furthermore, the danger of resection of deep channels into the adenomatous tissue also is reduced, because the tissue is resected over a wide field and the sector of operation is often changed.

Fig. 18 Positioning of the patient (sec text).
The patient's buttocks should extend about 10 cm over the lower edge of the operating table (to facilitate rectal palpation and the surgeon's upright position).

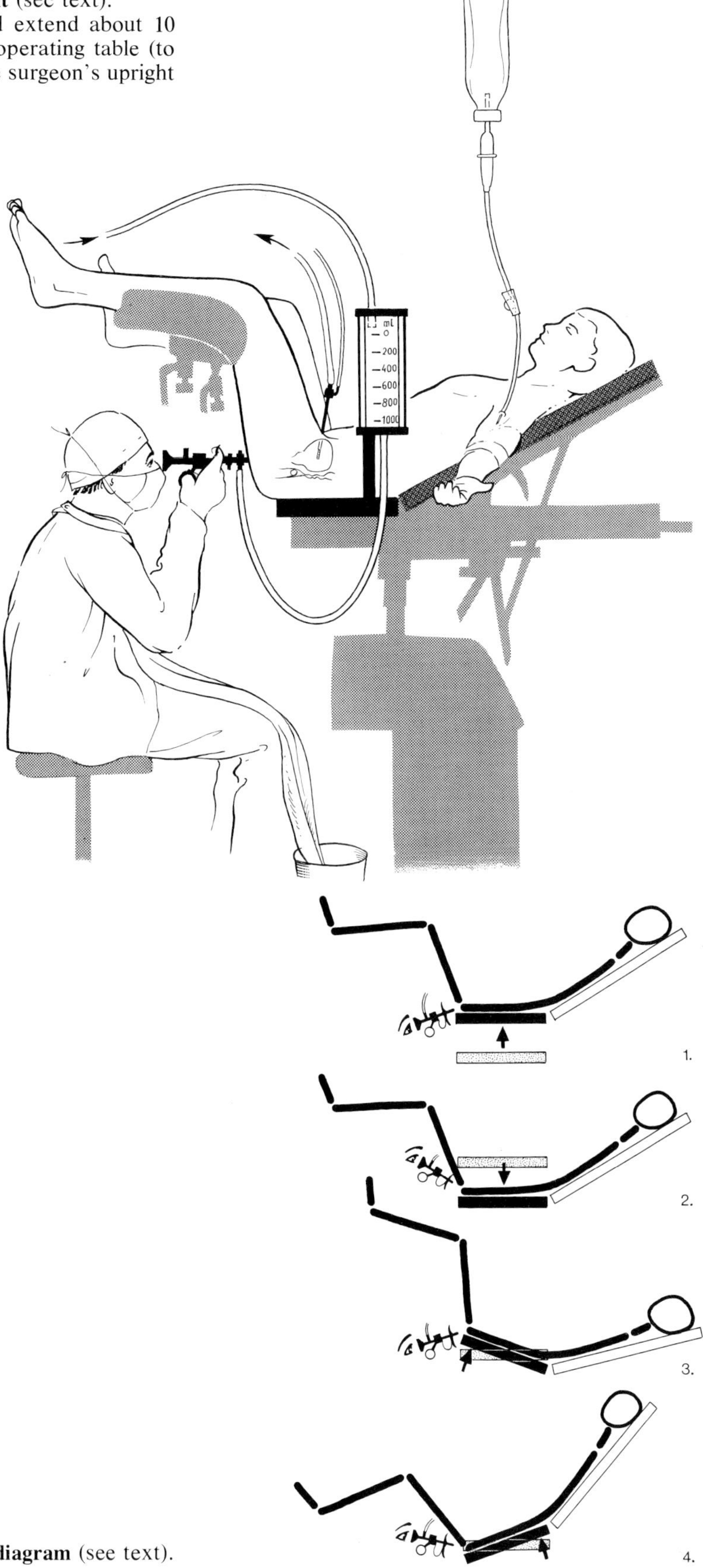

Fig. 19 Positioning; schematic diagram (see text).

Vasotomy

During TUR the seminal vesicles or the ejaculatory ducts often are cut, and epididymitis frequently develops. Therefore, a vasotomy is performed under peridural anesthesia before TURP.

Vesiculography

The position and condition of the genital tract and its possible infiltration by disease can be demonstrated by routine vesiculography, which is easily performed in conjunction with vasotomy. The extension of prostatitis or carcinoma into the adnexa can be demonstrated. This is especially useful in differential diagnosis. Carcinoma of the bladder or prostate cannot be demonstrated as easily and exactly by any other technique (Goldberg).

Demarcation of the Prostatic Capsule by Dye (Fig. 92, b)

The colors of prostatic tissues (capsule, adenoma, fat and muscle) differ only slightly, making it difficult to distinguish one from another. For example, infiltration into the destroyed capsule cannot be differentiated from adenomatous tissue. This is the most frequent cause of perforation of the prostatic capsule.

Differentiation of color is even more difficult when fiberoptics are used, because the bright light tends to equalize the shades. The different tissues can be better contrasted by transrectal injection of indigo carmine into the capsule (see Fig. 91, b). The effect is most striking in the small prostatic adenoma. When dye is injected into the seminal vesicles, the blue liquid can be seen flowing off the ejaculatory ducts adjacent to the verumontanum. A few minutes after the injection, blasts of blue urine from the ureteral orifices can be seen, because the solution is rapidly resorbed in the prostate. This illustrates the mechanism of extravasation of irrigant with quick resorption. In addition, if the seminal vesicle is cut, blue dye comes out.

Coloring of the bladder muscles below a papillary bladder tumor by injection under the base of the tumor can be of help to the beginner. Here the needle is introduced above the symphysis (see Cryosurgery, p. 185) or through the urethra, the vagina or beside the urethra.

Biopsy of the Prostatic Capsule (Fig. 20)

Histology of the resected adenoma provides no information regarding the state of the remaining capsule. Therefore, transrectal needle biopsy of the prostatic capsule is performed immediately before TUR. We found carcinoma of the capsule in 6.1 per cent of our patients (379 cases) when the histologic diagnosis of the resected material had been benign. In 8.3 per cent of the cases, cytologic examination produced uncertain findings of carcinoma (Papanicolaou III). In the group with malignant histology of the resected tissue, in only 2.9 per cent was cytology of the capsule negative; in 2.3 per cent the cytology was undecided (Pap. III).

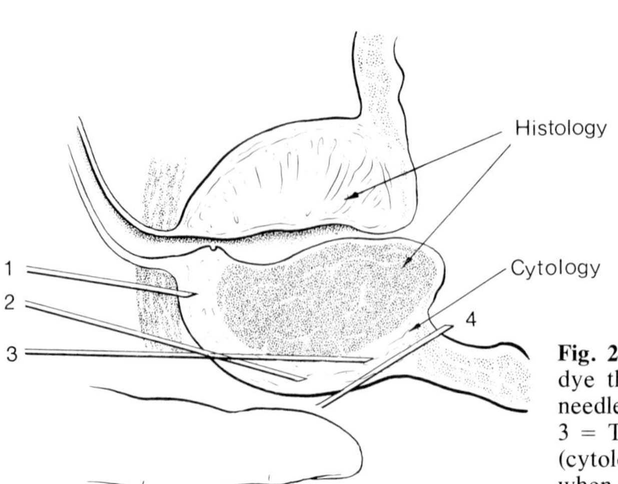

Fig. 20 1 = Marking of the prostatic capsule by dye through a needle such as that used for fine needle biopsy (compare Figs. 32, 94, 110, c). 2 and 3 = Transrectal fine needle biopsy of the capsule (cytology). 4 = The needle pierces the bladder when inserted too far into the rectum.

Irrigation During TUR (Figs. 21–31)

Irrigation of the prostatic fossa and bladder is a major part of TUR. The well-being of the patient and the smooth performance of TUR depend on its proper function. The relatively simple physiology of irrigation has been totally neglected since the first cystoscopy about a century ago, even though every rise in pressure above physiologic values is dangerous.

The physical principles of irrigation often are insufficiently considered. The TUR syndrome is a subsequent effect of this neglect. Therefore, we will repeat the following:

Physiology of Prostatic Fossa and Bladder Irrigation

Two different pressures are effective in the prostatic fossa: the dynamic pressure at the tip of the resectoscope and the static pressure in the bladder and prostatic fossa.

(1) *The dynamic pressure* is caused by the flow of irrigant into the prostatic fossa. It depends on the speed of flow of the irrigant, which is determined by the pressure gradient — i.e., the relation of bladder pressure to the height of the water column in the irrigant reservoir over the bladder. The force of dynamic pressure is illustrated when a small gap or a perforation is torn into the prostatic tissue by the irrigant flow (see Fig. 93).

Extravasation and paravesical irrigant depots are probably caused by this pressure (Fig. 21). The dynamic pressure in the prostatic fossa is related to the hydrostatic pressure in such a way that it decreases when the hydrostatic pressure increases, because the pressure gradient from the irrigant reservoir to the bladder decreases.

(2) *The static pressure* in the bladder and prostatic fossa increases with the bladder volume. It also depends on the tension of the bladder muscles and on the intra-abdominal pressure. In the atonic bladder, the pressure is lower, as in the normotonic bladder at equivalent volume. The filling of the bladder is completed when the intravesical pressure corresponds to the height of the water column in

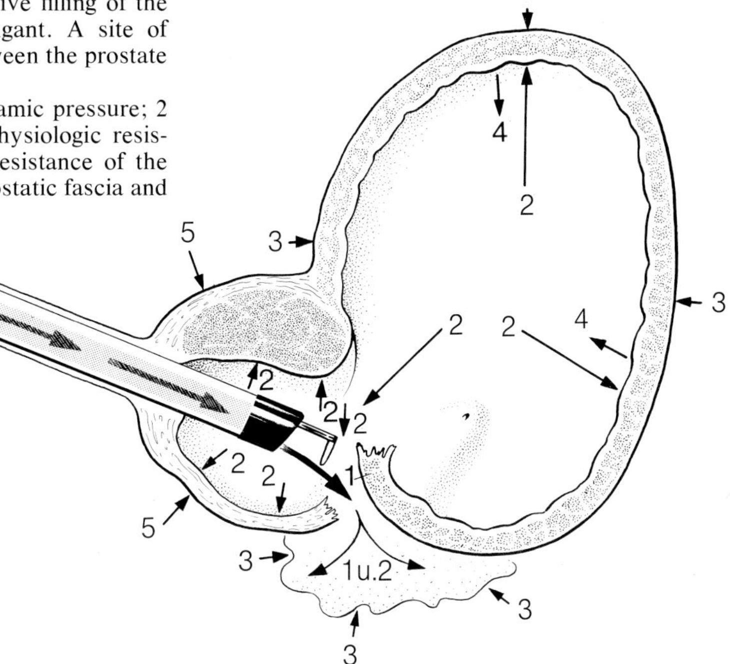

Fig. 21 High pressure irrigation with separation of bladder neck and prostatic fossa.

The unphysiologic dynamic pressure caused by too high elevation of the irrigating reservoir and the high static pressure due to excessive filling of the bladder causes absorption of irrigant. A site of predilection is the connection between the prostate and trigone (compare Fig. 93).

Irrigation: 1 = direction of dynamic pressure; 2 = static pressure; *Tissue:* 3 = physiologic resistance of the tissue; 4 = elastic resistance of the bladder wall; 5 = resistance of prostatic fascia and capsule.

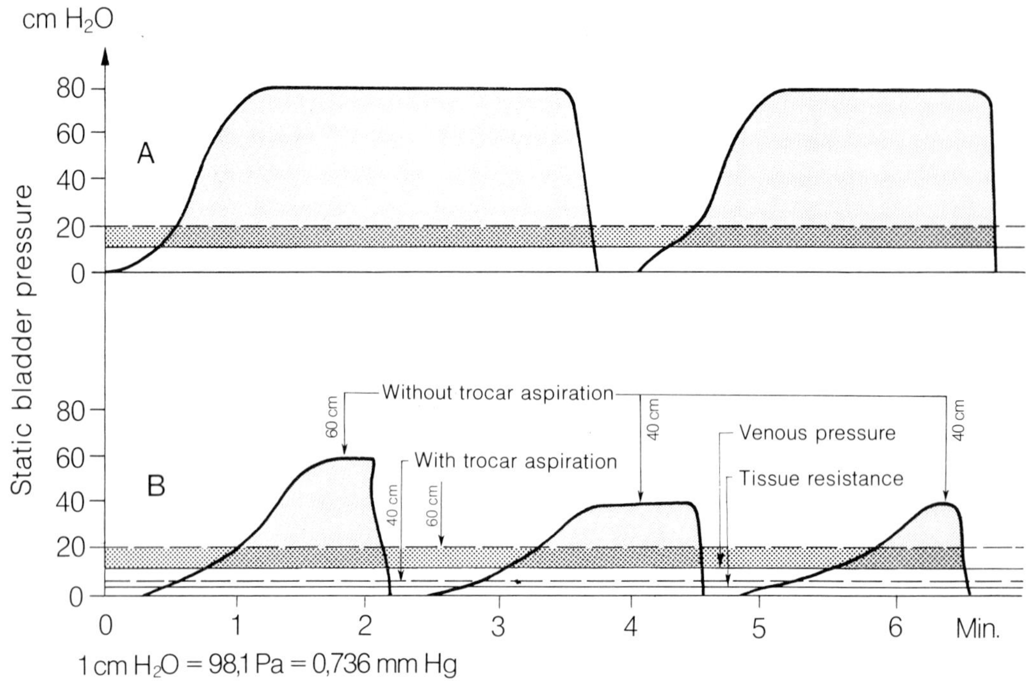

Fig. 22 (A–B) Intravesical pressure (after Madsen).
A = During high pressure irrigation (irrigating reservoir elevated 80 cm but without trocar aspiration), after 1.3 to 3.5 min the bladder is filled and the intravesical pressure corresponds to 80 cm water following irrigation. B = Low pressure irrigation with the reservoir elevated 40 cm and 60 cm and with trocar aspiration (horizontal dashed lines); no irrigating intervals are needed, and there is no increase in intravesical pressure above average venous pressure. Without trocar aspiration and with irrigating intervals, the pressure rises more slowly than in *A* but not over, respectively, 60 and 40 cm of water.

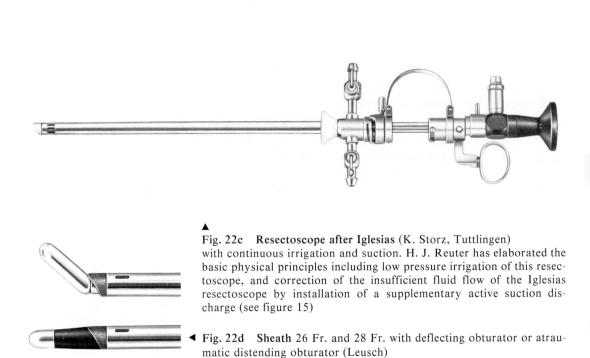

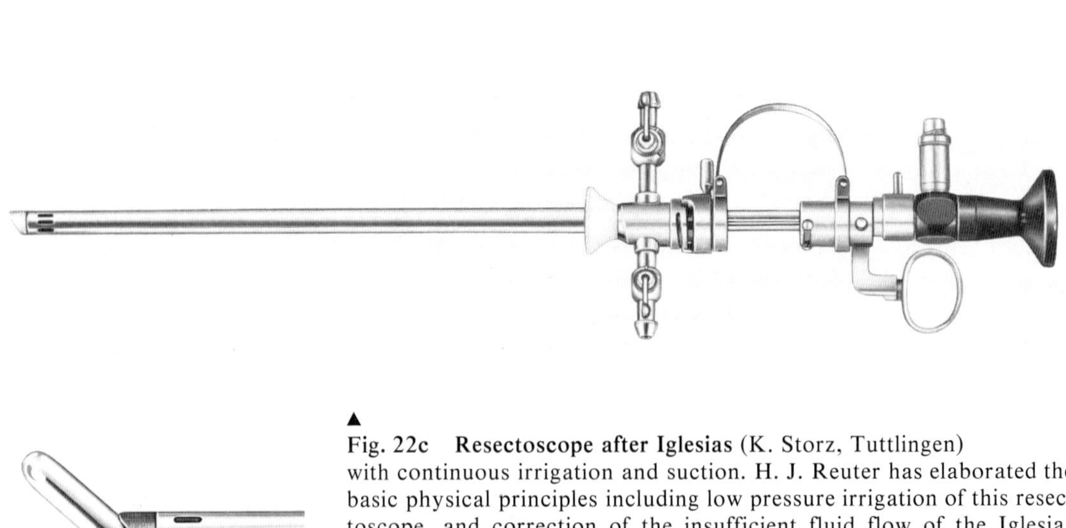

▲
Fig. 22c Resectoscope after Iglesias (K. Storz, Tuttlingen) with continuous irrigation and suction. H. J. Reuter has elaborated the basic physical principles including low pressure irrigation of this resectoscope, and correction of the insufficient fluid flow of the Iglesias resectoscope by installation of a supplementary active suction discharge (see figure 15)

◀ **Fig. 22d Sheath** 26 Fr. and 28 Fr. with deflecting obturator or atraumatic distending obturator (Leusch)

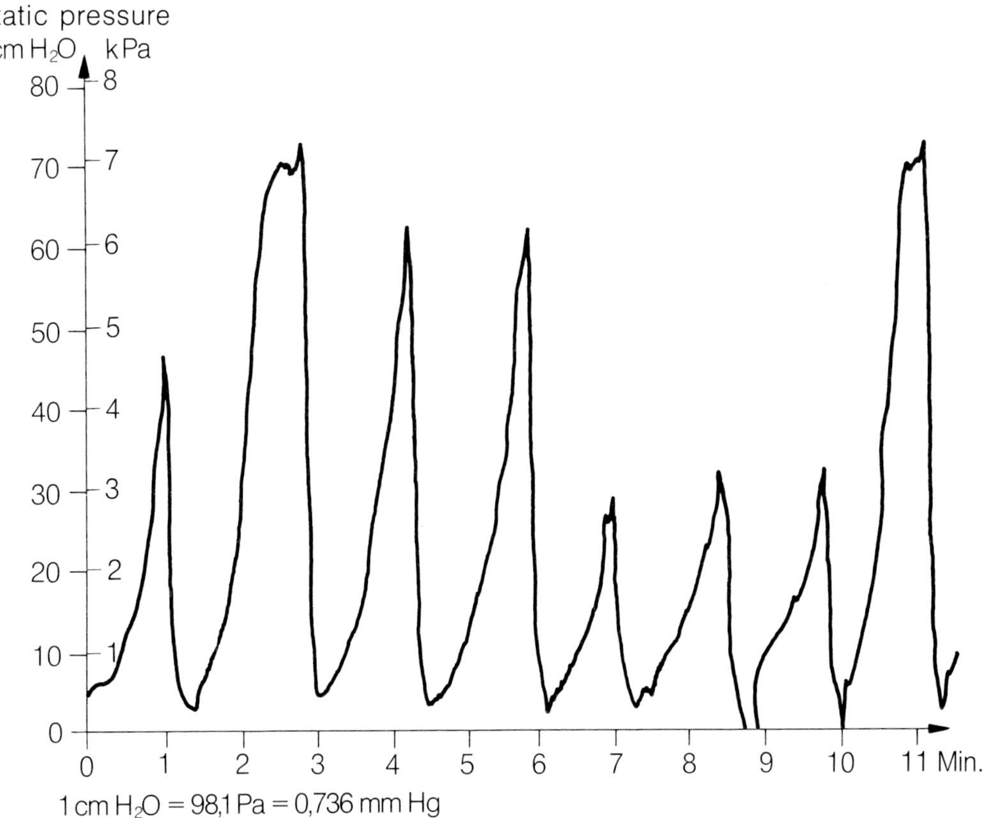

Fig. 23 Determination of bladder pressure during TUR with high pressure irrigation (80 cm elevation of the irrigating reservoir over the prostatic fossa) with short filling times (1 to 2 min) and frequent intervals for voiding of the bladder (drawing by M. A. Reuter). Compared to Fig. 22, *A* the bladder is voided after approximately one minute inflow, whereas in the Madsen diagram voiding occurs after about 1.5 to 2.5 min. The bladder pressure always rises above the physiologic level of the venous pressure, 10 to 15 cm water (0.98 to 1.47 kPa = 7 to 11 mm Hg).

the reservoir over the bladder: the pressure gradient equals zero. In the normal bladder, a volume of about 600 cc is then reached; in an atonic bladder, 1000 to 2000 cc may be necessary (see Figs. 22–24).

The hydrostatic pressure is useless and therefore harmful for TUR. Dynamic pressure, however, is useful in TUR. For example, it washes hemorrhage away and transports chips of tissue into the bladder. Dynamic pressure in the prostatic fossa therefore should be kept within tolerable physiologic limits. Static pressure should remain as low as possible. This is realized when the reservoir is only about 30 cm above the bladder (28 Fr. resectoscope) and the bladder volume remains minimal (below 50 cc).

The TUR syndrome can be avoided only when these principles are observed. This is achieved by low pressure irrigation with continuous aspiration of irrigant (Fig. 25).

Conventional Irrigation and Its Complications (Tables 1–3, p. 232)

The irrigating reservoir is elevated 80 to 120 cm above the bladder during TUR. The higher it hangs, the faster the irrigant flows into the bladder. Dynamic pressure rises; the bladder volume and, therefore, the static pressure increase and the intervals between the bladder fillings become shorter. Absorption of irrigant starts when the reservoir is placed 60 cm above the bladder. TUR is thus complicated by the following:

Atonic bladder, overdistention of the prostatic fossa (see Fig. 62).

Overhydration of the tissue (see Fig. 93).

Perforation; dehiscence (see Fig. 71).

Ureteral reflux with ascending pyelonephritis; urosepsis by direct and indirect extravasation of bacteria; hydremia; hyponatremia; crush-kidney; uremia; general reactions (TUR syndrome).

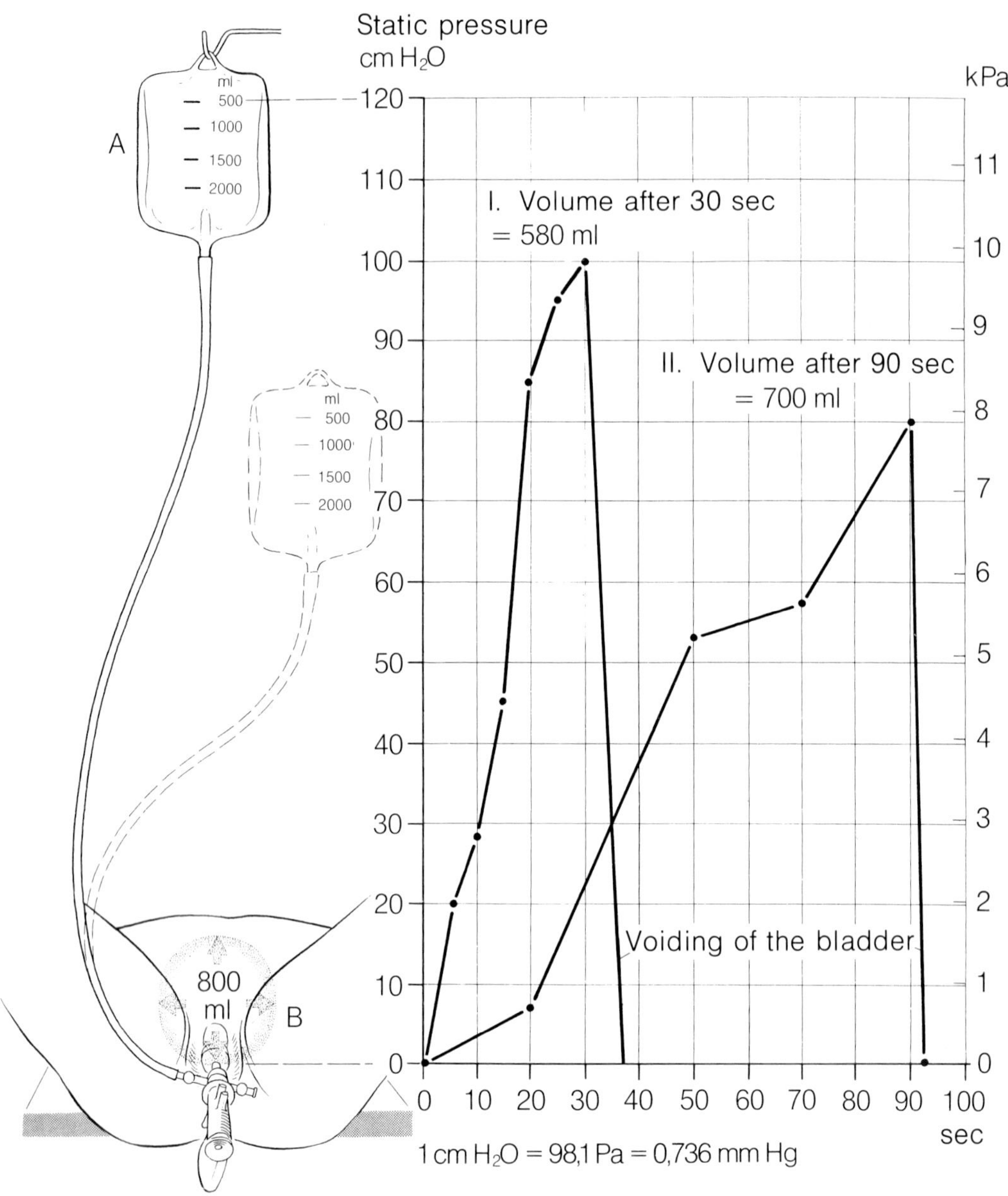

Fig. 24 High pressure irrigation.
Schematic representation of unphysiologic high pressure in the fossa and bladder (elevation of irrigating reservoir is 80 to 120 cm above the fossa). Further disadvantages are the interruption of irrigation and the frequently overdistended bladder (see Figs. 22, 23). A = irrigant bag (2-L). B = Overdistended bladder and fossa with 100 cm water static pressure = 9.8 kPa; volume is 800 to 2000 cc.

Left side: Irrigation of the bladder with reservoir elevated 120 cm.

Right side: Representation of the intravesical pressure in relation to time in two patients (I and II). The bladder pressure of Graph I already exceeds physiologic venous pressure 5 sec after the start of irrigation; after 30 sec, the bladder is overdistended, with an intravesical pressure of 100 cm water (= 9.8 kPa = 74 mm Hg) with a volume of 580 cc. The declining line demonstrates the fall of pressure when the normotonic bladder is voided. Graph II shows the pressure rise in the bladder with the irrigating reservoir elevated 80 cm. After 30 seconds the bladder pressure is 20 cm water (= 1.96 kPa = 15 mm Hg); after 90 seconds the volume is 700 cc; the intravesical pressure is almost 80 cm water (= 7.85 kPa = 59 mm Hg).

Physiologic Low Pressure Irrigation with Continuous Aspiration of Irrigant (Figs. 25–30 and Tables 2 and 4, pp. 232, 233)

(1) *Here, the height of the water column* in the irrigant reservoir over the prostatic fossa is about 30 cm. This limits the dynamic pressure to a tolerable force (1–2 cm water, Fig. 29) and the static pressure in the fossa to below 30 cm water from the beginning. In addition, the bladder volume can be controlled exactly with the aid of the graduated one-liter reservoir (irrigant dosimeter). We limit the bladder volume to 200 cc during TUR in order to prevent overdistention of the prostatic fossa and the bladder.

(2) *Active, continuous aspiration of irrigant* from the bladder significantly improves low pressure irrigation because the bladder is not filled and interruptions for evacuation are not necessary. All the dangers of high pressure irrigation are eliminated. For elastic and efficient aspiration we use a simple water jet vacuum pump, which is equal to if not better than an electric vacuum pump. The passive syphon effect of a one-meter tube is often adversely affected by bubbles; its pressure is not sufficient, and it cannot be easily regulated. The vacuum is adjusted by an air inlet valve to minus 1 to 2 m of water. Suction functions well only when the system is airtight. Continuous low pressure irrigation is achieved by two systems — the suprapubic trocar and the return flow resectoscope (Fig. 15). Both instruments were brought to their present state by the author; precursors of both systems proved to be neither efficient nor reliable.

(3) *The suprapubic trocar* (Fig. 33) is preferred for more extensive and difficult TUR (prostates weighing over 20 gm). Its capacity of flow (Fig. 29, b) is large enough (16 Fr. diameter). Its function is reliable and is maintained by a self-cleaning mechanism.

(4) *The returnflow resectoscope* has a channel for returning the irrigant (see Fig. 15). Its small diameter does not allow a capacity of

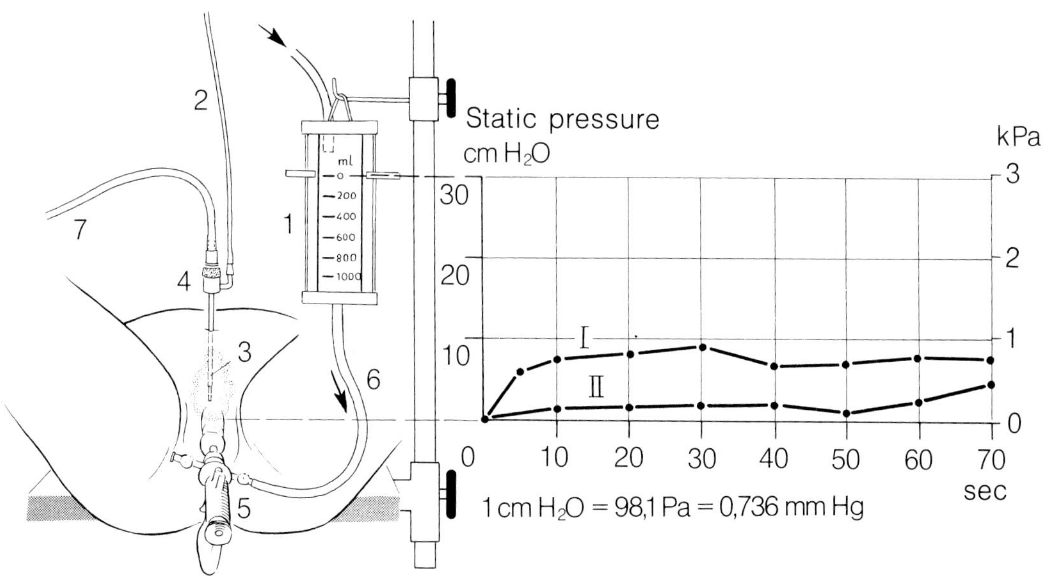

Fig. 25 Low pressure irrigation (after H. J. Reuter).
Physiologic low pressure irrigation effectively prevents the TUR syndrome (30 cm elevation of irrigating reservoir). The bladder always remains nearly empty (volume 10 to 15 cc) owing to continuous suprapubic aspiration.

Left side: 1 = Dosimeter (after Reuter) with 1-L content (graduated irrigating reservoir mounted on the operating table); 2 = gauge for bladder pressure determination (ascending tube); 3 = bladder and fossa (pressure below 15 cm water = 1.47 kPa = 11 mm Hg; contents below 50 cc); 4 = suprapubic trocar (14 Fr.); 5 = resectoscope; 6 = inflow of irrigant; 7 = outflow of irrigant (aspiration with water jet suction pump).

Right side: Rise of bladder pressure to up to 9 cm water = 0.88 kPa = 7 mm Hg with elevation of the irrigating reservoir at 30 cm and continuous aspiration. The bladder content does not exceed 25 cc. Graphs I and II were obtained in different patients (in II, a bladder atony is present).

flow (Fig. 29, b) comparable to that of the suprapubic trocar. Here in particular the bladder pressure should be monitored continuously to avoid overfilling.

(5) *Advantages of continuous low pressure irrigation*

(a) The physiologic conditions of the irrigation efficiently prevent all the complications that occur with high pressure irrigation.

(b) TUR can be prolonged to 100 minutes without risk of the TUR syndrome and its generalized patient reactions. Adenomas of 200 gm and more can be resected in one session (see Fig. 2). Even TURP of the huge adenoma or radical TUR does not — in our experience—carry increased patient risk (unlike TURP with high pressure irrigation or open prostatectomy; see above and Table 8, p. 234).

(c) Venous bleeding is reduced by the aspiration of irrigant from the bladder. The bladder is not distended, avoiding compression of the prostatic veins and increased venous pressure. The veins remain collapsed. Arterial bleeders can be observed more readily, since the blood is constantly removed from the site. Coagulation of all vessels is facilitated by a consistently clear view.

(d) Teaching is fundamentally simplified. The student learns TUR in about half the time thanks to an uninterrupted view of the well irrigated operating field. The instructor has more time and patience to offer the student because the TUR syndrome does not occur. He controls and corrects the TUR by means of the teaching attachment.

(e) Investigations by Madsen and M. A. Reuter have confirmed the accuracy of our conception. Clinically significant extravasation was not demonstrated (Figs. 22, 29).

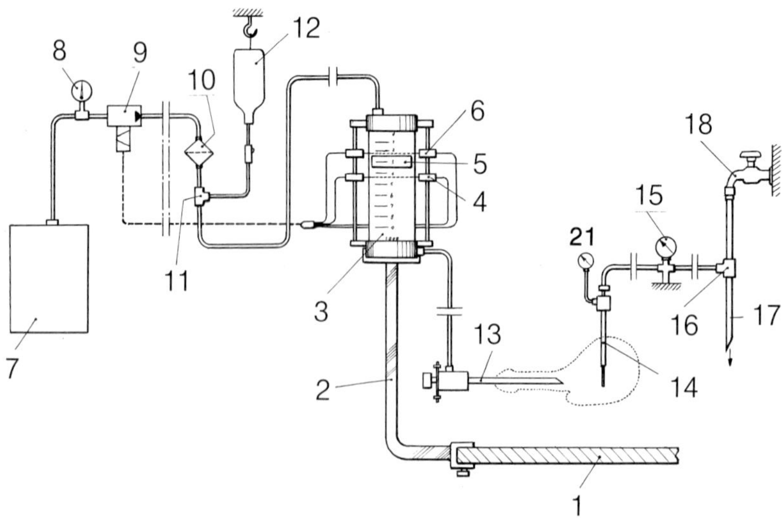

Fig. 26

Figs. 26 and 27, a–b Irrigant conditioning from tap water; inflow and outflow of irrigant during TUR.

Fig. 26 shows diagrammatically the pipes used for irrigant conduction in low pressure TUR (after H. J. Reuter).

Fig. 27, a, Dosimeter with irrigant reservoir; height adjustable.

Fig. 27, b, Suprapubic trocar with self-cleaning mechanism.

1 = Operating table; 2 = support of the dosimeter (3) mounted on the operating table; 3 = dosimeter (after Reuter) with water level adjusted to about 30 cm over the resectoscope (13); 4 = lower light gate switch for automatic start of filling with irrigant; 5 = float for interruption of light gates; 6 = upper light gate switch to stop filling; 7 = water-boiler (10-L, 30° C); 8 = thermometer; 9 = magnetic valve; 10 = sterile filter (R. Wolf); 11 = suction pump; 12 = 50% glucose solution; 13 = resectoscope sheath; 14 = trocar aspiration; 15 = pressure gauge for suction pump (control of negative suction pressure); 16 = water jet pump with drainage (17) and stopcock (18); 19 = electronic control gear for light gate switches and magnetic valves (4 and 6); 20 = self-cleaning-mechanism of the trocar; 21 = manometer for control of intravesical pressure; 22 = reservoir filling line; 23 = line to resectoscope; 24 = outflow line from the trocar; 25 = measuring channel inside the trocar sheath (for bladder pressure determination = 21).

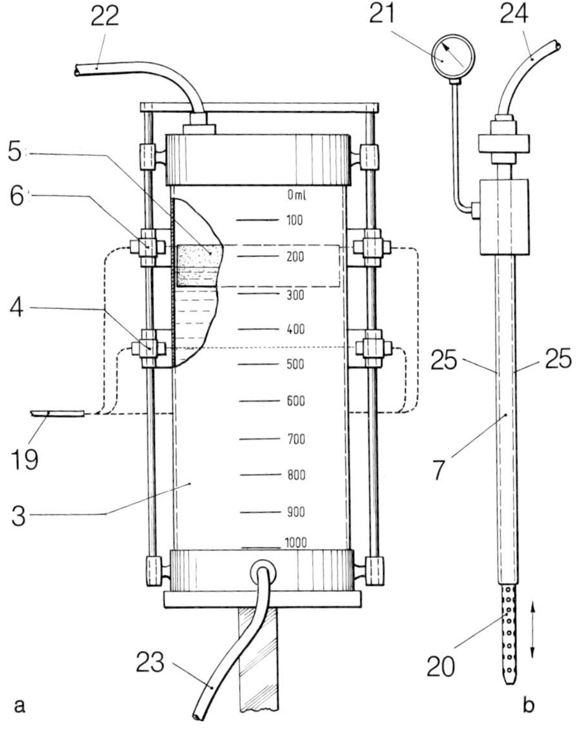

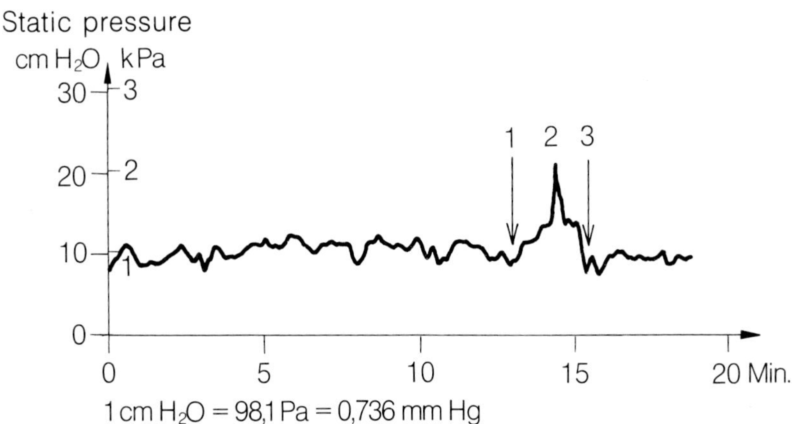

Fig. 28 TUR with low pressure (drawing by M. A. Reuter).

The static pressure in the bladder is determined through the measuring channel of the suprapubic trocar. The pressure in the prostatic fossa stays at about 10 cm water (= 0.98 kPa = 8 mm Hg). At (1), the aspiration through the trocar is stopped; the pressure rises immediately. At (2), the surgeon's hand is pressed on the lower abdomen. At (3), the pressure quickly falls down to 10 cm water when aspiration is resumed.

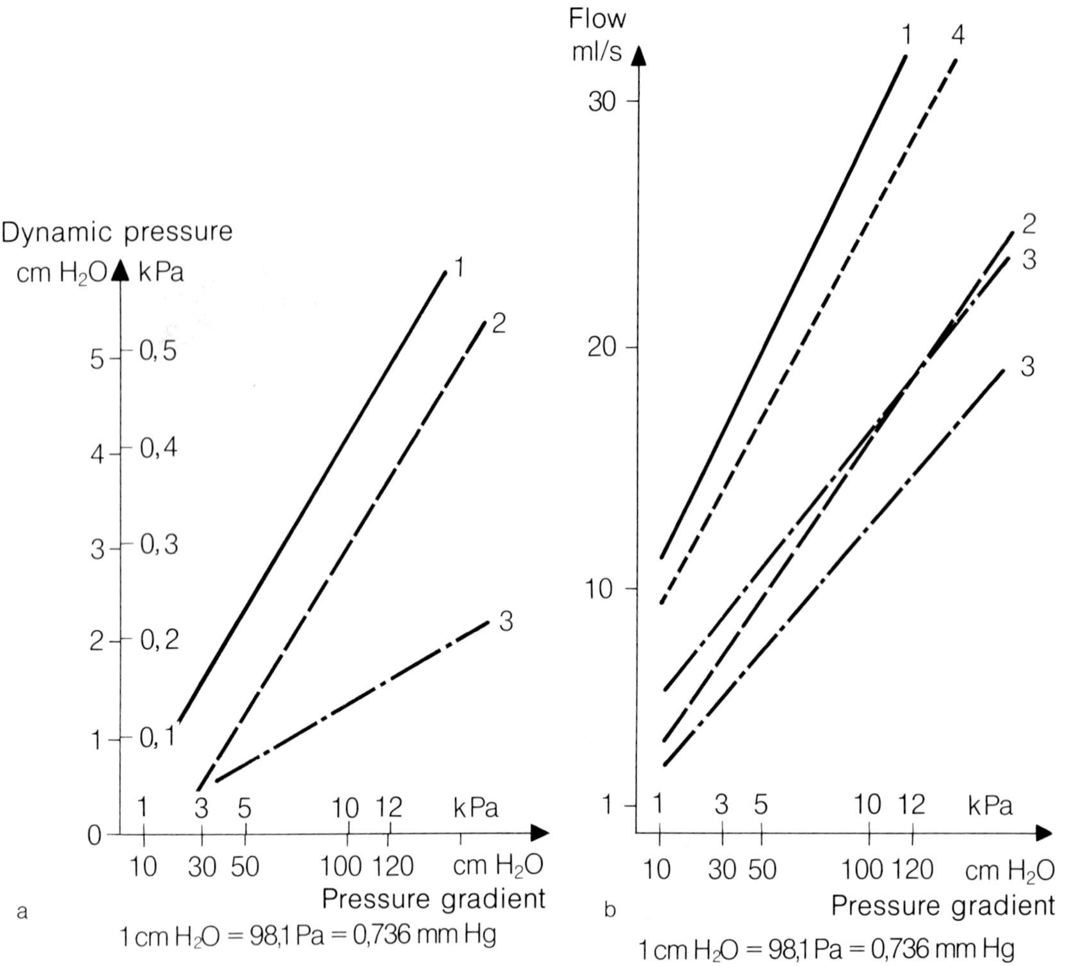

Fig. 29, a–b Dynamic pressure and flow of irrigant in the prostatic fossa in different types of resectoscopes (1–3) and in the suprapubic trocar (4) (after M. A. Reuter).

(a) The dynamic pressure in the prostatic fossa depends on the pressure gradient (i.e., height of the water level in the irrigating reservoir over the prostatic fossa minus static intravesical pressure) and on the type of resectoscope (1–3).

This graph demonstrates the relatively small amount of dynamic pressure produced by the flow of the irrigant at the tip of the resectoscope sheath. However, dynamic pressure may, together with intravesical static pressure, cause irrigant absorption.

(b) Inflow and outflow depend on the pressure gradient and on the type of instrument used (resectoscope: 1–3; trocar: 4).

This graph shows the different relations of inflow and outflow of the resectoscopes, the trocar and the return-flow sheath. The 28 and 24 Fr. resectoscopes provide a good relation of inflow to the outflow through the trocar (4).

The relation of inflow (upper line 3) and outflow (lower line 3) through the return-flow resectoscope is inadequate insofar as the inflow is 30 per cent greater than the unobstructed return flow. This explains the occurrence of unintentionally high bladder fillings and pressures during TUR, when the inflow is fully open. Reduced inflow and bladder pressure monitoring therefore are obligatory during TUR with the return-flow resectoscope. The balance of flow through the return-flow resectoscope must still be improved.

1 = Conventional 28 Fr. sheath (resectoscope of R. Wolf; compare Fig. 14); 2 = conventional 24 Fr. sheath (resectoscope of Winter and Ibe); 3 = return-flow resectoscope with 27 Fr. (resectoscope after Reuter of R. Wolf; compare Figs. 14/6, 15, c); 4 = suprapubic trocar 14 Fr. (after Reuter from R. Wolf; compare Figs. 27, b, 33, 43).

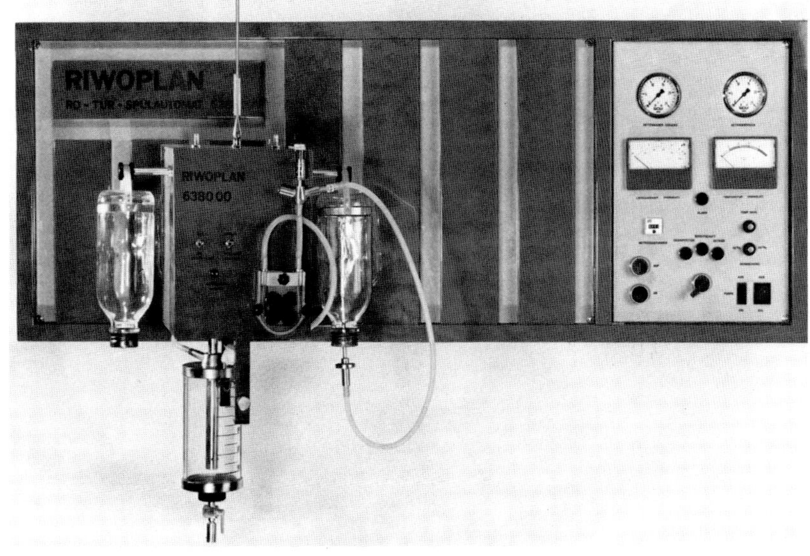

Fig. 30 RO-TUR automatic irrigating system (after Brühl, with dosimeter after Reuter; compare Fig. 27, a).

It produces pyrogen-free, low-salt, sterile water by conversion osmosis (R. Wolf).

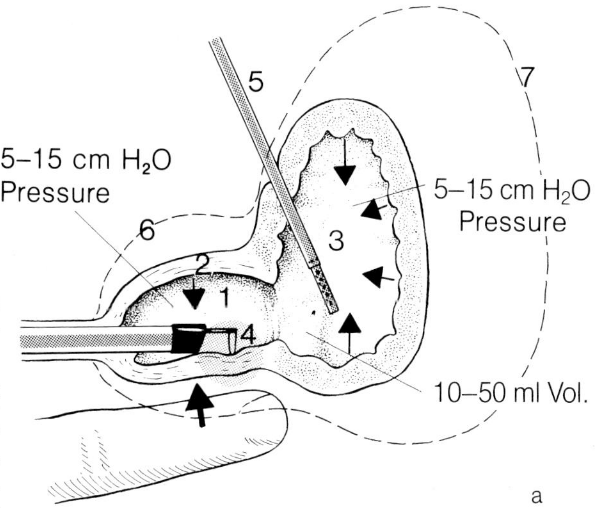

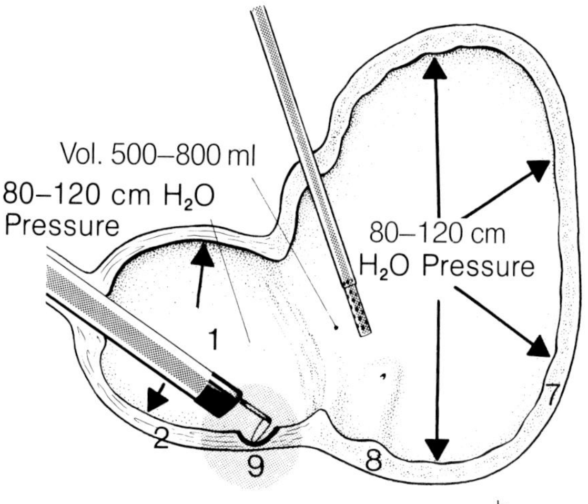

Fig. 31, a–c Response of bladder, bladder neck and prostatic fossa to physiologic low pressure and unphysiologic high pressure irrigation during TURP.

(a) Low pressure irrigation. The prostatic fossa (1) is relaxed; a low physiologic pressure of 5 to 15 cm water is in the almost empty, collapsed bladder (3; volume 10 to 50 cc). The relaxed capsule (2; true prostatic tissue) — unlike adenomatous tissue — evades the cutting loop (4); its contractability is not reduced by overdistention (dashed lines; 6). The same is true for the bladder wall (e.g., in TUR of bladder tumors). The finger in the rectum easily lifts (arrow) the fossa or bladder floor. Even in the nearly collapsed bladder (contents near O) TUR is performed without danger to the bladder wall because the trocar (5) protects it. On the other hand, the return-flow resectoscope aspirates the bladder wall, risking perforation. 7 = outline of the full bladder.

(b) High pressure irrigation. Bladder and prostatic fossa (1) are overdistended during unphysiologic high pressure irrigation (see pp. 21–24). The elastic fibers of the capsule (2) and muscular bladder wall must resist a pressure of 30 to 120 cm water. The bladder floor (8) is pressed more and more toward the rectum, changing the topography. The tension in the prostatic fossa (1), which is blown up like a balloon, can be felt by the finger in the rectum, and there is danger of perforation.

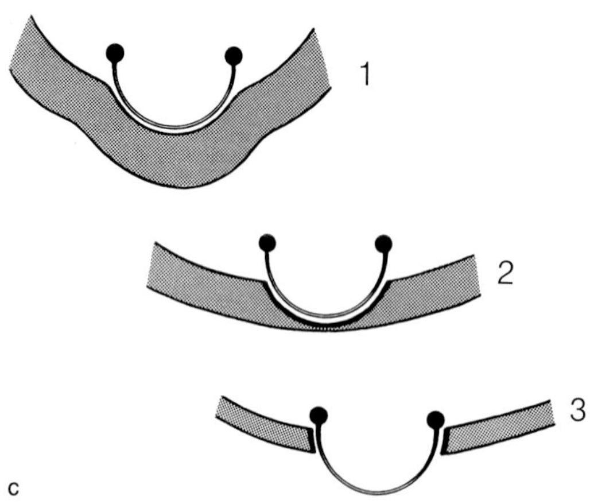

Fig. 31 *Continued* (c) The prostatic capsule (true prostatic tissue or the bladder wall) during TUR. 1 = The relaxed capsule (or bladder wall) evades the cut during low pressure irrigation. 2 = The capsule or bladder is stretched by high pressure and cannot evade the cut; perforation is imminent. Contractility of the fossa and bladder is disturbed by overdistention and irrigant absorption, and healing and hemostasis of the damaged tissue are impaired (see Fig. 62). 3 = Perforation of the capsule (or bladder) overdistended by high pressure (see Figs. 94, d, 138).

Insertion of the Suprapubic Trocar (Bladder Puncture) (Figs. 32, 124, 125)

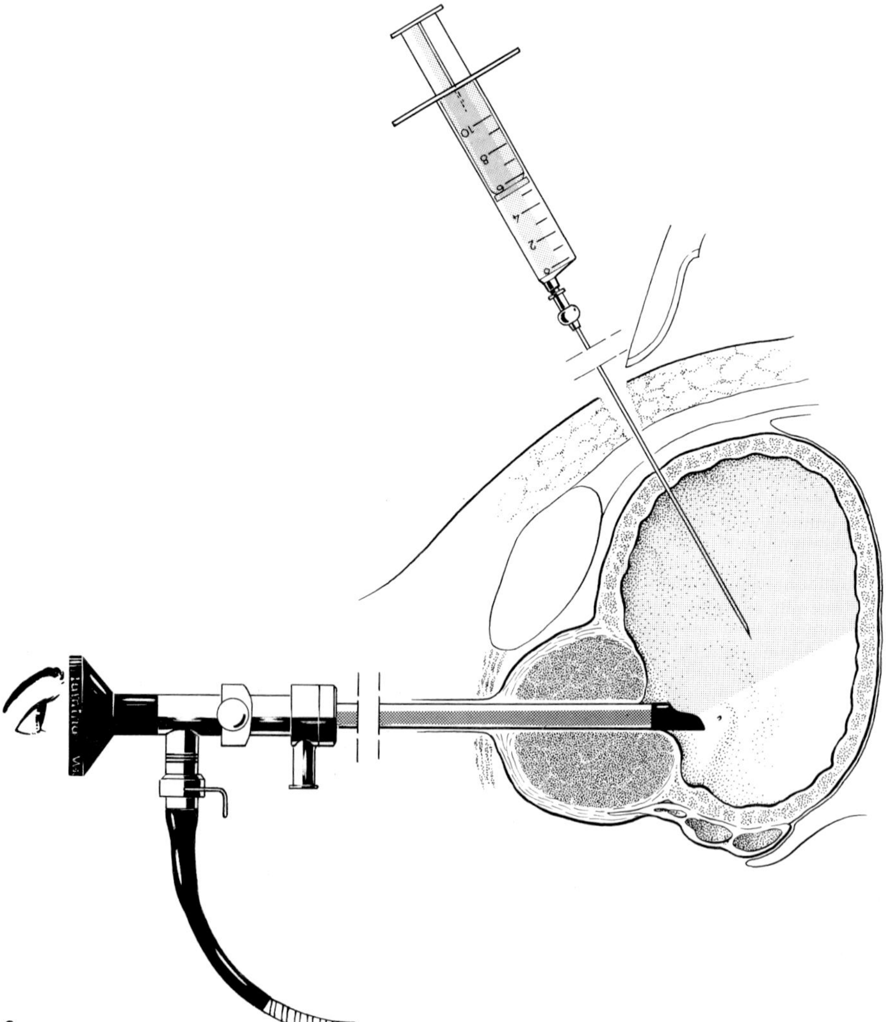

a

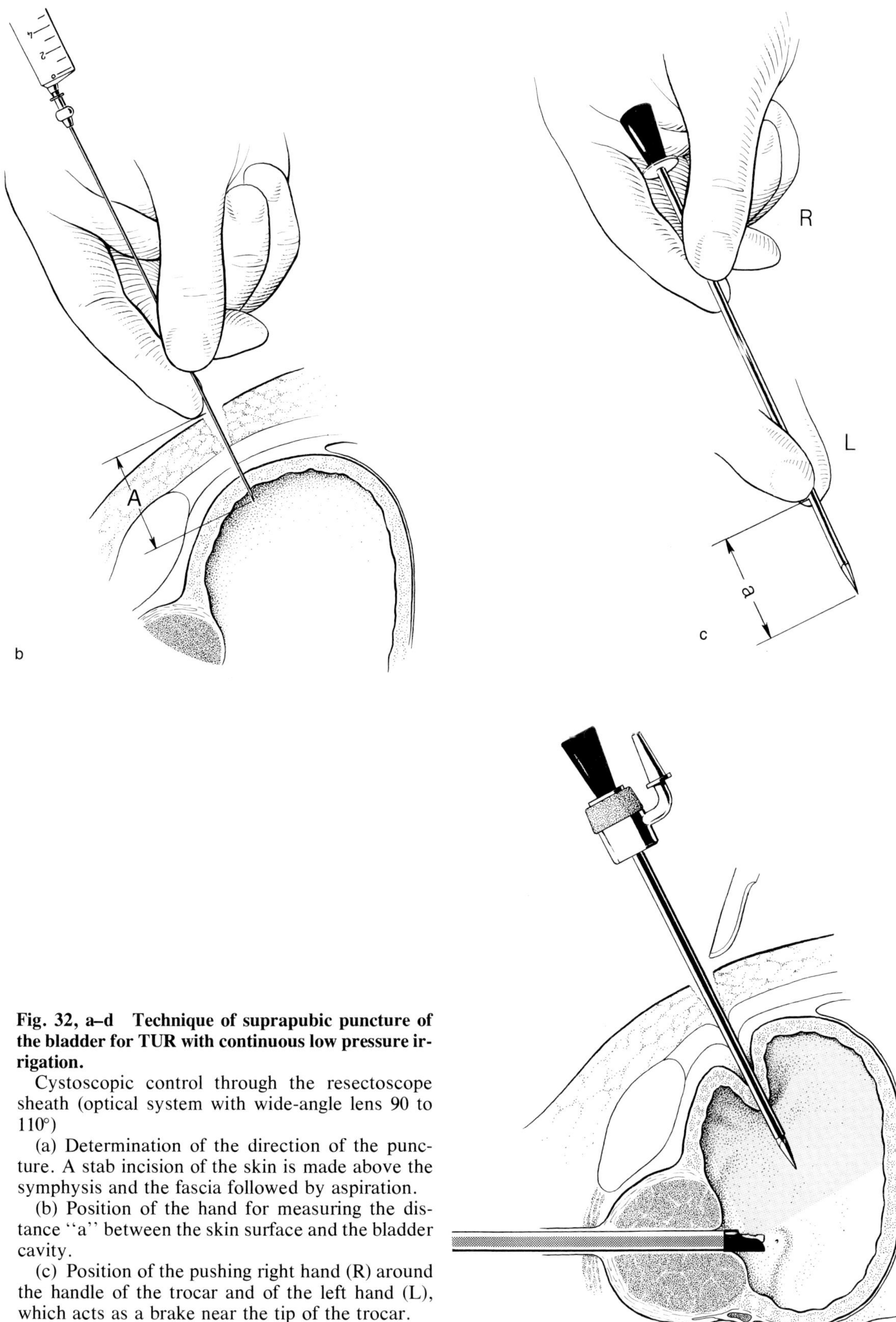

Fig. 32, a–d Technique of suprapubic puncture of the bladder for TUR with continuous low pressure irrigation.

Cystoscopic control through the resectoscope sheath (optical system with wide-angle lens 90 to 110°)

(a) Determination of the direction of the puncture. A stab incision of the skin is made above the symphysis and the fascia followed by aspiration.

(b) Position of the hand for measuring the distance "a" between the skin surface and the bladder cavity.

(c) Position of the pushing right hand (R) around the handle of the trocar and of the left hand (L), which acts as a brake near the tip of the trocar.

(d) The trocar is pushed forcefully with a jerking motion into the bladder (see Fig. 125).

Technical Disturbances of Trocar Irrigation

(1) The trocar is introduced too far into the bladder and the tip lodges in the pile of resected chips on the bladder floor. Aspirated chips occlude all the holes of the trocar (Fig. 33, a). *Correction:* Under endoscopic control of the resectoscope position the tip of the trocar. The sheath of the trocar should not be drawn off the bladder.

(2) The trocar is not inserted deep enough into the bladder. Therefore, the sheath slides out of the bladder when the insert is retracted. This can be avoided by endoscopic control during or after suprapubic insertion of the trocar.

(3) The bladder is not emptied well; aspiration is insufficient, even though the insert of the sheath was moved for cleaning (self-cleaning mechanism):

(a) The insert is obstructed by slime, coagula or fibrin. This occurs when the prostatic tissue is very slimy or when the flow through the trocar is too slow. Insert must be replaced.

(b) Loss of pressure in the aspirating system. Aspiration breaks down when the system is not air-tight. This may be discovered when many air bubbles are seen moving within the transparent plastic tube. Entirely air-tight connections should be used.

(c) Defective vacuum pump. The negative pressure is controlled with a pressure gauge. Excess pressure (over minus 2 m water) sucks the bladder wall or chips of tissue onto the trocar. A negative pressure less than 1 m water is not sufficient. The optimal negative pressure range is between minus 1 and 2 m water, which is hand-regulated with an air inlet valve.

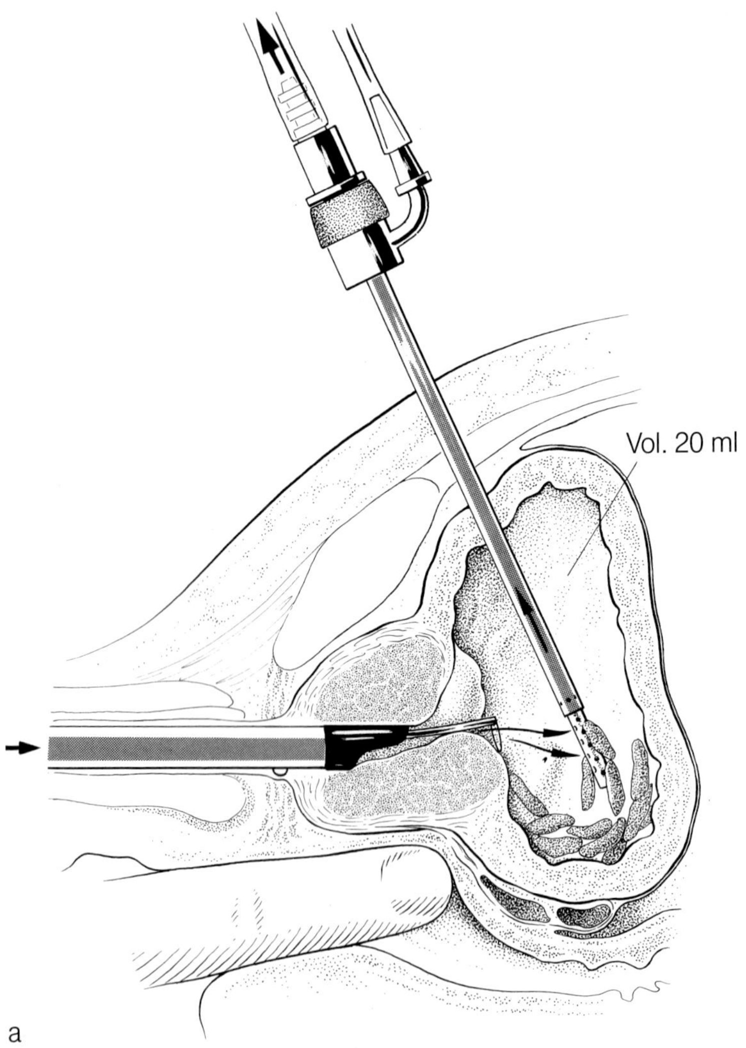

a

Fig. 34, a–d Transurethral introduction of the resectoscope.

(a) The penis is stretched forcibly with the left hand while the resectoscope sheath passes through the penile urethra.

(b) Then the tip of the sheath is felt directly behind the scrotum at the perineum. This is a site of predilection for traumatic urethral strictures.

(c) Next the tip of the obturator is bent by pressure on the knob (thick arrow), the penis is deflected to a horizontal position, and the resectoscope sheath is guided by the finger in the rectum through the prostatic urethra and into the bladder.

(d) The beak of the resectoscope sheath lies within the bladder when the urine flows out freely.

The bladder wall stops the outflow when the sheath is introduced too deep; in this case the beak is retracted to the bladder neck (the control knob at the apex facilitates orientation; see Figs. 13, 41).

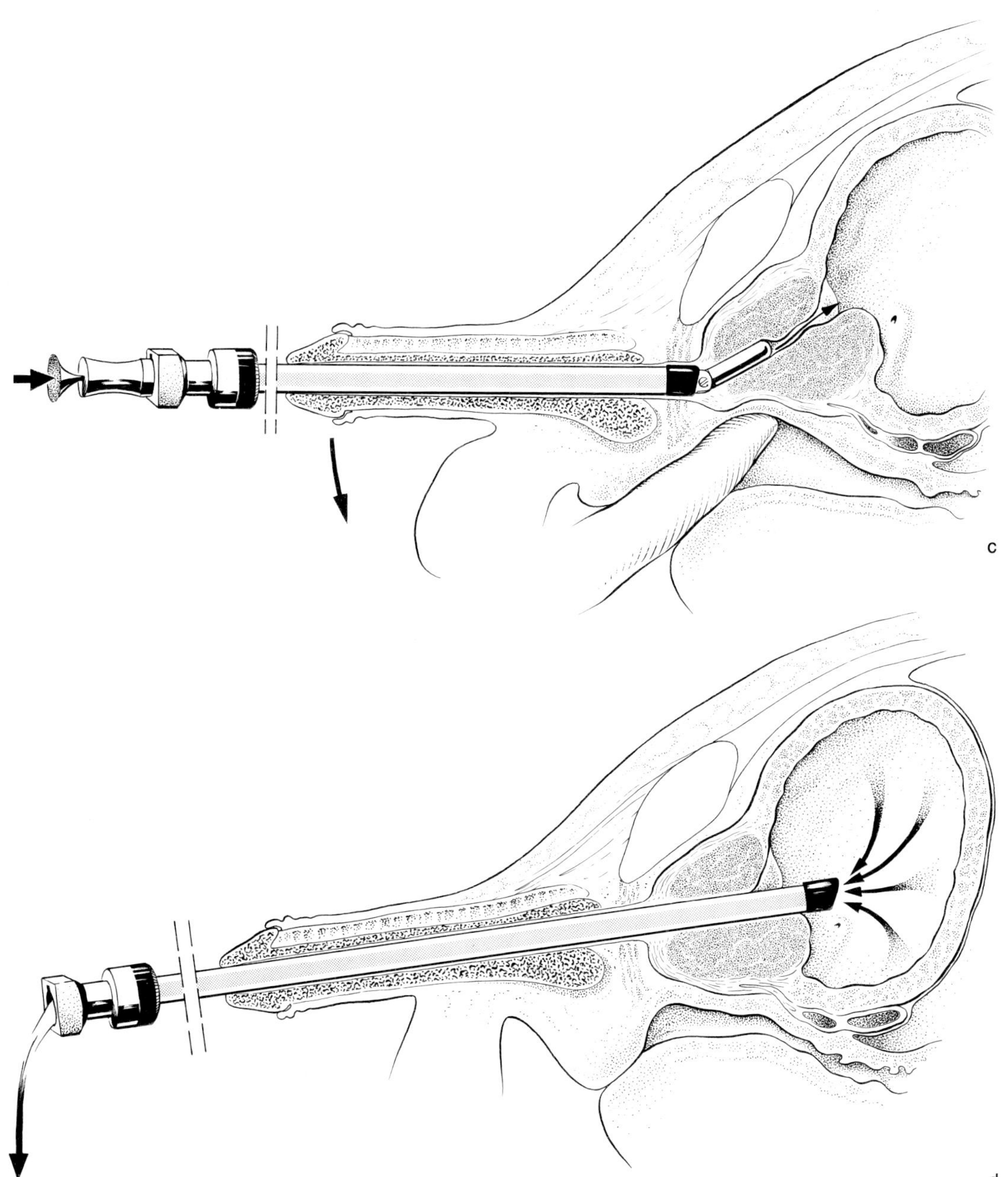

(3) *The transurethral passage* of the resectoscope (see Fig. 21). The sheath is introduced into the penile urethra at an angle of 30 degrees to the body axis. It glides by its own weight more or less passively down to the bulbous urethra, where its tip can be felt behind the scrotum under the perineum. During the introduction of the scope, until this point is reached, the penis is extended forcibly. Now the sheath is slowly lowered into a horizontal position and guided as passively as possible through the prostatic urethra into the bladder. The pliable tip of the obturator facilitates passage. The urogenital diaphragm, a prostatic adenoma and the bladder neck each exert a characteristic resistance to passage. The sheath is guided along its path as easily as a feather; each attempt at forced passage increases the risk of perforation and stricture (see Fig. 123).

We strongly recommend control of the passage of the sheath through the middle and posterior (prostatic) urethra by rectal palpation. All obstructions are inspected with foroblique optics (urethroscopy with the resectoscope or, in a major obstruction, with the thinner urethroscope). Using either the (cold) cutting loop of the resectoscope or the urethroscope, the obstruction can be sounded. Polyps are resected with the cutting loop; urethral valves and strictures are incised with the urethrotome. If necessary, TUR may be postponed. The view can be improved by passing a ureteral catheter alongside the resectoscope sheath or through the channel of the urethroscope to drain clouded irrigant from the operating field. This problem is avoided by using the return-flow resectoscope, urethroscope or urethrotome (see Figs. 15, 53).

In any case we avoid causing stress to the urethral lesion with unphysiologically high pressure (irrigating reservoir over 30 cm of water above the bladder, see p. 23). If the passage of the urethra is forced by high pressure, direct intravasation of septic irrigants into the urethral vessels is inevitable. That fatal complications can follow the intravasation of tetracaine is well known; other local anesthetics (with gel) also are dangerous.

The amount of irrigant flowing through the endoscope is controlled with the 1-liter reservoir (irrigant dosimeter, Fig. 27) to avoid overdistention of the bladder (over 400 cc). The sheath of the resectoscope lies well within the bladder if urine flows spontaneously after removal of the obturator. Bloody urine indicates undesirable traumatisation of the urethra. The beak of the resectoscope is not within the bladder if, when the obturator is removed, air is sucked in, causing a smacking sound. The beak lies in a perforated excavation if a small amount of blood but not urine passes the sheath.

Perforation of the Urethra (Fig. 123)

In general, the extent of the urethral lesion is determined by the diameter of the endoscope. Urethral cystoscopes with a diameter of less than 21 Fr. perforate the wall of the urethra, creating a hole of varying depth (via falsa). This does not interrupt the continuity of the urethra; therefore, a catheter with an elbow tip usually passes the lesion without difficulty. These instruments typically perforate the urethra in the bulbous and medial sections.

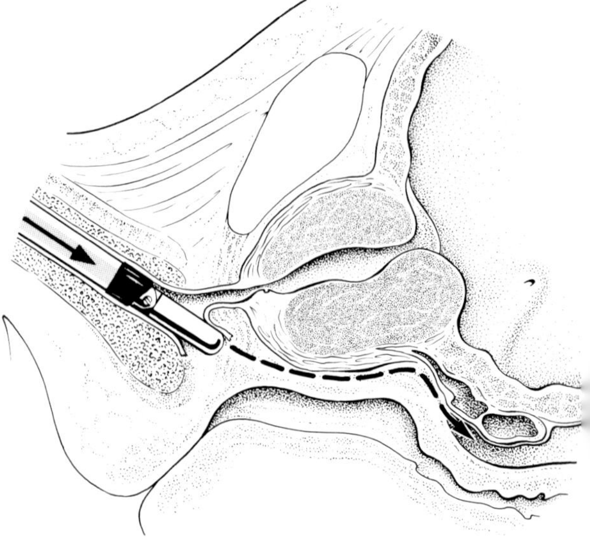

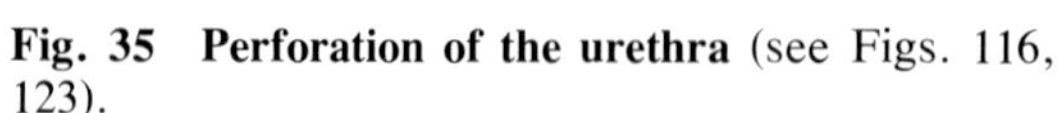

Fig. 35 Perforation of the urethra (see Figs. 116, 123).

Perforation of the bulbous and middle portion of the urethra is shown. The tip of the sheath can be felt at the inner rim of the rectal sphincter. The arrow shows the course of the tip from the perforated middle urethra between the prostate and rectum into the peritoneum (see Fig. 96).

Fig. 36, a–c Perforation of the urethra.

(a) Perforation of the urethra between the middle and prostatic urethra (inside the external sphincter). The tip of the endoscope glides between the capsule and the adenoma (within the false capsule); it finally stops beneath the trigone when it touches the capsule. The short arrow shows the course of the tip toward the bladder; the long arrow shows how it may progress into the subvesical space and the peritoneum (see Cleft Formation, Fig. 93).

(b) Perforation of the prostatic urethra into the adenoma. Often this goes unrecognized — especially when the tip of the endoscope finds its way back into the bladder.

(c) Perforation of the prostatic urethra above the tumor. Only seldom is the capsule perforated into the retropubic space; most often the sheath perforates into the bladder.

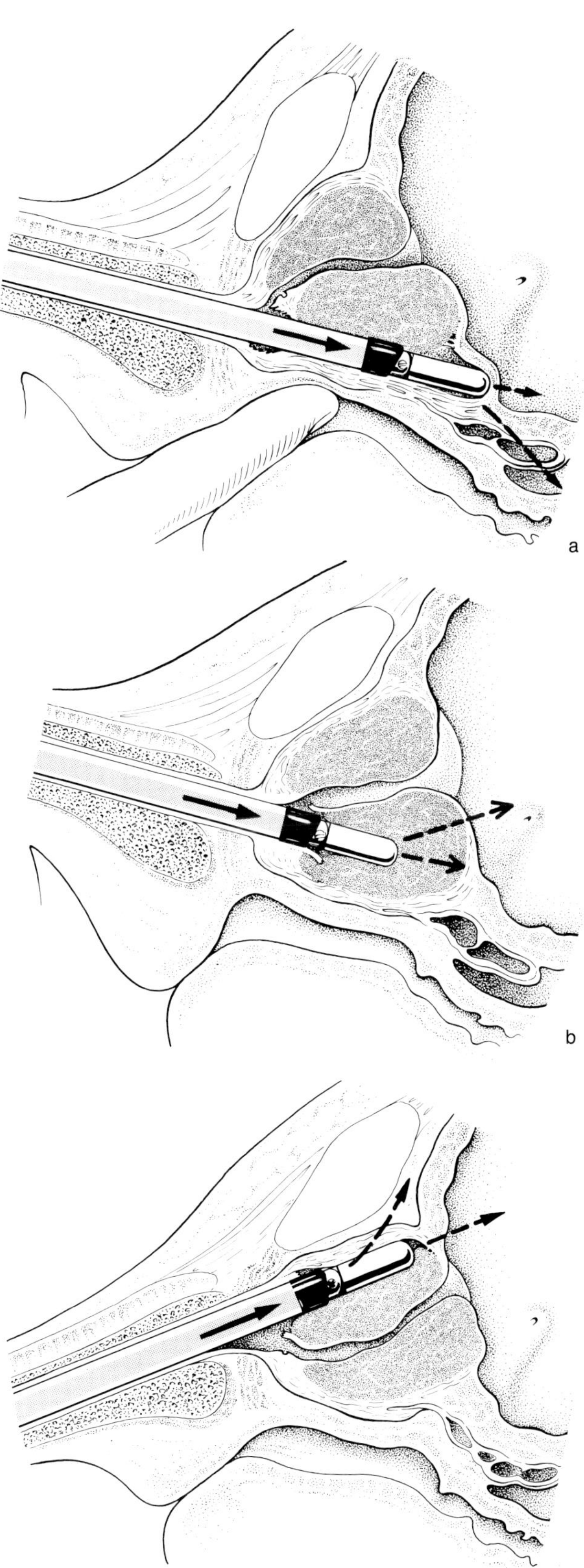

Such a lesion can be treated conservatively by a permanent catheter or by cystostomy (see Figs. 32, 48). Even intraperitoneal perforation can be treated successfully in this way. On the other hand, perforation of the anterior urethra by thick endoscopes, such as the resectoscope, leads to (partial) disruption. This situation is seen in pelvic trauma (fracture). The proximal end of the disrupted urethra is displaced and difficult to find. When searching for the perforation by urethroscopy, the irrigant infiltrates the paraurethral tissues. Therefore, the use of physiologic low pressure irrigation (see p. 25) with isotonic irrigant and a return-flow mechanism (built-in channel; ureteral catheter alongside the sheath) is obligatory. Several typical locations for perforations of the urethra are known:

(1) *Perforation of the middle urethra at the edge of the prostatic urethra, i.e., at the external sphincter* (See Fig. 35). This is the most frequent location. The false passage created leads posteriorly under the adenoma. Even the experienced surgeon cannot always avoid it. Often the perforation is due to deformities of the urethra: most frequently a stricture, but also adenomatous or carcinomatous nodes or unusual inflammatory enlargements and alterations of the tissue may occur. These deformities cause a slight resistance to the passage of the endoscope. To overcome this resistance, the operator pushes forward the endoscope automatically with increased force. This causes its tip to perforate the thin wall of the urethra, usually between capsule and adenoma.

This situation is well known from open prostatectomy: in this layer, the tissue is easily impressed by the finger for the enucleation of an adenoma. Much like the finger, the beak of the instrument protrudes between the adenoma and capsule (in the false capsule) until it is stopped by the internal sphincter. Seldom the median lobe is perforated into the bladder (Fig. 36). There is imminent danger of perforating the capsule below the bladder (trigone) or into the peritoneum when great force is applied.

Our observations by trocar cystoscopy show that unnoticed perforations of the lateral or median lobe of the adenoma into the bladder occur more frequently than had been realized previously. Perforation below the adenoma is easily recognized. The first sign that a false path has been established is an elastic resistance to the advance of the instrument. By rectal palpation, the endoscope sheath is felt too distinctly through the thin prostatic capsule and the rectal mucosa (Fig. 36). In such a case, the sheath should be retracted from the prostatic urethra until its tip is felt in the middle urethra between the anus and apex. Now the finger in the rectum guides the prostate ventrally and corrects the curve of the urethra through the urogenital diaphragm. This finger also serves as guide for the endoscope from the middle into the prostatic urethra (Fig. 34). If this manipulation fails, we terminate the operation and introduce a stiff Foley-catheter with elbowed tip (18 to 20 Fr.) into the bladder. Only an experienced operator should attempt to find the right path by means of the urethroscope or resectoscope. Cystostomy is recommended when the situation is too complicated.

(2) *Ventral perforation of the prostatic uretha.*

(a) The tip of the endoscope glides upward between the adenoma and the capsule. No resistance like the trigone is felt, and the instrument easily perforates the bladder. By rectal palpation the prostate is abnormally prominent. From the ventral perforation the adenoma can be resected toward the back. Thus, one can try to find the prostatic urethra again (see Fig. 36, c).

(b) The tip of the endoscope perforates the capsule and enters the retropubic space. Here, the instrument points upward at an unusually steep angle. The situation is readily recognized by trocar cystoscopy. It is best to terminate the session if this happens.

(3) *Lateral perforation of the prostatic urethra* is similar to ventral perforation (2 a). The attempt to resect back into the natural urethra requires great skill. It is better to find the right way with the help of trocar cystoscopy.

(4) *Perforation of the fibrous capsule,* i.e., into the periprostatic space, seldom occurs. Since this very often leads to perforation of the peritoneum, it is dangerous. The entire sheath glides into the urethra without resistance. Intestinal loops are seen through the optics. Urethroscopy shows a hole in the middle urethra. The more distal the perforation from the bladder, the better the prognosis. Laparotomy is indicated only when the bladder cannot be voided reliably by transurethral or suprapubic drainage. Perforation of the rectum or the bladder wall during introduction of the endoscope has never happened in our hospital.

Treatment of Perforations of the Urethra

Instrumental perforation of the urethra seldom has severe complications when the following rules are observed:

The kind of perforation (localization, extent, direction, etc.) must be diagnosed exactly. This indicates therapy. If necessary, the diagnosis should be proved by x-ray or laparoscopy. Transrectal ultrasound also may be a diagnostic aid.

Drainage of the urine from the bladder must be guaranteed.

All therapeutic interventions — especially local manipulations, such as urethroscopy, sounding, radiographic contrast studies and surgical procedures—must be restricted to an absolute minimum.

The programmed TUR has to be interrupted and postponed. The surgeon can decide otherwise, as an exception, in uncomplicated cases.

If there is the slightest suspicion, the diagnosis of intraperitoneal perforation must be established. Careful soundings with a urethral catheter and filling of the area with contrast medium, illumination of the perforation by urethroscopy and laparoscopy are appropriate diagnostic measures (see Figs. 93, 96, 123).

Primary open surgical treatment of the instrumental perforation of the urethra is not indicated except in two situations:

(1) Direct communication of the bladder with the peritoneal cavity.

(2) Extended disruptions of the urethra.

We have seen neither of these two extreme possibilities. The establishment of a suprapubic bladder fistula assures micturition when transurethral catheterization has been unsuccessful.

Instruments Facilitating the Passage of the Urethra

(1) Elbowed metal sounds for dilatation (12 to 30 Fr.). The bougie indirectly shows us the correct path of the endoscope.

(2) A thin sound or catheter is introduced into the bladder. The sheath of the resectoscope is put over it and thus guided into the bladder (principle of the guiding bougie; secure insertion of a catheter through the sheath over an extended perforation also is practicable).

Trocar Cystoscopy

The bladder neck is observed by suprapubic cystoscopy through the aspiration trocar. If an instrument is introduced through the urethra the wrong way, its tip is clearly seen lifting the bladder neck. Its position can be corrected and the tip centered into the internal urethral orifice. The urethra also can be sounded retrograde, pushing through a trocar cystoscope with an operating channel. The sound also can be introduced through a thick cannula pushed into the bladder at the side of the trocar cystoscope.

Endoscopy of the Bladder

As the resectoscope sheath passes through the prostatic urethra, a certain resistance is felt. When the tip enters the bladder, this resistance ceases noticeably. The sheath now lies almost on the horizontal; it is moved with ease a few centimeters back and forth. The bladder is quickly emptied after retraction of the obturator (Fig. 34). The following observations and examinations are performed:

(1) *Impurities of the urine:* blood (from trauma to the prostatic urethra); coagula (fresh or old); stones or gravel; mucus; fibrous material; shreds of tissue; discharge of air (intestinal fistula); fetor; pus; dislocation. These impurities suggest tumor, calculus, abscess, infection *(E. coli)*, diverticula, necroses, intestinal fistula (fistula of the small intestine with food particles), intake of drugs, etc.

(2) *Scraping of the instrument* in the proximal urethra suggests stone, hard stricture, calcified necroses, foreign body or tumor.

(3) *Abnormal capacity of the bladder:* The graduated 1-L irrigating reservoir permits exact measurement of bladder volume (irrigant dosimeter, see p. 26). A volume of below 100 cc (up to 300 cc) shows a (beginning) contracted bladder. A spastically contracted bladder should be ruled out, however. An atonic bladder is easily missed. Here, the bladder can be filled without resistance with 500 to more than 1000 cc of irrigant (cystometry).

(4) *Displacement of the bladder by external influences.* The position of the bladder changes, depending on its volume and the position of the patient and the endoscope. External influences, such as putting the hand on the lower abdomen, wiping the rectal sheath, coughing, straining, etc., act on the bladder and can disturb the TUR procedure.

(5) *Appearance of the trigone:* the distance of the ureteral orifices from the bladder neck, the shape and doubling of the orifices at the trigone, the interureteral crest and the recess on the bladder floor are examined.

(6) The *thickness of the bladder wall and its condition* are judged (trabeculation, paper-thin bladder and irradiation effects on the bladder, infiltrations and tumors).

(7) Inflammatory changes (catheterization) and secondary results of urinary retention (reflux, stones, diverticula, etc.) are noted.

(8) The length of the urethra corresponds to

the distance between the bladder neck and urethral meatus, which can be judged from the length of the resectoscope sheath that remains outside the body. The endoscope thus can be positioned at the bladder neck without the aid of optics. The left eye is kept open to observe the sheath. Thus, the danger of involuntary movements of the sheath can be prevented. These relatively gross controls require easy movement of the instrument within the urethra.

(9) *Diverticula* are examined in the filled bladder (size, stones or tumor in the diverticulum).

(10) *The bladder roof* between the bladder neck and the air bubble requires special attention. This part of the bladder is frequently not examined in quick cystoscopy. Bladder tumors are easily overlooked here.

(11) Pathologic changes in the bladder can be secondary to disorders in adjacent organs (infiltrative cystitis in tumors of the genitals or rectum; metastases of melanoma; tuberculosis; etc.).

Endoscopy of Bladder Neck and Prostate

Water is not always the optimal medium for cystoscopy (it may be clouded by blood, stone debris, purulent matter, etc.). Such gases as helium, nitrous oxide and carbon dioxide may be preferable in certain situations — e.g., suprapubic trocar cystoscopy (examination of TUR, see Figs. 107, 119 d and e; trocar litholapaxy, see Fig. 126; cryosurgery, Figs. 161 ff). The following four optical perspectives can be chosen (1, 2 and 3 are transurethral; see Fig. 10):

(1) The lower perspective with prograde optics (160° to 180° — "Foroblique" and "Directvision") is used for the resectoscope and the urethroscope.

(2) The plane perspective with angular view optics (prism with a diffraction from 90° — right angle — to 110° — obliquely forward vision). It is in general use for cystoscopy.

(3) The retrograde perspective (retrograde optics after Schlagintweit). Diffraction is extreme and enables the observer to look backward to the bladder neck (comparable to the side-mirror of an automobile).

(4) The perspective from above with (suprapubic) trocar cystoscopy. The bladder neck can be judged objectively. In particular, the size of an endovesical adenoma and its surroundings are viewed without distortion, as in transurethral cystoscopy. Trocar cystoscopy is routinely employed in cryosurgery, litholapaxy, and trocar irrigation (during TUR). The prograde optics (see above) are used for inspection of the urethra. Functional diagnosis of the sphincter mechanism is important. The verumontanum and the external sphincter form a functional unit, the operation of which must be observed, especially during TUR (see Fig. 103). The average distance between them is about 1 cm (7 to 17 mm according to Barnes, 1943). The lateral lobes of an adenoma often extend 1 to 2 cm distal to the verumontanum, although never distal to the external sphincter. Even a prostatic carcinoma respects this border, often to its final stage.

Differentiation of Various Tissues During TUR

Total extirpation of an adenoma (TURP) or a carcinoma (radical TUR) requires exact knowledge of the various kinds of tissue of the prostate and its surroundings (bladder, urethra, periprostatic space and pelvic muscle).

Mucosa (Figs. 103–107)

The mucosa of the prostatic urethra is characteristically altered by adenoma. It can show atrophy, vascular degeneration, inflammation, edema, hemorrhage, abnormal folding, etc. Therefore the extent of the adenoma (toward the bladder and middle urethra) often can be recognized by mucosal changes. The resected fossa is of course lined by mucosa, providing an important landmark for orientation during TUR. Superficially or obliquely cut blood vessels in the mucosa of the prostatic urethra bleed heavily and are difficult to coagulate. From the beginning, the experienced operator cuts deeply into the adenoma, thus avoiding this problem.

Adenoma (Fig. 91, a)

The tumor consists of pale, ivory-white amorphous tissue. Changes in its position and configuration during TUR occur without notice upon cutting, owing to internal tension. Incorrect technique can produce a rough cutting surface (too quick, superficial resection), overhanging lateral lobes (too deep resection), formation of channels (false urethra) or wavy cuts (wrong insert of the cutting loop and insufficient pressure during cut). The adenomatous tissue tends to protrude convexly from the cut surface; this is in significant contrast to the capsule, which *always* forms a concave surface. Protruding fat (after perforation of the capsule) and the dissected spherical seminal vesicles are not to be confused with the adenoma (see Fig. 106).

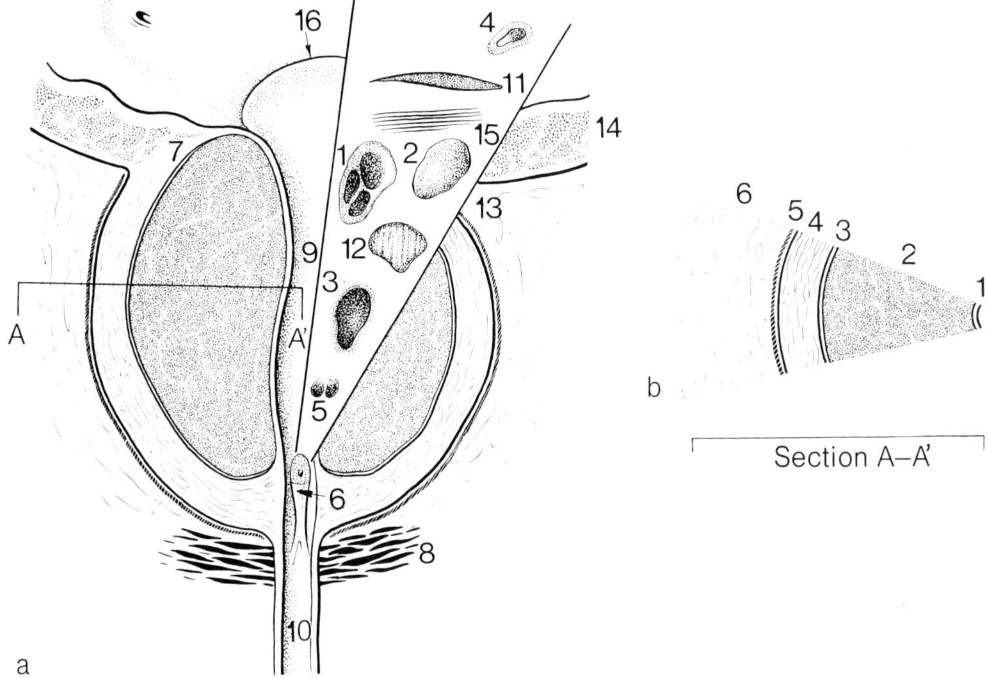

Fig. 37, a–b The tissue layers of the prostate.

(a) Longitudinal section: 1 = cut lumen of a seminal vesicle (see Fig. 94, f); 2 = spherical surface of a seminal vesicle (see Fig. 106, a); 3 = prostatic diverticulum; 4 = partially resected ureteral orifice (see Fig. 97, a); 5 = ejaculatory ducts (see Figs. 103, 108); 6 = verumontanum (see Fig. 88, f); 7 = internal sphincter (see Fig. 91, h); 8 = external sphincter (see Fig. 86, c); 9 = prostatic urethra (see Fig. 85); 10 = middle urethra (see Fig. 86); 11 = perforation into the peritoneum (see Fig. 96); 12 = perforation into the rectum (see Fig. 116); 13 = cleft between capsule and bladder with periprostatic tissue (see Fig. 93); 14 = bladder wall (see Figs. 90, 134); 15 = cleft formation between trigone and prostatic capsule (see Fig. 93); 16 = median lobe.

(b) Frontal section through the prostatic fossa: 1 = mucosa of the prostatic urethra; 2 = adenoma; 3 = false capsule; 4 = true gland; 5 = true prostatic tissue (capsule); 5 = true fibrous capsule; 6 = periprostatic tissue.

Carcinoma (Fig. 109)

Typical carcinomatous tissue differs from the adenoma by its hard consistency, gray color and immobile cut surface, which bleeds only slightly. TUR of the deeper layers, especially the peripheral capsule, is, on the other hand, mostly impeded by vigorous and profuse bleeding. Rectal palpation is obligatory in radical TUR. This makes possible a sensitive, fine resection of the fossa. Mobilization of the rectum can be controlled (see Fig. 110) after resection of the rigid tissue.

Extensive infiltration of the bladder floor causes a reduction in bladder capacity (below 300 cc). In such a case, "radical TUR" has lost its meaning.

Prostatic Capsule (Fig. 94)

If the term "prostatic capsule" is used in connection with TUR, the true prostatic tissue is always meant. However, the differentiation between the false and true capsule is also important. Therefore, we specify the tissues in the order in which they come into view during TUR (Fig. 37):

(1) The mucosa of the prostatic urethra.

(2) The false capsule is the hypothetic layer between the adenoma and true prostatic tissue. The false capsule is important in open surgical prostatectomy, where it guides the finger that enucleates the adenoma. During TUR it is recognized only indirectly when fibers of the capsule are freed of adenomatous tissue by resection.

(3) The adenoma (paraurethral glands).

(4) The true prostatic gland, "the capsule." The original prostatic gland is composed of three hypothetic layers: the superficial layer with delicate dense fibers; the middle layer with rough fibers; and the peripheral layer of

loose mesh adjacent to the fibrous capsule (see Figs. 91, 99).

(5) The fibrous capsule (true capsule; see Fig. 113, e). The fibrous layer between true prostatic tissue and the periurethral connective tissue often is recognized by its smooth metallically shining surface. The true capsule often is incorrectly referred as to the "true prostate" (see 4).

(6) The internal sphincter (see Fig. 91, h). Its circular muscle derives from the bladder muscle and distinguishes the bladder neck from the adenoma and the capsule. These circular fibers are an important landmark during TUR; they connect the prostate and bladder.

(7) The external sphincter (see Fig. 101). It extends about 1 to 2 cm distal to the utriculus of the verumontanum and marks the transition from prostatic to middle urethra. The verumontanum is its landmark at the distal rim of the fossa. Laterally and above, the bulging lateral lobes indicate the border of the prostatic urethra. The external sphincter usually is recognized by its function — seldom by its anatomy.

(8) The colliculus seminalis (verumontanum) (see Fig. 103). This marks the distal end of the prostatic fossa; as a rule it is recognized by the utriculus. The ejaculatory ducts are recognized (like the ureteral orifices) by the ejection of seminal fluid, especially if dye was injected into the seminal vesicles (see p. 20).

(9) The bladder musculature can be distinguished from the capsule only by its rough structure (see Fig. 134).

(10) The seminal vesicles are difficult to cut; by palpation they often resemble carcinomatous infiltration (see Fig. 106).

(11) The periurethral tissue consists of connective tissue, fat and long fibers of the levator ani muscle. It rarely bleeds and is not easily cut.

Appearance and Reaction of Different Tissues During TUR

The *mucosa* resists the cutting loop to a certain degree. The loop therefore should be inserted "behind the mountain" (see Fig. 42).

The *adenoma* is easy to cut, protrudes convexly into the lumen of the fossa and changes its structure during TUR (displacement of tissues). Cut blood vessels retract into the surrounding tissue. This complicates coagulation. For this reason one should coagulate only in the capsule (see Fig. 92).

The *true prostatic tissue* (the capsule) has an obvious fibrous structure (like nylon stockings). It can be distinguished from the adenoma by its reddish color (meat-colored). Its wall is always convex; it evades the cutting loop (like a rubber fabric) and floats freely in the irrigating stream (see Fig. 91). Inflammatory or tumorous infiltration destroys this structure.

The *fibrous (true) capsule* is as smooth as the skin; its surface often has a metallic shine. Small air bubbles collect in the capsule — particularly on its surface (see Fig. 91, m).

The *circular fibers* of the internal sphincter are easily verified (see Fig. 91, h). Thus, we resect the adenoma extensively and free the internal sphincter between the 4- and 8-o'clock positions. When the lesion is resected too far, the tissue is undermined in a typical manner, forming a cleft (see Fig. 93).

The *external sphincter* is not exposed. The action and shape of its opening at the transition from the middle to the prostatic urethra are the functional expression of its existence (see Figs. 101–103).

The *bladder muscle,* apart from the internal sphincter, appears during TUR only when surgical mistakes are made (over-resection; perforation). In radical TUR, the tissues frequently are resected down to the ureteral orifices (see Fig. 133, b).

Formation of Clefts in the Prostatic Fossa

Seminal vesicles (see Fig. 106) have a characteristic shape and localization. They are found below the trigone and the adjacent prostatic urethra. When their thick-walled lumen is cut, they discharge milky seminal fluid.

The *ejaculatory duct* (see Fig. 108) connects the seminal vesicle on both sides with the colliculus seminalis. Therefore, their lumina, which resemble small blood vessels, always are cut together on the floor of the fossa.

The *prostatic diverticulum* (see Fig. 37) is a pathologic enlargement of the prostatic glandular ducts. Its shape and localization vary enormously, and it often contains stones or purulent material. The wall is thin; unlike a seminal vesicle, it is not septated.

The *venous sinus* (see Fig. 98) usually is found in the deepest layer of the capsule (true prostatic tissue). Most often it is cut because of errors in judgment (too deep resection of the capsule). The venous sinus may be found anywhere in the fossa, although it usually is located at the apex and in the lateral fossa. The lumen of the sinus often is not verified. Hemorrhage from the sinus often appears to be critical, but in most cases can be controlled by using a correct technique of coagulation in combination with low pressure irrigation and continuous aspiration. A compression catheter (30- to 50-cc balloon) seldom is necessary (see pp. 55, 59).

Perforation (Figs. 35–36, 40; 45; 93–96; 123)

We distinguish between covered and open perforation. The distinction between "near" and "complete" perforation is not made as frequently as in the past because we use continuous low pressure irrigation (see Figs. 31, 92–94). The radical TUR technique employed in prostatic and bladder cancer requires, by definition, extensive, complete and intentional perforation.

The surgeon without endoscopic experience has difficulty in distinguishing between endoscopic and surgical perforation. The latter always is a dangerous condition, and immediate operative closure is obligatory. Endoscopic perforation often can be treated conservatively.

Covered perforation tends to occur at four sites:

(1) The lateral wall of the fossa near the bladder (see Fig. 93). Here, the longitudinal fibers of the levator ani muscle regularly appear (see Fig. 94).

(2) The bladder neck between the internal sphincter and the prostate. At the trigone, perforation causes the so-called lift-off of the bladder from the prostate (see Fig. 93); laterally, it causes a cleft (see Fig. 94).

(3) The floor of the fossa close to the bladder. The seminal vesicles are exposed (see Fig. 94, f); further distally, a circular defect is caused (comparable to the hole in a cloth burned by a cigarette). Here the longitudinal muscle of the rectum or underlying connective tissue is seen (see Fig. 95, a).

(4) The roof of the fossa. Here perforation is rare; it is recognized when the tough tissue of the symphysis is exposed. Perforation into pericapsular fat most often occurs in the proximal third of the prostatic fossa, usually in the upper hemisphere (see Fig. 95, e, f). The dangers of covered perforation are reduced by physiologic low pressure irrigation, because the experienced resectionist notes them early enough in the procedure. TUR almost always can be continued because physiologic low pressure irrigation prevents grave complications (infiltration and destruction of tissue). On the other hand, high pressure irrigation often leads to premature termination of TUR, since traumatization of the perforation causes subperitoneal irrigant absorption. This is recognized by a rise of blood pressure, peritoneal pain (often epigastric pain as well) and subsequent shock (see Fig. 93, d).

Rules for the Diagnosis and Treatment of the Covered Perforation

The perforation is examined endoscopically to exclude open perforation of the peritoneum. Bleeding vessels of the rim of the capsule are coagulated meticulously. Endoscopy and coagulation are without risk only when physiologic low pressure irrigation is used. Covered perforations are treated conservatively (permanent catheter) when isotonic irrigant (5 per cent glucose) is used (see Fig. 71).

Open perforation of the peritoneum and rectum can occur (see legends of Figs. 96, 116).

(1) Microperforation into the peritoneum (or rectum) is rare. It is localized at the bladder neck and closes when the bladder shrinks after voiding. It therefore heals spontaneously when constant urinary drainage of the bladder is maintained.

(2) True perforation of prostatic capsule or bladder wall into the peritoneum (see Fig. 96).

(3) Perforation into the peritoneal recessus reaching abnormally low (rectovesical pouch).

(4) Perforation into the rectum (see Fig. 116). This is extremely rare, because the elastic intestinal tube evades the cutting loop. This effect is useful during radical TUR of prostatic carcinoma (see Fig. 95). The diagnosis is evident when the irrigant comes out of the anus; the patient does not respond to rectal perforation. The site of predilection is near the trigone in the region of the seminal vesicles. Surgical suture is attempted immediately.

Over-resection is in certain cases the first step toward perforation of the bladder (see Fig. 97). The protruding bladder neck in this case is mistaken for adenoma (incorrect positioning of the resectoscope, i.e., exaggerated angulation of the sheath; see Fig. 39). In most cases, perforation of the bladder is dramatic when high pressure irrigation is applied because the fast flow of irrigant opens a large defect in the bladder wall, causing perivesicular absorption of irrigant with acute symptoms. Low pressure irrigation prevents these acute disturbances; TUR can, if necessary, be interrupted deliberately.

Gas explosions in the bladder cannot occur with continuous irrigation because the bladder is nearly empty and developing gas is aspirated constantly. We never have experienced a harmful explosion (Baumrucker 1968). *Warning:* Plastic tubes used instead of the specific trocar insert—in an inadvertent position—may not remove the gas, risking an explosion (Fritjofsson).

Surgical intervention is necessary to close defects in the bladder caused by an explosion. It is recommended that the retroperitoneal space be opened and drained well. Double drainage of the bladder (cystostomy and permanent catheter) secures the sutures. When the defect in the bladder is extensive, catheters are inserted into both ureters and the abdomen is also drained to prevent peritonitis.

Diagnostic Aids for Proof of Perforation

(1) The irrigant flowing into and out of the bladder is measured with the *dosimeter* (see Fig. 27). More than two thirds of the irrigant returns from the bladder when the perforation is covered. On the other hand, an open perforation of the peritoneum causes most of the irrigant to disappear within the abdomen.

(2) *Contrast endoradiography*: The bladder is filled with 50 to 100 cc of contrast medium and examined by x-ray monitor. Extravasation through the covered perforation can be seen. The contrast medium diffuses into the abdomen through an open intraperitoneal perforation. It is better to introduce a catheter into the perforation hole through the resectoscope sheath or the urethroscope (ureter catheter). The contrast medium then can be injected into the perforation under control.

(3) Transrectal and transurethral ultrasonic scanning.

(4) *Laparoscopy*: Evidence of irrigating fluid within the abdomen; inspection of the perforation hole.

(5) Surgical intervention.

Warning Signs of Imminent Perforation

When TUR is performed under epidural anesthesia the patient can communicate symptoms that indicate the danger of perforation.

(1) *Peritoneal pain.* The electric current produces an aching pain a few millimeters before the peritoneum is perforated.

(2) *Local tension* of the lower abdominal muscles combined with uncomfortable sensations indicates liquid infiltration of the extraperitoneal space (covered perforation). The patient can point to these sensations with his finger.

(3) *Acute jerks* of the pelvic floor and adductor muscles. The obturator nerve is irritated by the electric current. This signals too-extensive resection when the bladder wall is mistaken for adenoma (over-resection).

(4) General reactions of the psyche, autonomic nervous system, blood pressure, etc., as known from the TUR syndrome, also are probable symptoms of perforation (peritoneal irritation, irrigant absorption, etc.)

(5) Electrical sensations felt in the surgeon's finger generally signal too much current (especially if mixed current is used), not a risk of perforation (e.g., during examination of the thickness of the capsule).

(6) The quality of the cut depends on the electrical current as well as the specific properties of the tissue. Adenoma and taut muscles (e.g., the internal sphincter) are easily cut. Normal capsular tissue (without inflammatory or carcinomatous infiltration) resists the cut. It is difficult to hook the loop onto the capsule for cutting. At this point, the cutting sector is changed.

The wall of the resected fossa is checked with the cold loop for thickness and mobility. Rectal palpation supports this test.

(7) The typical behavior of tissue before perforation should be recognized. The structure of the capsule becomes loose and disorganized (see Fig. 93a); the metallic fibrous capsule is the last warning layer (see Fig. 91l). The wall of the fossa floats in the irrigating stream. Blue ink injected into the capsule facilitates verification of the nature of the tissue (see Fig. 92, b).

(8) The correct irrigating technique (low pressure irrigation with continuous aspiration, see p. 25) reduces the risk of perforation. If resection is performed in an empty bladder, with the wall of the bladder and the prostatic fossa not under tension (see Fig. 31), the relaxed capsule can thus evade the cut and warn the surgeon of imminent perforation.

Basic Technique of the Transurethral Resection

Technique of TURP

The technique of TUR is determined by two factors (see Fig. 12):

(1) The design of the resectoscope. The cutting loop moves only in one dimension (back and forth). The colliculus seminalis is the distal limit of the cut. From there, a cone is resected by one-dimensional cutting into the prostate. The result is a partial TUR.

Transformation of this cone-shaped figure into a hollow sphere (total TUR, TURP) requires complex movements whereby the resectoscope and the cutting loop are moved synchronously, guided by the finger in the rectum (Fig. 41).

(2) The topography of the operating field. This is determined by the consistency, extension and shape of the adenoma, as well as by pathologic alterations in the anatomy of the bladder neck by the adenoma. Further artificial alterations occur during TUR (unphysiologic pressure due to the irrigation, bladder overdistention, irrigating fluid absorption, distortion of tissues, etc.).

The borders of the prostate are indicated by several landmarks. The most important is the colliculus seminalis, which marks the external sphincter below. Another is formed by the swollen adenomatous lobes: a fold connecting the internal and external sphincter at 12 o'clock. The transition from the prostatic to the middle urethra at the distal end of the adenoma is recognized by changes in the appearance of the mucosal blood vessels and by the function of the external sphincter. The normal length of the prostatic urethra from the verumontanum to the bladder neck is 1 to 2 cm (average: 1.7 cm).

For the resection of a hollow sphere, the operating field (fossa) is divided into several sectors (see Fig. 38):

(1) Resection of an irrigating channel between the colliculus seminalis (external sphincter) and the bladder, including extensive TUR of the median lobe until the internal sphincter is bare (between 4 and 8 o'clock). This channel is necessary to ensure irrigation between the resectoscope sheath and the return flow channel, allowing the aspirating trocar to function unhindered (see Fig. 38).

(2) Resection of the lateral lobes (sparing the apex; see Fig. 91).

(3) Resection of the apex (see Fig. 103).

(4) Resection of the roof of the fossa (see Fig. 119, c)

(5) Clearing of the external sphincter (see Fig. 101).

The beginner has two important aids at his disposal:

(1) Low pressure irrigation with active aspiration of irrigant from the bladder (through the suprapubic trocar or the return flow resectoscope sheath). This allows orientation and patient progress with TUR without the hindrance of intervals for bladder evacuation (see p. 25).

(2) Rectal palpation, together with use of the control knob of the resectoscope sheath at the apex. This makes "blind" orientation possible if optic orientation is lost (see Fig. 41). The control knob represents an absolutely reliable fixing point at the apex, helping to prevent unintended TUR of the bladder floor or the distal urethra due to false orientation (see p. 101 f).

Opening of TUR

First the colliculus seminalis and the ureteral orifices are inspected. The instrument is held horizontally within the body axis. Angulation is not correct.

I. Basic Cut

(1) The beak of the sheath is slipped into the bladder with the cutting loop retracted.

(2) The resectoscope is then slowly pulled back over the trigone until the median bar (or the median lobe) is in the center of view.

(3) Now the cutting loop is extended to its full length.

(4) The control knob is set onto the apex "blind" (by rectal palpation); the sheath now covers and protects the verumontanum. The same determination is made endoscopically. The verumontanum is viewed and the sheath is then slipped forward over its proximal edge. Adjustment is not possible by endoscope. When the irrigation of the prostatic urethra is reduced by the adenoma blocking the beak of the resectoscope (see irrigating channel, Fig. 85), optical control of the cut cannot be maintained.

(5) The cutting loop is retracted cold, until it hooks onto the bar (median lobe). Then the current is started and the loop cuts.

(6) The quality of the cut depends not only on the current and the size of the loop but also on the following factors:

(a) Deep insertion of the loop (behind the mountain) at the bladder neck;

(b) Sufficient pressure of the resectoscope on the tissue with opposing pressure of the finger in the rectum to keep the loop from emerging (see Figs. 41, 42).

Text continued on page 50

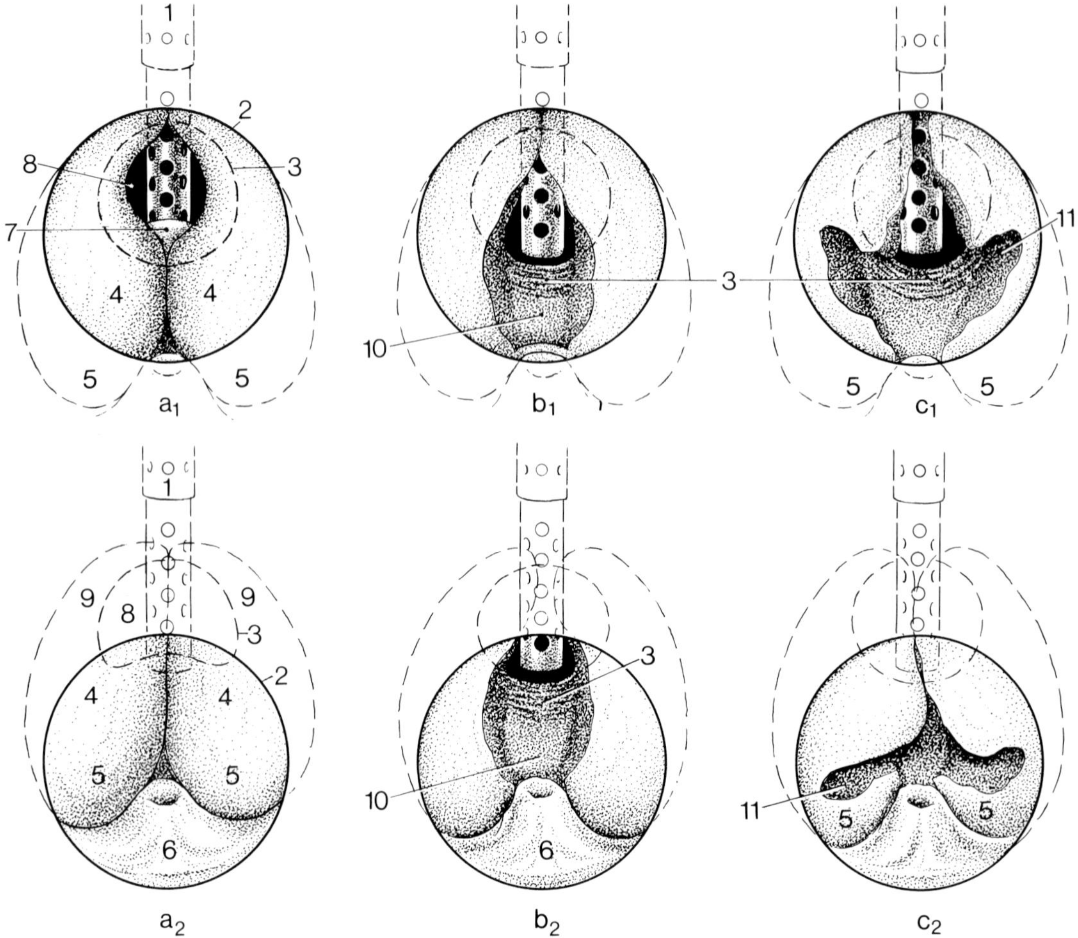

Fig. 38, a–g Technique of TURP (frontal section; modification of the technique of R.W. Barnes and R.M. Nesbit; see Figs. 101–105).

a_1–f_1: The inner position of the resectoscope permits a view of the lateral lobes, which form the typical fold above at 12 o'clock. The verumontanum (below) is just out of sight.

a_2–f_2: Alternatively, the resectoscope may be retracted until the external sphincter and verumontanum are seen. Above, the bellies of the lateral lobes meet. The internal sphincter with the median lobe and the upper third of the lateral lobes are indicated by dashed lines.

a and *b* show the resection of an irrigating channel from the verumontanum to the internal sphincter. The finger in the rectum must be used to lift the adenomatous tissue in *a–c, e* and *f* (see Fig. 13).

In a_1, the resectoscope is positioned at the distal end of the prostatic urethra (see Fig. 85, c). The irrigation pushes the lateral lobes aside (8). The view is unobstructed over the median lobe (7), into the lumen of the bladder and onto the suprapubic trocar (1). The internal sphincter is marked with a dashed circle (3). Below the view (2), the verumontanum and the bases of the lateral lobes (5) are indicated by dashed lines.

a_2: The resectoscope is retracted into the middle urethra until the apex with the verumontanum (6) and the distal faces of the lateral lobes (4, 5) are seen (see Fig. 85, d).

b_1 and b_2: The median lobe and the adenoma at the fossa floor are resected. The irrigating channel (10) ends directly in front of the verumontanum (b_2, 6). The internal sphincter (dashed circle) is prepared between 4 and 8 o'clock (3). The irrigating channel now insures that irrigant will flow from the resectoscope directly into the trocar. This is the first step in a systematic TUR.

(*c*) Lateral enlargement of the irrigating channel. The lateral lobes (5) are resected in their lower third, beginning the cut at the internal sphincter (3). However, far lateral resection must be avoided, because a false urethra (11) is formed by the overhanging residuals of the lateral lobes (see Fig. 40). The lower third of the prostatic fossa now is resected almost to the capsule. Adenomatous tissue remains only at the apex (c_2, 5). The internal sphincter (dashed circle; c_1, 3) is dissected between 3 and 9 o'clock.

(*d*) Cutting of the lateral lobes in the upper third of the fossa. At 2 to 3 o'clock, broad channels (12) are cut into the upper lateral base of the lateral lobe; thus, the mass of the adenoma (4) falls down. It can now be resected easily from above. This reduces stress to the surgeon's spine.

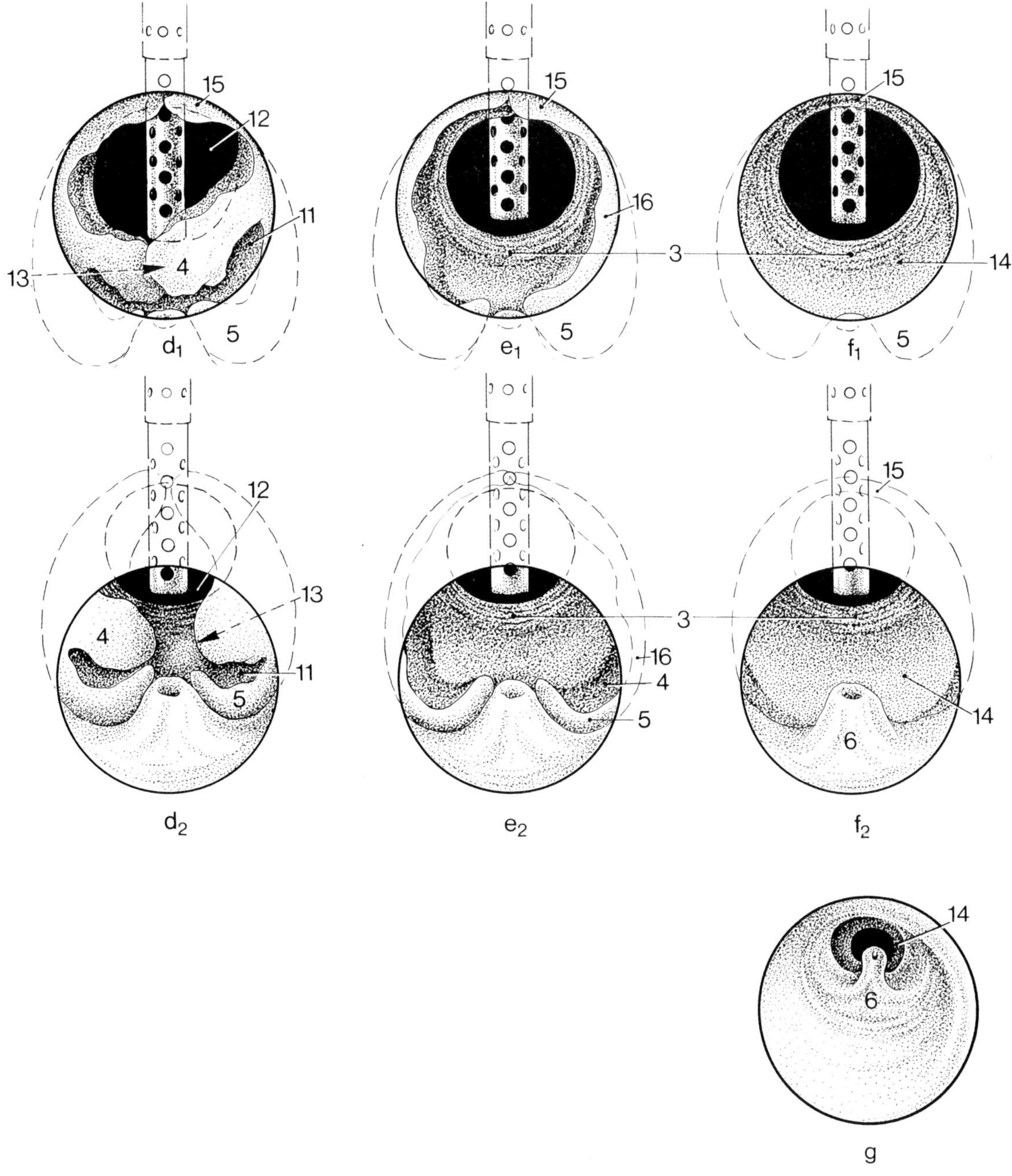

(*e*) Reduction of the lateral lobes. The lateral lobe (*d,* 4) now is cut at its most prominent point (*d,* 13), reducing its mass from the center toward the periphery. This makes cutting of larger pieces unnecessary, and there is no danger of perforation.

f–g: 1. Resection of the bladder roof; 2. cleansing of the fossa from adenomatous remainders; 3. resection of the apex with molding of the external sphincter.

f_1 and f_2: The fossa (14) is resected to a hollow sphere; its roof (15) is freed of the lateral lobes. The internal sphincter now is a smooth circle of annular fibers (3). At the apex, all adenomatous remainders (*e,* 5) are resected over the finger in the rectum. Only seldom do so-called "columns" remain (*e,* 16); these should consist mainly of capsular wall and mucosa.

(*g*) The middle urethra now communicates through a circle with the fossa (14). If the resectoscope is retracted farther back into the middle urethra, the retraction and contraction of the external sphincter and verumontanum can be observed (see Fig. 103). The verumontanum (6) stands isolated like a tower on a cliff.

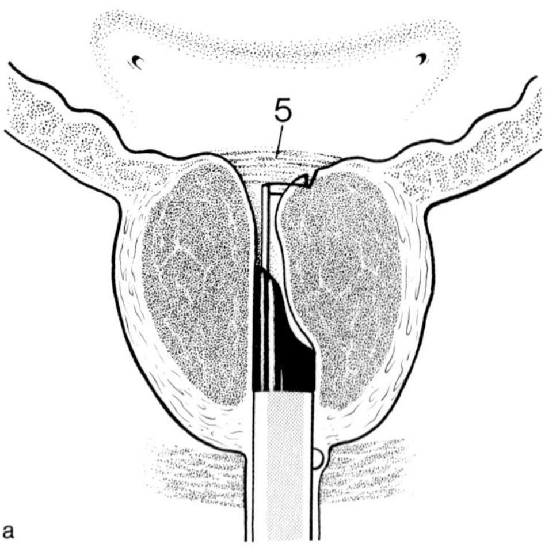

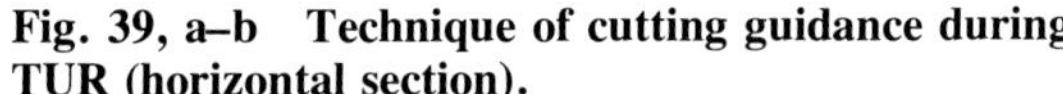

Fig. 39, a–b Technique of cutting guidance during TUR (horizontal section).

(a) Correct cutting guidance. The control knob is positioned at the apex; the verumontanum is just covered by the resectoscope sheath. The loop is hooked blindly on the lateral rim of the adenoma at 3 o'clock inside the internal sphincter. The middle lobe is resected; already, fibers of the internal sphincter (5) are exposed.

(b) Incorrect cutting guidance. The resectoscope (3) is introduced too far into the bladder; this leads to a pseudoresection of the bladder neck (see Fig. 97, b). The resectoscope (4) is angled far to one side (arrow). The adenoma is deformed and seems to tug the bladder neck into the prostatic urethra. This causes over-resection of the lateral lobes at 3 o'clock. 1 = Distortion of the bladder wall; 2 = control knob too far advanced into the fossa.

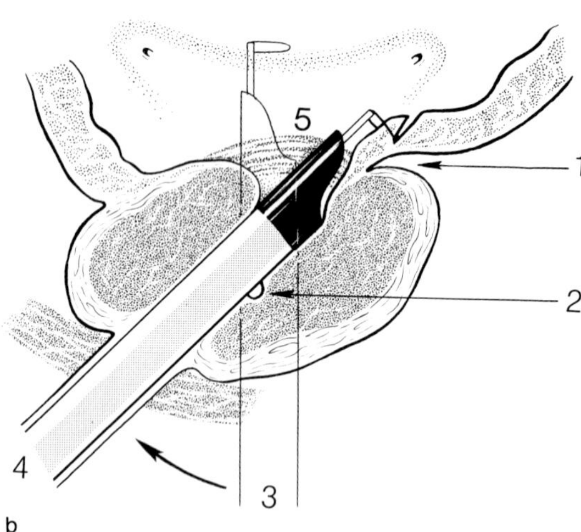

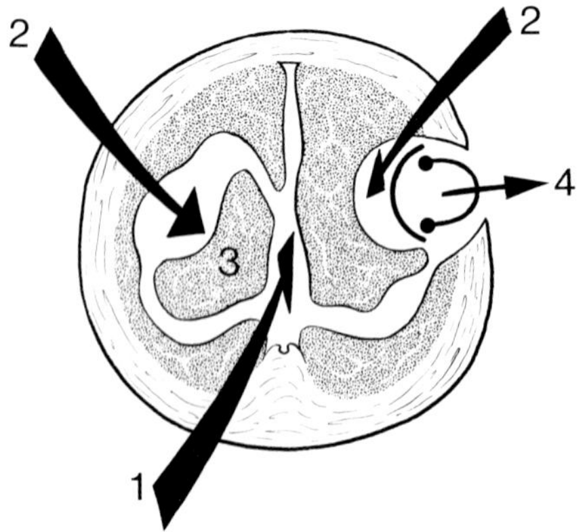

Fig. 40 Undermining of the lateral lobes with resection of a false urethra (2, frontal section; see Figs. 38, c, d, and 101, c).

With correct technique, the cuts are laid out broadly, one next to the other. Here, incorrectly, one cut was made below the other, forming a deep groove. Continuation of TUR in this groove leads to the creation of large, freely mobile pieces of adenoma (3) or to perforation of the capsule (4). 1 = Prostatic urethra; 2 = free piece of adenoma.

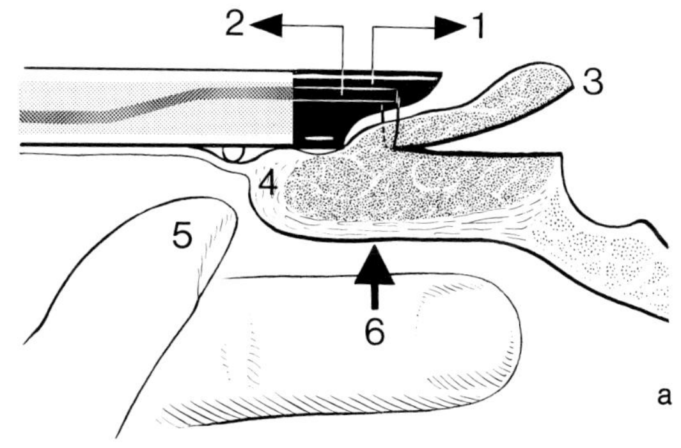

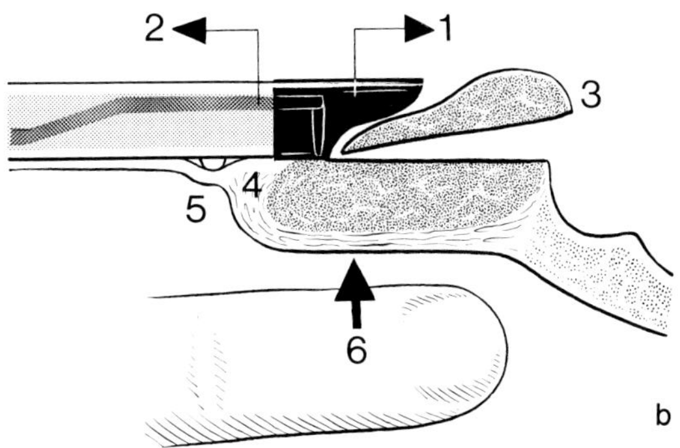

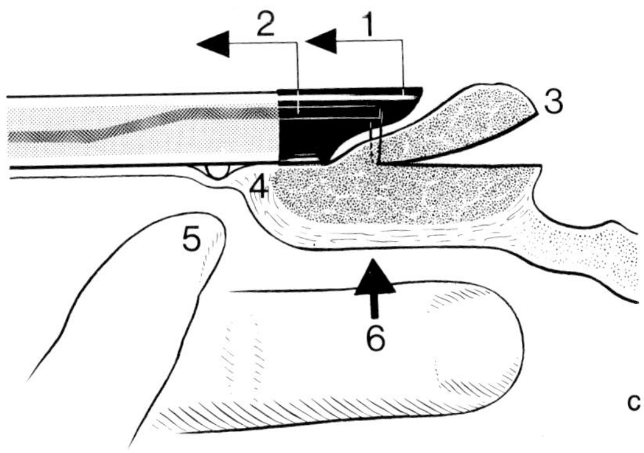

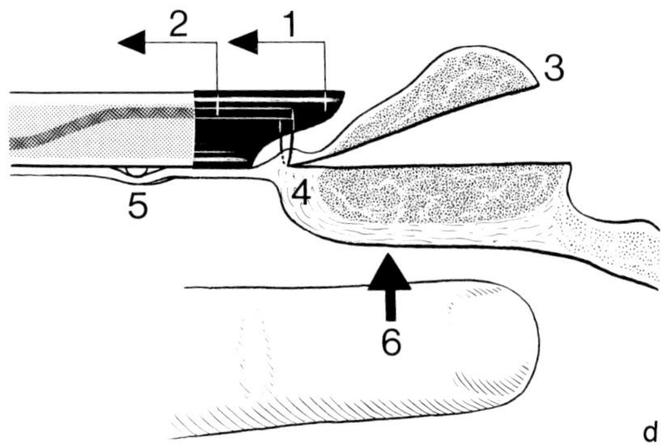

Fig. 41, a–d Correct and incorrect cutting of the tissue chip.

(a) Correct shearing movement of the sheath's window against the loop (first phase). The sheath is moved a few millimeters toward the bladder (arrow 1). Simultaneously, the loop is retracted into the sheath (arrow 2). This cuts the chip (3) off smoothly; the colliculus seminalis (4) is spared. The index finger is used to adjust the control knob at the apex (5) and to lift the prostate (arrow 6).

(b) In the second phase, the chip (3) is cut. The loop (2) has disappeared into the sheath. The control knob is positioned at the apex (5). The colliculus seminalis (4) is unharmed. The index finger has straightened the curve of the capsule (6).

(c) Incorrect shearing with simultaneous movement of sheath (1) and cutting loop (2) in the same direction. First phase: distal retraction of the sheath (1) is unknowingly performed by the beginner.

(d) Second phase: while retracting the sheath (1), the cut ends too near the sphincter. This cannot be controlled by direct vision. The damage to the external sphincter (mainly at 9 o'clock) or the colliculus seminalis (4) therefore comes as a surprise. Correct positioning of the control knob at the apex (*a*, 4, 5) helps one avoid this mistake.

(c) A complete cut is only possible without optical control;

(d) Speed of the cut (1 cm/sec).

(7) Endoscopic control of the cut channel by slipping the resectoscope forward and coagulating the arteries.

(8) Subsequent cuts enlarge the first channel sideways. Simultaneously the internal sphincter between 4 and 8 o'clock is prepared (see Figs. 89, 90).

II. Resection of the Lateral Lobes

(1) Basic cut (see I.1 above) on the most prominent part of the lateral lobes (between 2 and 4 o'clock and 8 and 10 o'clock, respectively).

(2) This cut must be extended from above to below, dissecting the internal sphincter between 2 and 10 o'clock perfectly.

(3) The operating site of the fossa is changed, often to prevent the formation of deep trenches and perforation due to inner distortion of the adenomatous tissue.

III. Resection of the Apex

The apex is (together with the external sphincter) palpated rectally as a hump around the sheath. After total TUR no hump formation can be felt. During TUR parts of the adenoma, including the apex, remain in the distal third of the fossa until the final stages of the operation; this can be explained by the adverse longitudinal movement of the loop (see p. 11). For resection, the finger pushes the "hump" into the window of the resectoscope sheath. In this way the concave (inner) curve of the capsule is straightened (see p. 13). The capsule now lies parallel to the movement of the loop, enabling resection of the elevated remaining adenoma. The thickness of the remaining capsule is estimated between the finger and the loop.

IV. Resection of the Roof of the Fossa

In the small adenoma a mucosal bridge is left untouched between 10 and 2 o'clock (prophylaxis of stricture). In the larger adenoma (over 50 gm), this often cannot be preserved because the adenomatous layer is too thick. The pistol grip and revolving sheath of the resectoscope facilitate TUR, particularly at the roof, in that they spare the surgeon awkward acrobatics (compare Figs. 14, 18, 76).

V. Correction on the External Sphincter (see Figs. 101–103)

The window of the resectoscope (beak of the sheath) now is retracted to the middle urethra. Thus, the function of the external sphincter can be observed (see Fig. 101). Adenomatous residuals deform the lumen of the sphincter and must be localized and resected. Only when the external sphincter forms a large round opening (see Fig. 103) can one be sure that the apex is totally resected. If one allows small columns of the lateral lobes (see Fig. 102) to remain, this should provide protection against incontinence in patients with cerebral sclerosis and when micturition has remained disturbed after a stroke. We have found that perfect TUR of the apex (III–V above) is the most difficult part of TURP, requiring frequent practice in many hundred resections. On the other hand, optimal postoperative progress — the complete cure of urinary infection and permanent good results equal to those of open prostatectomy — are guaranteed only when there is no residual tissue in the fossa, including the apex.

Incorrect Technique

Beginning resectionists experience difficulties of both technique and topography. The prostatic urethra, for example, may resist endoscopy when the median and lateral lobes reduce irrigation flow or if the colliculus seminalis is covered by fibrin coagula.

Forceful high pressure irrigation will solve this problem, but at a cost to the patient, who must suffer the consequences of the water syndrome. However, it is simple to perform TUR under physiologic conditions (low pressure irrigation with an average height of the water level in the irrigating reservoir of 30 cm; see p. 25). First, a channel for irrigation is cut into the middle lobe from the bladder down to the colliculus seminalis (see p. 45), thus marking the borders for further cuts — proximally, the internal sphincter at the bladder neck; distally, the colliculus seminalis. Following are some typical mistakes:

(1) Over-resection (see Figs. 97, 119, h)

Here, it is mainly the proximal third of the fossa — i.e., the bladder neck — that is resected, and the resectoscope is held at a sharp angle to the body axis. This angulation pushes the adenoma below the bladder neck, and the elevated bladder neck is mistaken for the adenoma. Resection continues far into the bladder, and perforation and bladder neck stricture result. Over-resection can be avoided if the resectoscope is kept horizontal along the body axis and the loop is inserted blindly into the adenoma (see p. 48).

(2) Cleft Formation
The prostatic capsule and bladder neck are separated by cutting too deep. The trigone retracts into the bladder, forming a cleft between the fossa and bladder neck (see Figs. 21, 93).

(3) Undermining of the Lateral Lobes (see Fig. 40)
When the lower part of the lateral lobes is resected too far, a false urethra forms, which in turn leads to further incorrect cuts. This happens when the cuts are not laid out beside each other covering different sectors, but instead are set only in one place. Often a large piece of the adenoma is cut off; it falls into the bladder and is difficult to remove. Often the capsule is perforated because of the altered topography.

(4) Formation of Grooves
The adenoma is under pressure within the elastic capsule. A few deep cuts are sufficient to cause enormous distortion of tissue. Only solid tissue (as in carcinoma, in secondary TUR or after cryosurgery) does not change position during cutting.

If, because of incorrect technique, orientation within the fossa is lost, TUR is continued in another sector. We recommend that a sector above the groove be chosen so that one can cut comfortably from above into it. Here the control knob at the sheath and the finger in the rectum often are better for orientation than the eye. If TUR is terminated before all adenomatous tissue is removed, inflammatory infiltrations indurate the wound within a few days. Mistakes now are easily recognized and corrected. *This is why secondary TUR is the best teacher of TURP.*

(5) Pseudo-TUR and Partial TUR
The real weight of the resected tissue is too low in relation to the clinical site of the adenoma. The prostatic fossa has delineated incompletely or not at all on the cystogram. This requires correction in the second operative session. Too many failures are the result of partial TUR; the surgeon harms the patient and discredits the technique.

(6) Incorrect Posture
Strong angulation of the sheath is the most common mistake. It always leads to an unnatural topography and complicates TUR (see Fig. 39). It is better to use the finger in the rectum to lift the capsule into the path of the cutting loop (see Fig. 41). The external sphincter is in danger of being split if the resectoscope is retracted unnoticed during the cut.

(7) Incorrect Cutting Guidance During TUR
A full cut requires complete extension of the cutting loop, insertion "behind the mountain" (see Fig. 42), horizontal positioning of the resectoscope, sufficient pressure of the loop on the surface with corresponding opposite pressure from the finger in the rectum, and restrained movement of the cutting loop (about one cut every three seconds). Further, the quantity and quality of the cutting current must be adjusted optimally. Cutting mistakes are made:

1. When inserting the cutting loop;
2. In guiding the cut;
3. When finally cutting off the chips;
4. In surface pressure.

Top Cutting of the Adenoma at the Bladder Neck (pseudo-TUR). The insertion of the cutting loop has an important effect on the course of the cut. If one tries to insert the loop under visual control (e.g., into the median lobe), the following mistake occurs: The optical window is positioned in the proximal fossa. Therefore, the cutting loop must be retracted halfway or further into the sheath, and the full length of the cutting loop is not utilized (see Fig. 42, a). Only the top of the "mountain" formed by the median lobe is cut (pseudo-TUR).

Undulatory Cutting. The loop is inserted on the top of the "mountain," not behind it, for fear of over-resection (see Fig. 97) or perforation. The consequence is undulatory cutting (see Fig. 42, b); i.e., the loop dives deep into the adenoma at the beginning of the cut but tends to come back to the surface because of insufficient pressure or the oblique posture of the resectoscope. The cut becomes more and more shallow toward the end.

Sawing Cut. Here, all kinds of possible mistakes are combined with different intensities. The sawing cut is characterized by the rough and irregular surface it creates. It results from cutting too quickly, from insufficient or excess pressure of the loop against the adenoma, and from inappropriate current quality. Pure coagulating current or incorrectly mixed current can cause a similar cut surface.

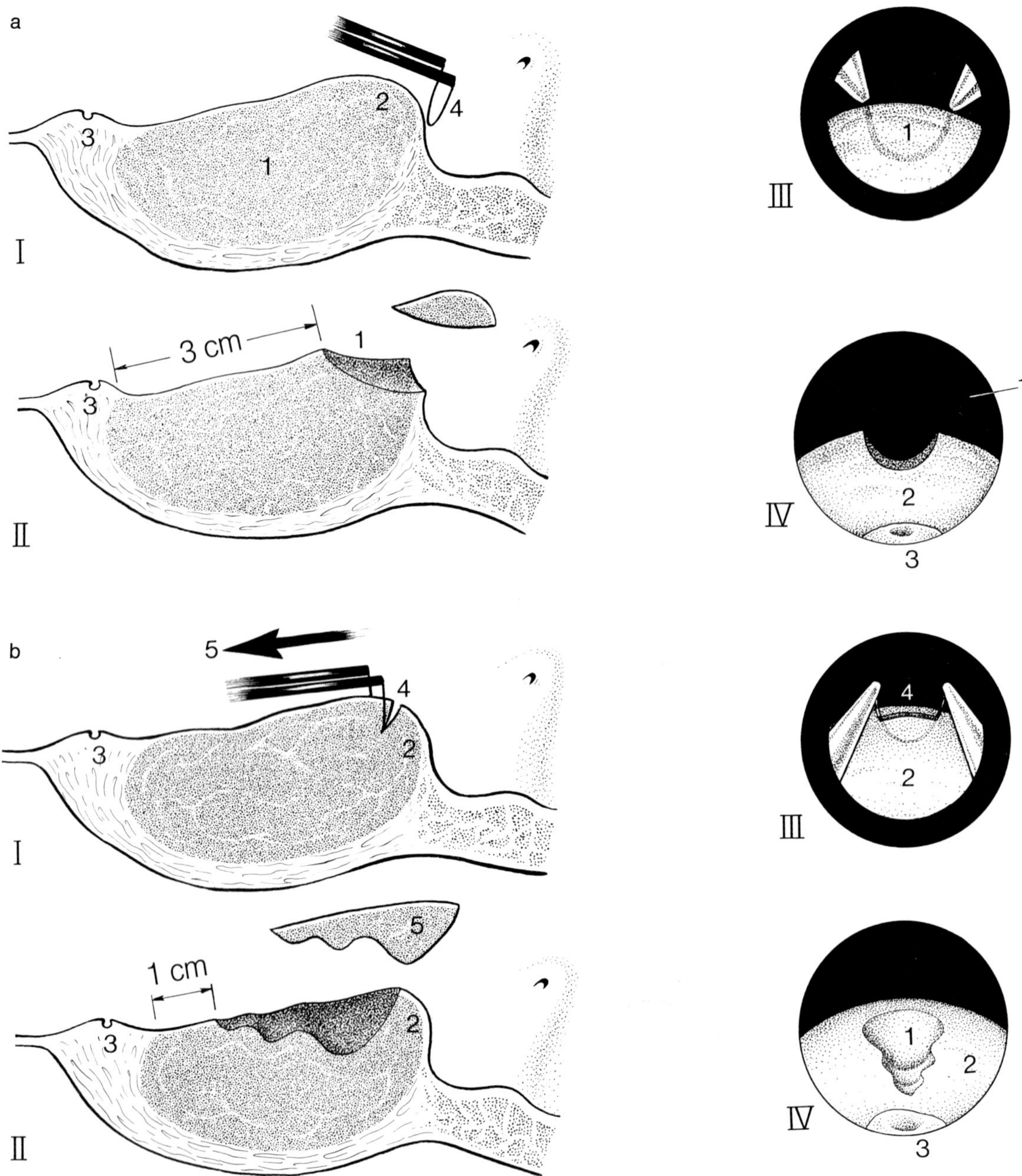

Fig. 42, a–d Incorrect guidance of the cut during TUR (longitudinal section).

(a) Resection of only the "hill-top" of the median lobe (pseudo-TUR):

I. Sagittal section through the lower half of the prostatic adenoma (1), the median lobe (2) and the verumontanum (3). The cutting loop (4) is inserted under direct vision (incorrect!) immediately behind the median lobe.

II. The loop (1) is utilized only to one third of its length, so that only the top of the median lobe (2) is cut. The sheath is held upward at a sharp angle (compare *b*, I). This also shortens the cut. 3 = verumontanum.

III. Endoscopic view of I: the cutting loop is not extended, although it disappears behind the median lobe (1, correct).

IV. Only a short groove is cut into the median lobe (2); this ends 3 cm before the verumontanum (3) is reached (compare II).

(b) Undulatory cutting:

I. The cutting loop (4) is placed too far distally on the median lobe (2): "on the mountain." The horizontal posture of the resectoscope is correct (arrow 5), although the surface pressure is not sufficient and the cutting velocity is too fast. 3 = verumontanum.

II. The cut surface (1) undulates; it flattens distally and ends about 1 cm before the seminal vesicle (3). The tissue chip (5) is short and thin. A bar-shaped part of the median lobe (2) remains.

c

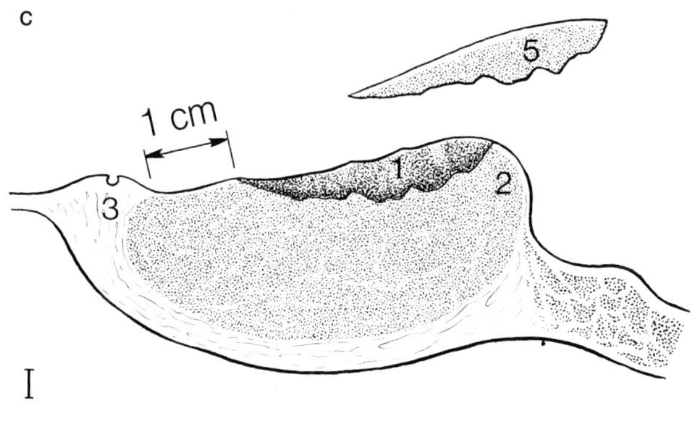

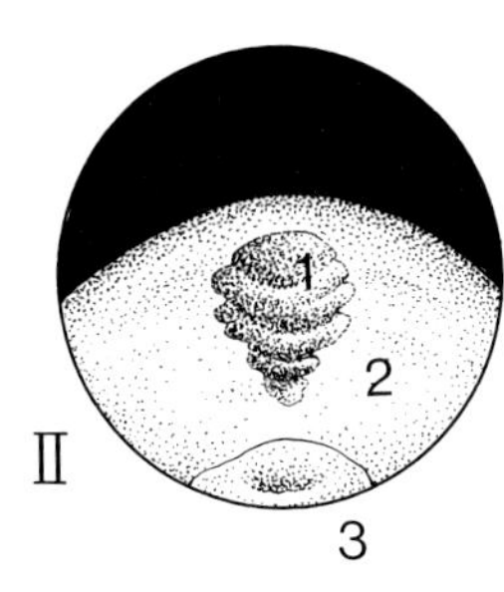

d

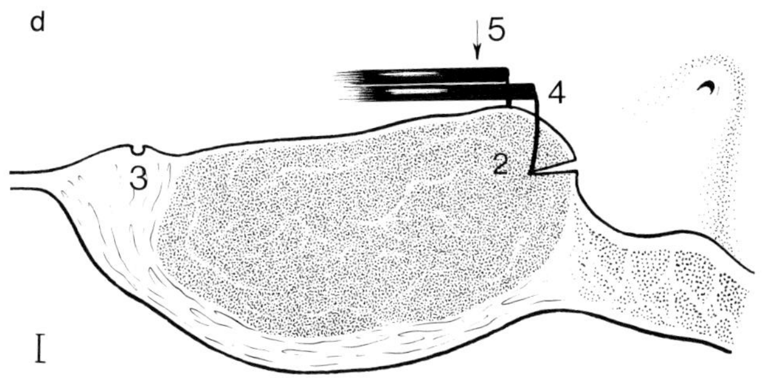

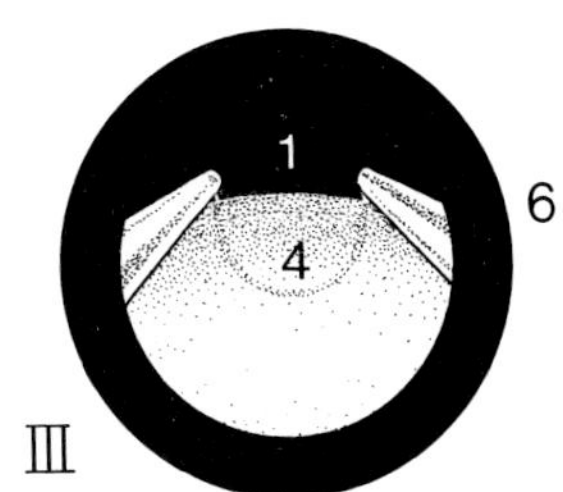

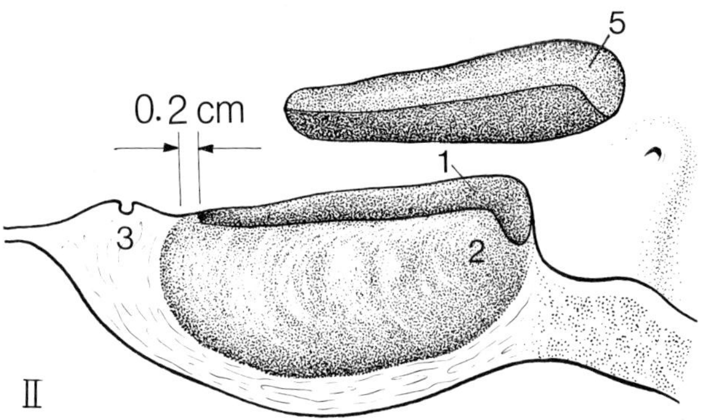

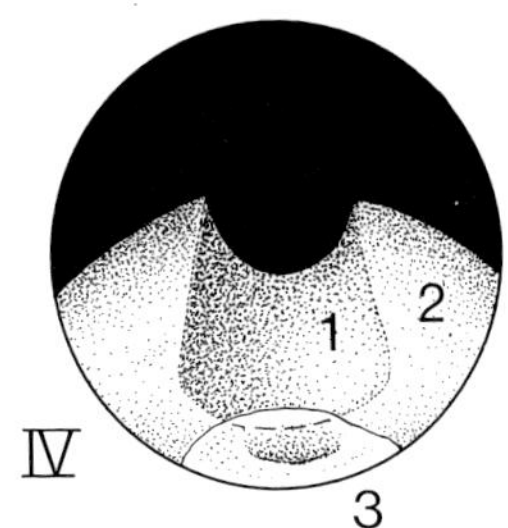

III. The endoscopic view demonstrates that the loop (4) is not incompletely immersed into the adenoma. 2 = median lobe.

IV. The cut, shortened by perspective (1) in the median lobe (2), does not reach down to the colliculus seminalis (3) and not beyond the "hill-top."

(c) Sawing cut (starting position of the loop as in *b*, I):

I. Rough, irregular cut surface (1). The tissue chip (5) is thin and narrow. 2 = Median lobe, 3 = colliculus seminalis.

II. Endoscopically, a superficial, irregular defect (1) is verified in the median lobe (2). 3 = colliculus seminalis

(d) Correct cut:

I. Correct insertion of the loop (4) without optical control (blindly) "behind the mountain" (2). Smooth blind cut down to the colliculus seminalis (3) with controlled movement (3 sec) and forceful surface pressure (5). The sheath is horizontal within the body axis; its control knob (see Fig. 41) is immobile at the apex.

II. The cut trench (1) is deep and broad; it reaches close to the colliculus seminalis (0.2 cm; 3). Thus, the tissue chip (5) is large. 2 = median lobe.

III. The extended loop (4) is inserted blindly "behind the hill-top." The wires of the cutting loop (6) are hardly recognized. The cut itself cannot be observed.

IV. Deep, broad cut trench (1) in the median lobe (3) reaching close to the colliculus seminalis (3).

(8) Positioning of Patient (see p. 19)

(a) The patient should always lie at the level of the head of the surgeon, who sits erect. The patient's buttocks should project 10 to 20 cm from the edge of the operating table.

(b) The patient's pelvic joints should not be bent too far; the calves should rest horizontally on a broad support.

(c) We perform TUR from a seated position. The surgeon's vertebral column should be comfortable; kyphosis and cervical syndrome can result from inadequate adjustment of the operating table.

(9) Misconceptions of Anatomy

An inadequate understanding of anatomy and topography can give rise to incorrect handling. Often the terms for "capsule" (see p. 40) and "prostate" are confused, being used for the adenoma as well as the prostate. The interureteral crest can be mistaken for the bar or the internal sphincter. By using the control knob on the resectoscope sheath and rectal palpation, lost orientation in the fossa can be regained quickly.

TUR Technique of the Small, Medium and Giant Adenoma (see Fig. 38).

The Small Adenoma

It is easy to resect a few chips off the bar of a small adenoma (up to 20 gm weight and 4 cm long; pseudo-TUR). Complete TURP is more difficult in these patients than in larger adenomas (30 to 50 gm). Many small, short cuts cause needless electric stress to the capsule. The prostate (true prostatic tissue) bleeds excessively, and electrocoagulation increases the electric trauma. This stimulates the formation of a bladder neck stricture. Therefore, it is recommended that a mucosal bridge be left in place between the 11- and 1-o'clock positions. If the patient's principal complaint is irritation because of sphincter sclerosis, prostatitis or adnexitis, we prefer cryosurgery because of its anti-inflammatory effect. In cases of doubt, conservative therapy is preferred to surgery. Preoperative vesiculography demonstrates the degree of the adnexitis more precisely. In neurotic and psychopathic patients, TUR is performed only in particular indications.

The Medium to Large Adenoma

A tumor with a weight of 30 to 50 gm and a length of 3 to 5 cm conforms well to the resectoscope. Therefore, the results of TURP often are decisively better in the larger adenoma. The distance from "trigone-to-apex" is made with one cut (by extension of the cutting loop). Only a rim of adenomatous tissue remains around the external sphincter, and this is resected at the end of TUR. At this point, the finger in the rectum is indispensable for lifting the remaining adenoma for resection.

The Large Adenoma

An adenoma weighing 50 to 100 gm and over 5 cm long requires a special technique of TUR. The endovesical part of the adenoma covers the bladder floor, including the trigone and the ureteral orifices. Here the loop is inserted blindly "behind the mountain" in the median lobe. If the loop is inserted under direct vision, the resectoscope must be withdrawn (blind). Only when the loop is extended to its full length is the tumor cut. The proximal portion of the adenoma then is resected until the internal sphincter between the 3- and 6-o'clock positions is freed (see Fig. 89). Then, in sequence, the distal part of the adenoma (near the apex) is resected, and the large lateral lobes are resected from above (Nesbit). We prefer to isolate the lateral lobe by drawing a groove at the 2- and 5-o'clock positions. Then resection of the lateral lobe is begun at its most prominent part (ridge technique). Finally, the apex is worked out (see p. 45).

The Giant Adenoma

In a tumor weighing 100 to 300 gm, both the length and the depth of the fossa must be divided into several operative stages. The adenoma always should be resected on a broad surface; deep grooves must be avoided. Often a change of sector will facilitate orientation. The dangerous rasping technique, where cutting back and forth under control of the finger in the rectum is used, should be restricted to fast TUR of large isolated nodules.

Physiologic low pressure irrigation with continuous aspiration solely (see p. 25) makes possible a low risk TURP of giant adenomas in one session that lasts one to two hours. Only one who masters the TURP of such giant adenomas can save high risk patients from the risks of mortality inherent in open surgical prostatectomy. When the correct technique is combined with sufficient experience, the surgical mortality of TURP is lowered significantly (see Table 2, p. 232).

Hemorrhage

Coagulation no longer brings dramatic crises, thanks to continuous low pressure irrigation (see p. 25). Even the beginner will recognize the advantages of the continuous vision and excellent irrigation provided by the new technique. The veins collapse in the bladder kept empty by suction. With increased bladder filling, as occurs in conventional irrigation, venous drainage is compressed, and the risk of hemorrhage increases.

Arterial Hemorrhage

Arterial bleeders are coagulated only in the capsule (true prostatic tissue), where they are recognized clearly. Coagulation is easy and positive (see Figs. 43, 44, 110). Bleeders in the adenoma are difficult to trace. The vessel retracts, and coagulation requires frequent applications of harmful current that must be repeated after each cut.

If the arterial blood jet is directed against the optical window, its source is difficult to find. Usually it originates from the proximal third of the prostatic fossa — frequently from under the trigone. The optic window must be directed from a different angle *toward* the jet (change the position of the patient; turn and angulate the resectoscope; see Fig. 46). Bleeders may be reflected symmetrically; i.e., the artery sprays on the opposite side, giving the hemorrhage an apparent false location. If the source of bleeding cannot be located, we recommend that the operating sector be changed and that one artery after another be coagulated there. Eventually one always finds the main site.

Coagulation of several arteries is difficult if they spray concentrically. Patience helps. The finger in the rectum can be especially helpful when:

(1) By lifting the prostate the direction of the blood jet is changed.

(2) The intensity of bleeding can be reduced (see Fig. 46).

No adenomatous tissue should remain near a coagulated artery. When such tissue becomes necrotic and is rejected, secondary arterial bleeding ensues. We have often seen this in partial TUR; after TURP, it is seldom seen. Coagulate can quickly cover a source of bleeding, impeding one's orientation. This is most easily removed by cuts; if this is impossible, it can be scratched away with the cold loop.

Venous Hemorrhage

Unlike arterial bleeding, venous hemorrhage flows with a pressure of only about 10 cm water (see p. 58). If the hydrostatic pressure in the fossa rises over 15 cm water, venous hemorrhage is suppressed. Then only arterial bleeders are seen.

In low pressure irrigation, however, venous bleeding flows toward the bladder. It therefore is easily recognized. In addition, the walls of the vessels collapse, stopping hemorrhage spontaneously.

Veins also are easily coagulated. The technique is the same as for the artery (see Fig. 44). Frequently the veins are plugged by thrombi (see Fig. 98). In high pressure irrigation, venous drainage is compressed by the overfilled bladder; venous pressure therefore rises, subsequently increasing bleeding. The spontaneous tendency toward hemostasis by contraction of the blood vessel and the prostatic capsule is thus impeded.

Hemorrhage from Venous Sinuses (see Figs. 47–49)

These are always localized in the deeper layers of the capsule (true prostatic tissue). Therefore, bleeding from a venous sinus often is due to accidental deep resection. The sinus bleeds heavily when the flow of irrigation is reduced. When the irrigation runs fully, bleeding disappears. Therefore, maintaining a balance between venous and static plus dynamic pressure is helpful in tracing the sinus. With patience, the sinus almost always can be coagulated. Sometimes it can be excised. If coagulation is not successful, bleeding can be stopped by a compression balloon catheter (30 cc filling of the balloon with a traction of about 150 gm on the catheter usually is sufficient). Frequently the bleeding ceases spontaneously. Postoperative continuous suprapubic irrigation is useful in these patients (see Fig. 48).

It should be mentioned that, after TURP, venous bleeders should be compressed by the balloon in the prostatic fossa, not at the bladder neck (our opinion here differs from that of Baumrucker). Arterial bleeding never can be compressed with a balloon; venous bleeding is best compressed following total resection of the adenoma (TURP).

Parenchymatous Hemorrhage

This bleeding usually is caused by fibrinolysis. It can be controlled with tranexamic acid and aprotinin (kallikrein-trypsin inhibitor). Such hemorrhage seldom occurs when low pressure irrigation is applied. Rarely, a blood transfusion is necessary (1.6 per cent of cases). Careful resection of the adenoma down to the inner surface of the capsule (false capsule, sparing the prostatic tissue) is, as in venous sinus hemorrhage, the best way of preventing this bleeding.

Text continued on page 60

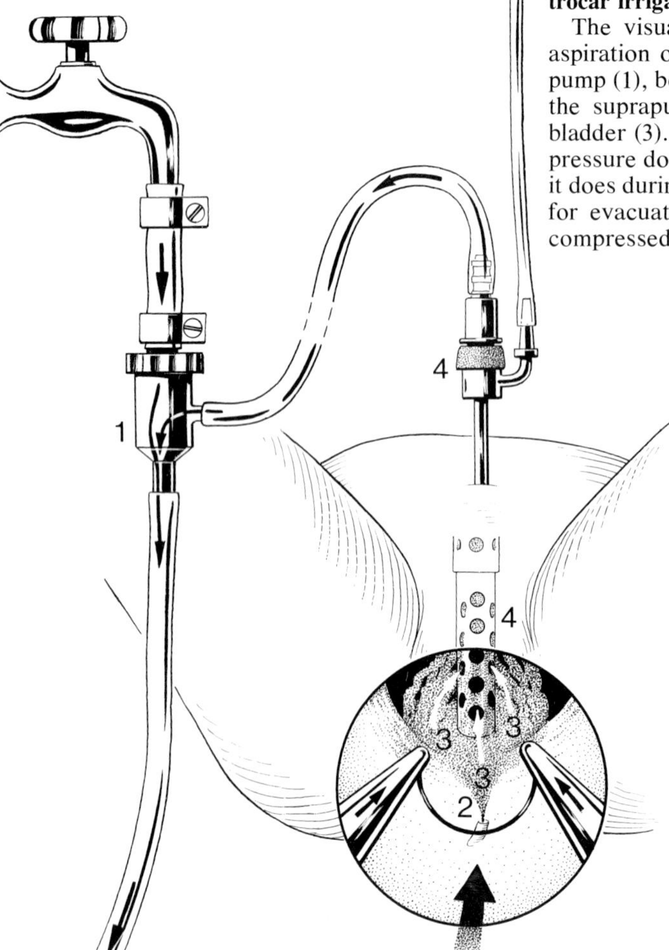

Fig. 43 Coagulation of arterial hemorrhage under trocar irrigation.

The visual field is clear, thanks to continuous aspiration of irrigant (water jet or electric suction pump (1), because the blood (2) is aspirated toward the suprapubic trocar (4) in the direction of the bladder (3). Coagulation is not interrupted and the pressure does not rise above physiologic values, as it does during high pressure irrigation with intervals for evacuation (see pp. 21–29). The artery (2) is compressed retrograde with the loop (arrow 5).

Fig. 44 Coagulation of an artery (1) with the returnflow resectoscope. The course of fluid (2) is not as favorable as with the suprapubic trocar; the efficiency of irrigation is reduced and the cutting loop (3) is smaller. 4 = Inflow; 5 = return-flow; 6 = prostatic capsule; 7 = almost emptied bladder; 8 = fossa.

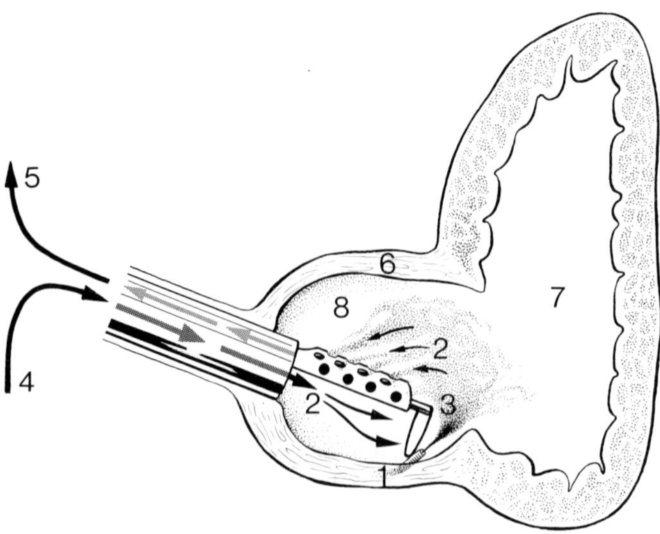

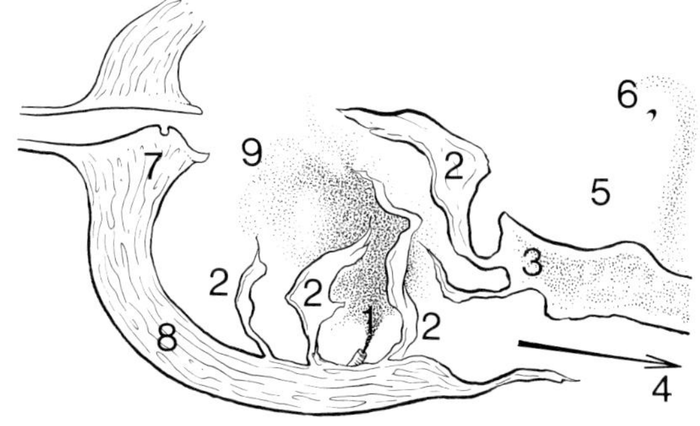

Fig. 45 Arterial bleeder (1) covered by pedunculated chips of tissue (2) in the fossa.

During TUR of a subvesical adenoma with a small median lobe, the trigone (5) is displaced upward toward the bladder by the tumor. During the resection, floating, pedunculated chips of tissue (2) can form by chance, covering the bleeder (1). The base of such a chip is narrow and difficult to find and cut. Often this condition is combined with cleft formation (see Fig. 93) and risk of perforation (4). 3 = Internal sphincter; 6 = ureteral orifice; 7 = verumontanum; 8 = capsule; 9 = fossa.

The chips are punched off with the cold loop and the bleeder is coagulated. This difficulty cannot always be avoided during TUR of a huge adenoma, even if the internal sphincter was prepared correctly.

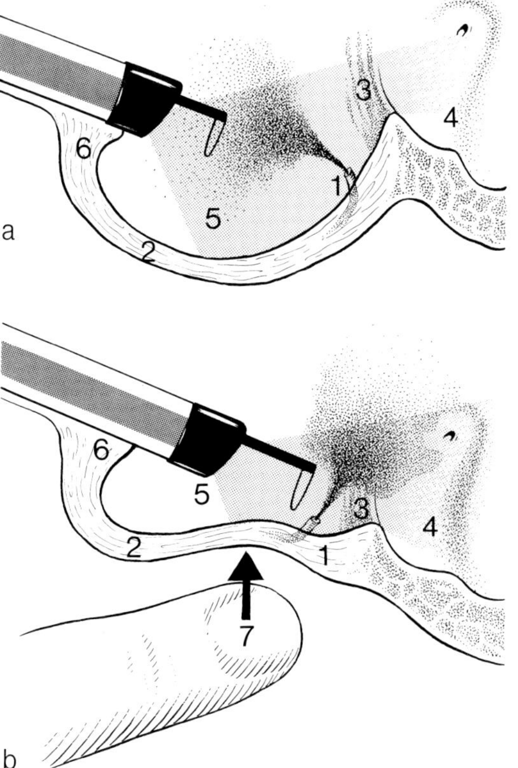

Fig. 46, a–b Arterial bleeder directed against the window of the resectoscope.

(a) Diffuse hemorrhage (1) against the window.

(b) Change of direction of the blood jet by lifting the capsule (2) with the finger in the rectum (arrow 7). 3 = Internal sphincter; 4 = trigone; 5 = prostatic fossa; 6 = verumontanum.

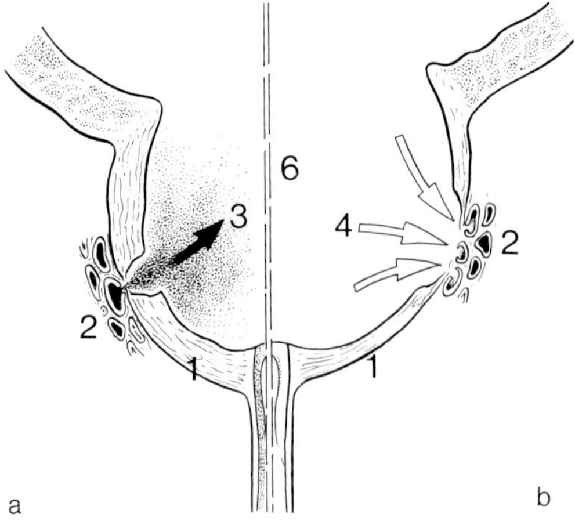

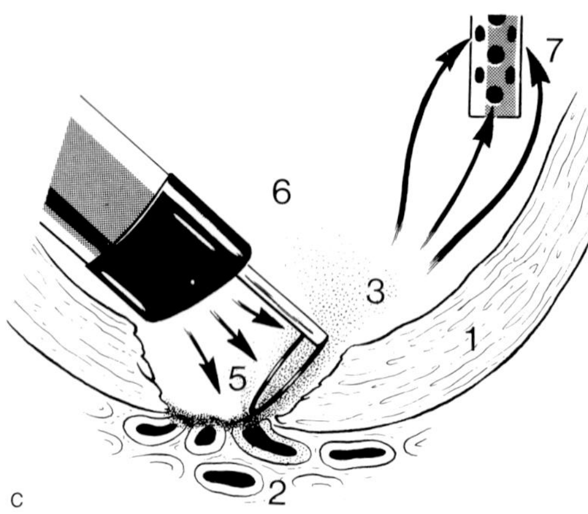

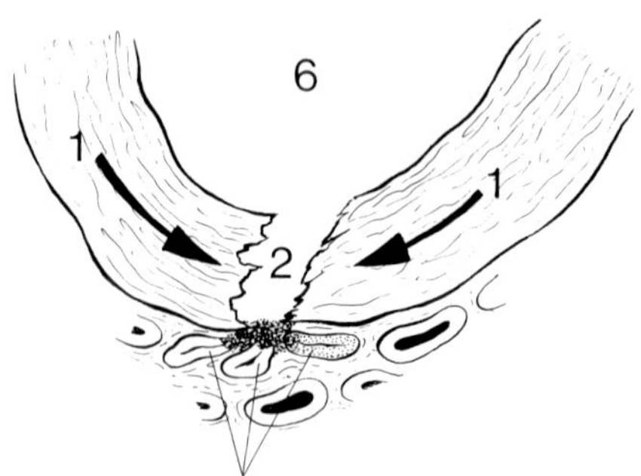

Fig. 47, a–d Venous sinus hemorrhage under high and low pressure irrigation.

(a) Hemorrhage during an interval of high pressure irrigation when the bladder is empty. The capsule (1) is resected too far, opening a sinus (2). When the pressure in the prostatic fossa falls by voiding the bladder during an irrigating interval, venous hemorrhage is increased (arrow 3) owing to previous obstruction of venous drainage by the full bladder.

(b) When the bladder pressure rises again (arrow 4), bleeding is stopped and irrigant (4) is forced into vessels and tissue. This way of reducing blood loss is dangerous (water syndrome); it should not be used for routine "coagulation" (so-called "hydraulic coagulation").

(c) Coagulation (5) under low pressure irrigation. The nearly empty bladder and fossa are under physiologic pressure. The capsule relaxes spontaneously.

(d) The sinus (2) collapses under the suction of the trocar. Bleeding ceases spontaneously. However, venous drainage into the iliac veins must be free. It may be obstructed by a full bladder (a) or reduced by cardiac insufficiency.

Fig. 48, a–c Postoperative continuous irrigation of prostatic fossa and bladder with low pressure (10 cm water)

(a) Continuous suprapubic irrigation (7). The trocar insert is replaced by a plastic tube (8) with its tip bent toward the fossa. The tube is left in place as a suprapubic fistula when the trocar sheath (9) is removed. The contracted bladder (10) and the relaxed fossa (6) now are irrigated continuously with an admixture of Braunol (povidone-iodine, 1:50–200). When the urine is clear, the transurethral catheter (11) is removed and the bladder is voided by the fistula only. 12 = 5-cc balloon.

(b) Transurethral continuous irrigation of the relaxed fossa (6) for treatment of sinus hemorrhage. The closed irrigating system consists of an infusion bag (0.9 per cent NaCl) elevated about 10 to 20 cm over the patient, a 20 Fr. three-way Foley catheter with 5-cc balloon (12) and a urinal (14). The draining tube (13) empties the prostatic fossa and bladder by siphon suction. The low irrigating pressure supports relaxation of the capsule and the vessels (2). The bladder (10) remains empty. The electronic catheter control device (14) above the urinal gives a signal when the flow of urine ceases.

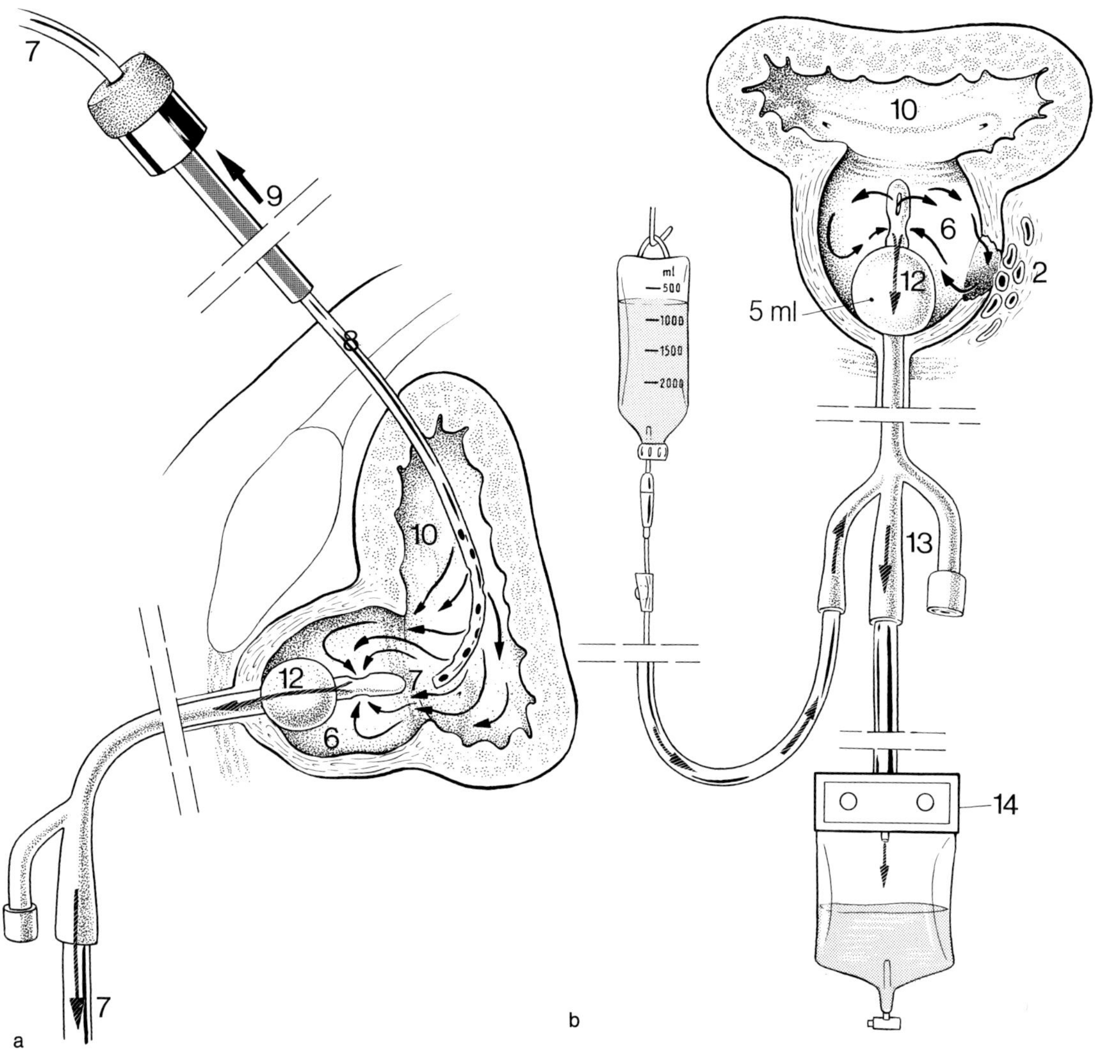

(c) Compression catheter for treatment of sinus bleeding. The big balloon (12) is filled with 30 to 100 cc. It may be under traction (arrow) of a weight of 250 to 1000 gm. We use it only exceptionally; e.g., when massive venous hemorrhage (2) persists.

Disadvantage: Distortion of the injured capsule. Natural hemostasis by contraction is prevented and wound healing is delayed.

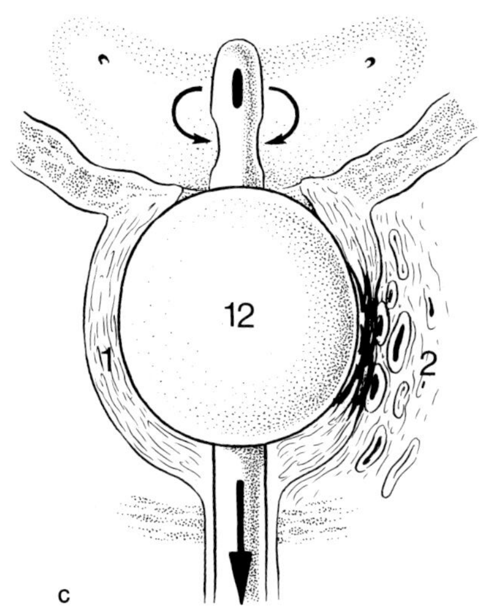

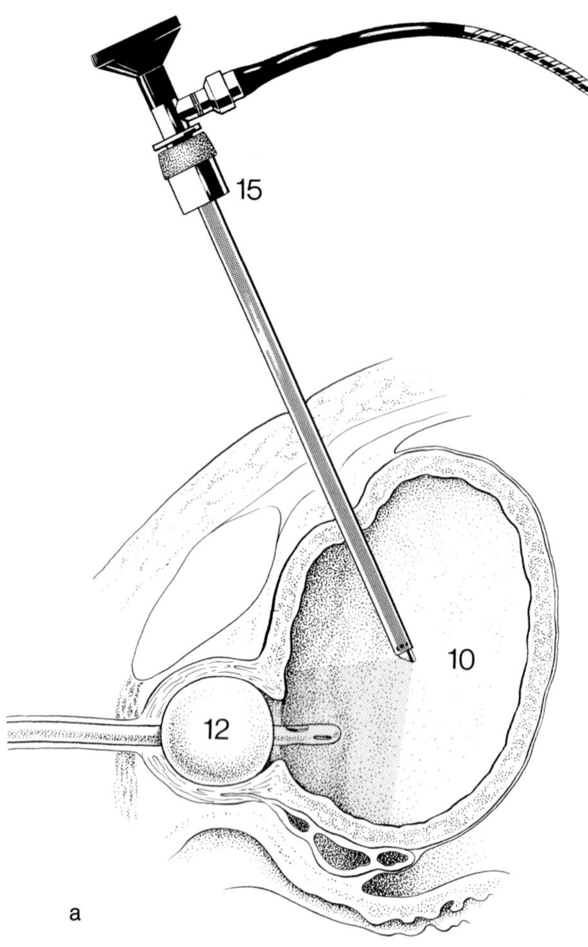

Fig. 49, a–b Trocar cystoscopy through the suprapubic trocar (15) for evaluation of the bladder neck.

(a) The bladder (10) is filled with air (150 to 200 cc. applied without pressure may be used without danger in our experience over several years). The balloon (12) is now filled in the fossa under direct vision until optimal compression is achieved.

(b) Lateral open guiding sleeve for inserting a suprapubic balloon catheter (12–14 Fr) after TUR, "Freiburg" model, as addition to the suprapubic trocar (Lesch) (see Fig. 48a).

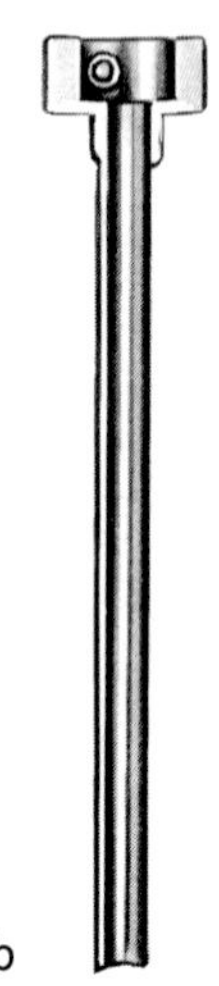

Hemorrhage and Hypertension

High blood pressure with systolic values of over 180 mm Hg usually causes increased arterial bleeding. Increase of the blood pressure during TUR — especially with high pressure irrigation — always indicates a water syndrome. Today this complication is avoided by using physiologic low pressure.

Hypotension and Hemorrhage

Since we use low pressure irrigation, we sometimes experience a decrease of blood pressure during TUR. This is further enhanced by drug-induced diuresis (furosemide). The reaction can be controlled with drugs that act on the peripheral circulatory system: 0.2 to 0.3 cc oxedrine IV in repeated doses is widely used. Hemorrhage is markedly reduced in hypotension (blood pressure below 120 mm Hg), facilitating coagulation. The systolic blood pressure should never fall below 100 mm Hg, because the central nervous system will be impaired, leading to subsequent regulatory disturbances and brain damage (respiratory and circulatory depression, cerebral sclerotic confusion, etc.). When the blood pressure rises quickly to systolic values of 150 to 200 mm Hg owing to high doses of antihypotensives, the chance of hemorrhage becomes markedly greater.

Summary

Any type of operating bleeding can be coagulated. Drug therapy acts only to support active coagulation. Except in fibrinolysis, its action is indirect (tranexamic acid; aprotinin; lowering of blood pressure; blood transfusion). The balloon catheter is suitable only for the compression of venous bleeding; it should be applied only in sinus bleeding. Postoperative continuous irrigation of the prostatic fossa through a suprapubic catheter often has a better hemostatic effect than does compression by the balloon (see Fig. 48). Low pressure irrigation permits complete coagulation, which previously was not possible with TUR.

Postoperative Hemorrhage

Postoperative hemorrhage following TURP occurs somewhat more frequently than after open surgical prostatectomy. Often it is triggered by discharge from the hospital and transport home and by straining to pass a hard stool. Sneezing, coughing and laughing are other initiating causes. Because of rejection of necrotic parts of the adenoma, partial TUR has a higher incidence of postoperative hemorrhage. Postoperative venous hemorrhage usually is without significance and needs only a permanent catheter (after clearing the bladder from the tamponade). Coagulated material must be totally evacuated from the bladder because a full bladder impedes venous drainage, thus increasing hemorrhage. Often evacuation is enough to stop hemorrhage spontaneously. In more difficult cases we prefer continuous irrigation with a 20 Fr. three-way catheter with 5-cc balloon.

Arterial hemorrhage always should be coagulated. This is done immediately, without attempting conservative therapy (catheter; medication). After mechanical scratching and evacuation of the coagulate in the fossa, tracing and coagulating the usual single artery is relatively easy. The patient recovers promptly after coagulation; further hemorrhages are extremely rare.

Bleeding at Intervals

Such hemorrhage is arterial, but it behaves like a venous hemorrhage, because it flows and stops spontaneously. It derives from relatively small arteries and collects below a layer of coagulate, and the irrigant flows clear over this layer. Therefore, for the sake of the patient, every bleeder should be verified endoscopically and coagulated early—in cases of doubt always before the end of the day. Often this is possible under local anesthesia of the urethra; necroses and small remaining parts of adenoma are resected at the same time.

Terminal Phase of TUR

Control of the Prostatic Fossa

The tissue chips are evacuated from the bladder. Then the prostatic fossa is evaluated. At the end of TURP, it forms a regular hollow sphere (see Figs. 87, 107) if the bladder is under slight tension (volume of at least 50 cc). When the bladder is emptied, the loose capsule (true prostatic tissue) forming the wall of the fossa collapses like the bladder, because its sustaining adenomatous shell has been removed. This shell remains in partial TUR (see Fig. 4).

When, under reduced continuous flow, the inflow is stopped or started, the shape of the fossa changes, and the motility of its wall can be tested. With the bladder empty, the finger in the rectum palpates the bulge of the external sphincter, its transition into the apex and the transition of the fossa into the bladder neck, where the hard seminal vesicles are felt. Adenomatous remnants and infiltration of the capsule can be felt as well. Then the fossa is searched for adenomatous tags. Aspiration (suprapubic trocar or return flow sheath) is stopped, and thc bladder is filled slowly with irrigant up to a maximum of 100 cc (easily determined with the dosimeter; see p. 27). This makes possible the ultimate correction and resection of all adenomatous remnants.

Control of Hemostasis

The intensity of hemorrhage can always be determined by the reddish color of the irrigant seen in the clear plastic tube used for suprapubic aspiration. Arterial hemostasis is controlled by viewing the great cavity of the fossa from the colliculus seminalis. Bleeding arteries are easily spotted. Bleeding veins, especially sinuses, are best seen when the inflow of irrigant is greatly reduced. Aspiration of irrigant (through the trocar or return flow sheath) often will stop otherwise uncoagulable hemorrhage from a sinus. We do not consistently coagulate each sinus. Often compression with a small balloon (5-cc balloon filled with 20 cc) is successful (see p. 59). Coagulation can be considered complete only when the irrigant at minimal flow is either clear or, at the most, bright rose in color. Ideal coagulation is routinely attainable only when continuous low pressure irrigation is used (see p. 25).

Control of the Internal Sphincter and the Bladder

The bladder neck and the adjacent part of the prostatic fossa are viewed with the resectoscope. Cleft formation and/or overresection can be verified and total resection of the adenoma controlled. The trigone, the interureteral crest, the orifices and the recessus are again controlled. It must be remembered that bladder tumors on the roof are easily overlooked.

Control of the External Sphincter and Its Function (Figs. 101–103)

The sheath of the resectoscope is retracted into the middle urethra. The external sphincter opens when the irrigation flows in at full force. It forms a circular opening, which, depending on the force of the irrigation and the distance of the beak of the resectoscope from the sphincter, becomes larger or smaller, like the pupil of the eye. If this opening is deformed, adenomatous remnants are left in the fossa. The same picture is found, when the ring of the sphincter is defective (see Fig. 102).

To control continence, we fill the bladder with 100 to 200 cc of irrigant (see dosimeter, p. 27). Then the resectoscope is removed. A slight pressure with the hand on the abdomen is enough to force a strong jet of water from the bladder. It stops at once when the hand is removed. Remnants at the apex, at the sphincter or in the fossa often are suggested by a helical stream. If, after TURP, the bladder does not empty under such pressure, a hypertonic sphincter or an atonic bladder is the cause. Only seldom does the bladder empty spontaneously (to the dismay of the surgeon) without manual pressure. However, incontinence should be expected only when the spontaneous voiding of the bladder is completed. If a residual of 100 cc or more remains in the bladder, continence is not jeopardized. Consistent voiding in a small stream or dribbling is more suggestive of incontinence.

Suprapubic Trocar Cystoscopy of the Prostatic Fossa

The view provided by this technique is particularly impressive because of the unusual perspective it affords (see Fig. 87). First, the bladder is filled carefully with 150 to 200 cc of air, either through the resectoscope sheath or through the channel of the trocar used for measuring bladder pressure. There is no risk of air emboli. Then a cystoscopic optical system is introduced into the bladder through the trocar sheath. The bladder and the fossa come into view. After TURP, the fossa has the shape of a hemisphere or a cut hollow sphere. Such technical errors as over-resection or remnants of adenomatous tissue can be recognized with precision from this "bird's-eye." Often the urethral stump and the verumontanum are seen (see Fig. 88, f).

Control of the Abdomen, Genitals and Rectum

The abdomen is completely relaxed after TURP because of peridural anesthesia. Localized pain and muscular spasm occur in the region of a covered perforation when irrigant is absorbed into the paravesical space. The pool of irrigant eventually flows back into the fossa when strong manual pressure is applied to the abdomen. It can then be evacuated through the catheter. For this reason, no compression catheter should be used that might close the perforation by chance (e.g., 5-cc balloon). We never treat a covered perforation surgically if an isotonic irrigant has been used.

Rarely, an open perforation into the peritoneum is not accompanied by the usual symptoms. Therefore, the endoscopic situation must always be clear. When it is certain that the prostatic fossa has not perforated into the open peritoneum, even severe abdominal symptoms, such as shock, pains and abdominal rigidity (TUR syndrome), can be treated conservatively. The patient then possibly may recover completely within a few hours. Only if the complaints persist, the diagnosis must be reviewed, and eventually surgical intervention is necessary.

Genital complications are rare after TURP. Penile edema or hematoma can occur following perforation of the urethra or prostate. Insignificant crepitation sometimes is noted after air-filling (cryosurgery).

Control of the Catheter

As a rule we use an 18 Fr. catheter with a 5-cc balloon. The soft catheter is introduced into the bladder with the aid of a stiff wire guide. This avoids the risk of trapping of the catheter in the fossa by the internal sphincter or an undermined trigone. In radical TUR, perforation of the thin rectal wall is avoided by directing the catheter tip in the fossa toward the bladder with the aid of the wire guide and the finger in the rectum (see Fig. 34).

The catheter is positioned properly when irrigant drains spontaneously and when air escapes from the emptied bladder. If the balloon is not in the fossa but in the middle urethra or in a perforated excavation, inflation of the balloon causes pain. Suprapubic continuous irrigation is begun at once (low pressure irrigation). This prevents formation of clots and irrigates the fossa directly (not the bladder; see Fig. 48). Continuous control of the irrigation is necessary because the bladder fills quickly when the drainage is blocked (electronic catheter control device; addition of povidone-iodine, 1:200).

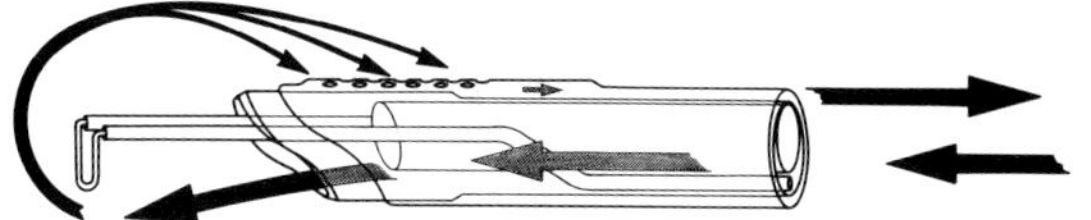

Fig. 49c Resection-instrument with returnflow-tube (Olympus Winter & Ibe). The channel for returnflow is in the space between resectionsheath and returnflow-tube and can easely be cleaned.

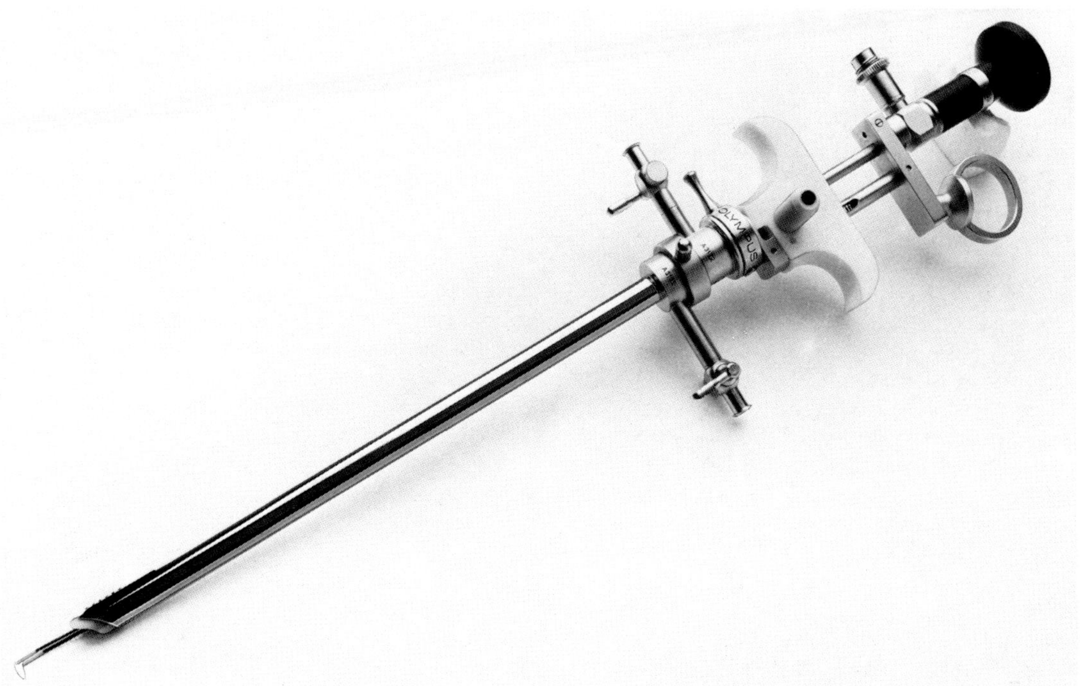

Fig. 49, d Resection instrument with continuous irrigation (Olympus Winter & Ibe). A standard resection instrument, 24 Fr, for intermittent irrigation or for suprapubic irrigation through trocar (Reuter) can be improved to a 26 Fr resection instrument for continuous irrigation by attaching an outflow tube.

Prostatic Carcinoma

Radical TUR is the alternative to radical open surgery in the stages T_1 and T_2. The patient is less stressed by TUR than by open prostatectomy.

The incurable stage T_3 can be treated palliatively by subradical TUR and by cryosurgery. Endoscopic methods of surgery (combined with estrogen therapy, orchiectomy and cytostatic therapy, such as estramustine phosphate, as well as radiation therapy) can produce respectable palliative results. In the high-risk patient these two methods are the only alternative. The (sub)radical TUR can be employed to advantage because of the following factors:

(1) Physiologic low pressure irrigation enables one to achieve an almost total TUR of the true prostatic tissue.

(2) The tumor is surrounded by a leukocytic infiltration, which enables one to resect periprostatic tissue.

(3) The TUR (and the cryosurgery) can be repeated in the recurrent cancer.

(4) Endoscopic surgery (TUR and cryosurgery) is feasible even in the high-risk patient.

(5) Incontinence, occurring in about 2 per cent of patients, can be corrected by endoscopic sphincterplasty: Teflon is injected into the defect transurethrally to produce a "cushion" around the urethra, thus repairing the defect. Radical TUR leaves (after resection of the true prostate) a large wound between the bladder neck and urethra, which in open surgery is sutured together (see Fig. 52, c). One to two months after TUR this wound is covered by epithelium; by chance, epithelium directly covers the longitudinal muscle of the rectum (see Figs. 110, 116).

Technique of Radical TUR (Figs. 109–120)

Radical TUR requires considerable experience. In the first phase of the procedure, the existing prostatic adenoma is resected down to the capsule. In this way the carcinomatous infiltration is traced; bleeding is conspicuously reduced on its surface but is increased at its base. Only in the periprostatic tissue — that is, the region of leukocytic infiltration — does bleeding cease.

In the second phase, the capsule (true prostatic tissue) is resected totally — at the very least to the farthest surroundings of the malignant lesion. The carcinomatous tissue is lifted by the finger in the rectum and is pushed against the cutting loop. The transition from the tough, gray-colored carcinomatous tissue of the capsule to the periprostatic tissue can be verified without difficulty (see Fig. 110).

During the third phase, the internal sphincter, external sphincter and the seminal vesicles are exposed. At this point, the trigone often must be resected back to the posterior bladder wall. If the ureteral orifice is infiltrated by tumor, a horse-shoe shaped cut is made around it; if necessary, this area is cut away. Subsequently, the fossa is reshaped and any remaining suspect tissue is resected. The lateral wall of the fossa can be resected relatively easily down into the periprostatic tissue (see Fig. 110). The tissue layer of the roof of the prostatic fossa often is thin; the tough tissue of the symphysis is not to be confused with cancer (danger of periostitis). The external sphincter, unlike the internal sphincter, is seldom infiltrated by carcinoma. We leave it as nearly untouched as possible; therefore, we have rarely seen permanent incontinence (see Fig. 101). Correct coagulation is possible only when low pressure irrigation is used. The dangerous complications of hemorrhage are thus avoided, as are the risks entailed in changing the catheter . The latter is dangerous because of possible perforation of the thin wall of the fossa (especially over the rectum). The recovery phase after radical TUR is delayed. For this reason, we leave the catheter in place in the bladder for six to ten days. The general condition of the patient is weaker than after TURP. Therefore, infusions, blood transfusions and other supportive measures should be given freely.

Fig. 50, a–c Radical TUR of prostatic carcinoma under low pressure irrigation (including total TUR of the accompanying prostatic adenoma; see Fig. 95).

(a) Frontal section of the adenomatous prostate (1) with carcinomatous infiltration (3) of the capsule (2). The periprostatic tissue is indurated by leukocytic infiltration (4; see Fig. 110).

(b) Frontal section through the verumontanum (5), open internal sphincter (6; see Fig. 38) and spheric fossa (7), after total TUR of the adenoma. Radical TUR of the carcinomatous infiltration causes a large defect (3) in the capsule. The suprapubic trocar (8) is directly behind the fossa. Continuous low pressure irrigation prevents infiltration of water into periprostatic tissue (4; see Figs. 94, 124).

(c) Frontal section with large defect of the prostatic capsule. In radical TUR the following tissues are exposed: muscle of the pelvic diaphragm (1; levator ani); longitudinal muscle of the rectum (2); lumina of the seminal vesicles (3); periprostatic fat hanging down at 3 o'clock (4; see Fig. 95).

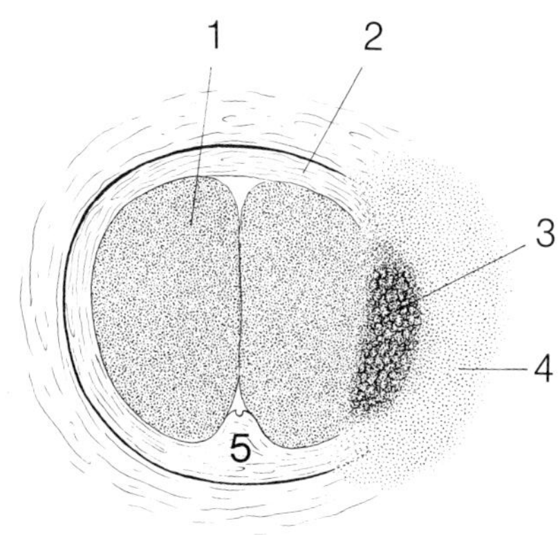

a

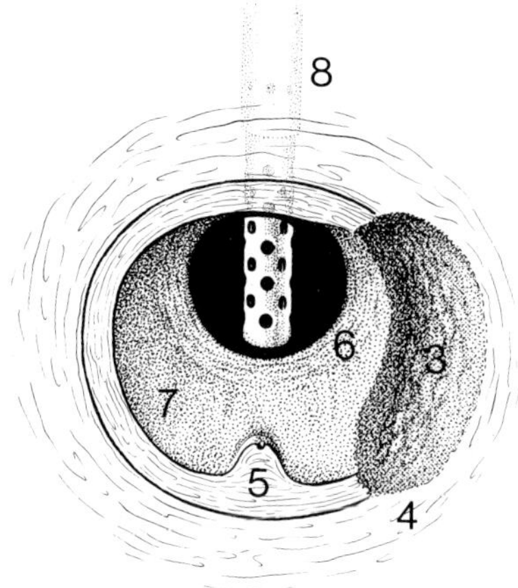

b

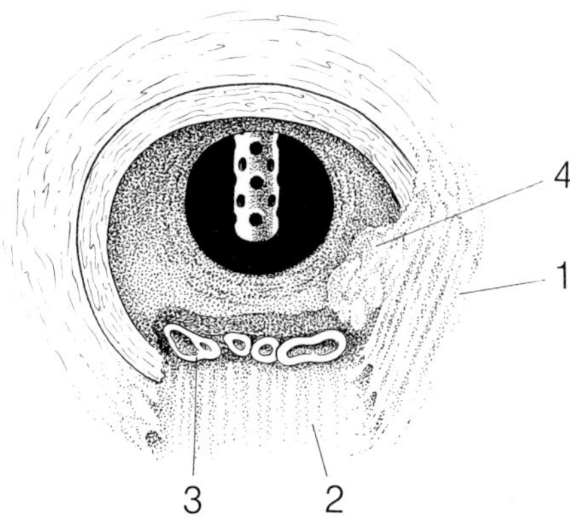

c

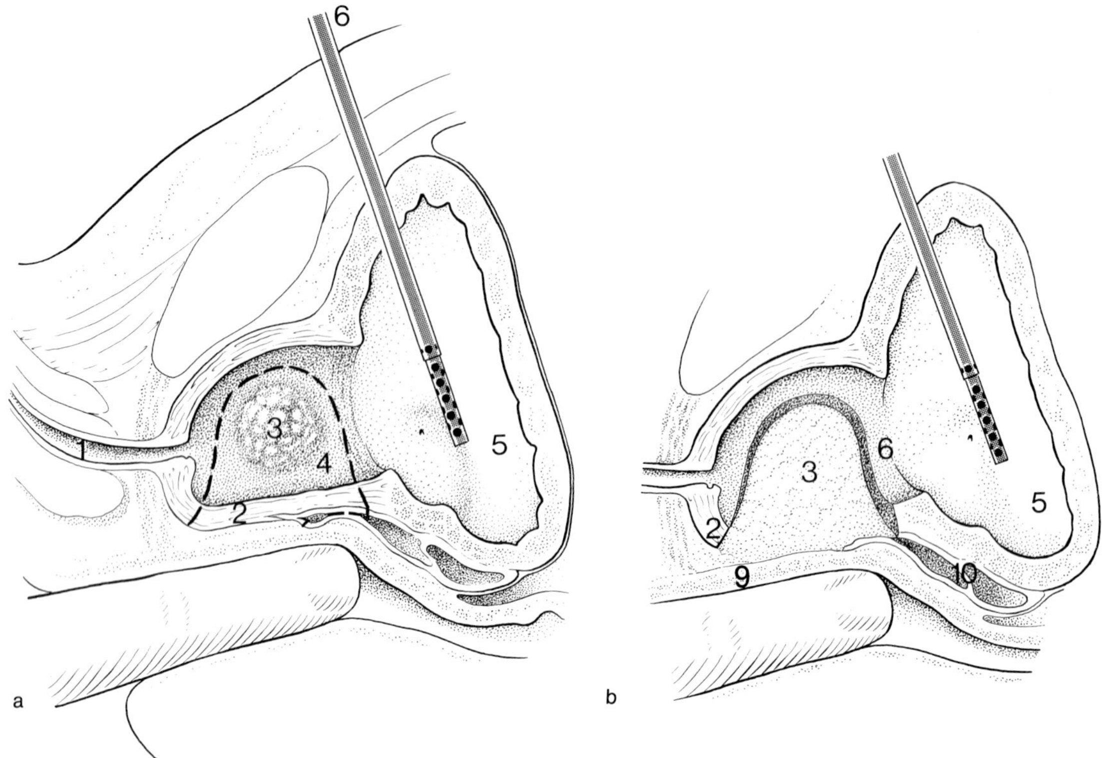

Fig. 51, a–b
(a) Sagittal section of prostate and empty bladder after total TUR of an adenoma with a carcinomatous node (3) in the capsule. Urethra (1); capsule (2); fossa (4); collapsed bladder (5); trocar aspiration (6). The floor of the fossa (2) is lifted by the finger in the rectum. Dashed lines mark the region of the capsule to be totally resected at minimum.
(b) Sagittal section of prostate and bladder (5) after radical TUR of the carcinomatous node (3) and partial TUR of the capsule (2). The longitudinal muscle of the rectum (9) and the seminal vesicles (10) are exposed (see Fig. 94, c). 6 = Internal sphincter.

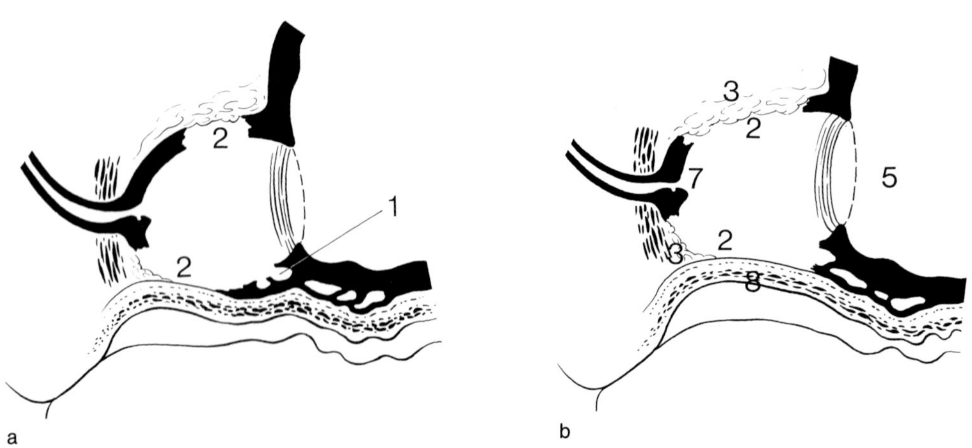

Fig. 52, a–c Sagittal sections of the prostatic fossa.
(a) Extensive TUR of the capsule and radical TUR of the carcinomatous infiltration (2). 1 = Cut seminal vesicle.
(b) Large wound between bladder (5) and urethral stump (7) after radical TUR of a carcinoma with extended (subtotal) TUR of the capsule (2) down into periprostatic tissue (3). This defect is masked by periprostatic tissue (3) and rectum (8).

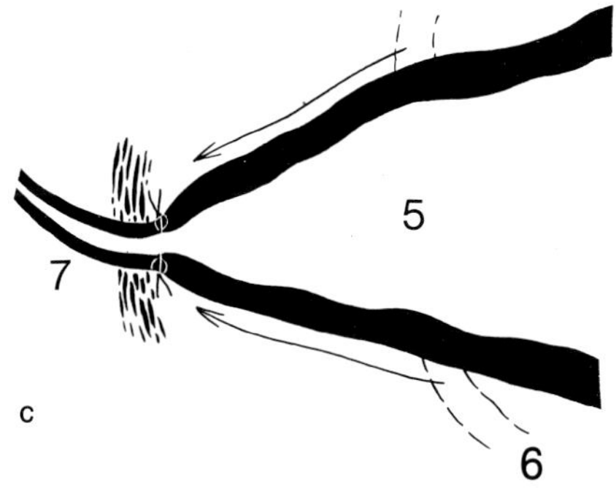

(c) Sagittal section of urethra (7) and bladder (5) after open radical surgical prostatectomy and suture of the stumps. 6 = Original bladder neck (dashed lines). In radical TUR, however, a large wound excavation remains between the bladder neck, apex and external sphincter. This heals spontaneously (a and b).

Strictures Following TUR

The narrowing of urethra and bladder neck seen after operations on the prostate has multiple causes. Strictures can be due to inborn disposition, trauma and chronic inflammation.

Stricture of the Prostatic Urethra (Figs. 120–123)

During TUR, mechanical and electrical trauma predominate. The prostatic capsule (true prostatic tissue) is very sensitive to electric current, as is the bladder muscle, which reacts to frequent electrocoagulation of papillomas (instead of TUR) by shrinkage and fibrotic degeneration. Adenomatous tissue, however, is relatively insensitive to electric current. Therefore, we must conclude that in partial TUR a mixed cutting and coagulating current can be used for cutting if need be. In TURP, however, cutting and coagulation require different qualities of current. Years ago in our hospital, mixed current resulted in a 6 per cent incidence of strictures of the prostatic urethra. This was reduced to 1 per cent when only the specific current was used (Table 7, p. 233).

Another factor leading to stricture is the time required for the operation in relation to the resected tissue and the size of the cutting loop. If only 10 to 30 gm of tissue per hour are resected with a relatively small cutting loop, more strictures are caused than when 50 to 100 gm are resected per hour. The tendency to form strictures is increased when the capsule is resected too deeply, causing perforations, and when a compression catheter is used (see Figs. 48, 49). These factors hinder spontaneous contraction of the fossa and increase the tendency of the capsule to shrink by chronic infiltrative-inflammatory processes. High pressure irrigation causes overdistention of the fossa, producing a similar effect (see Fig. 31).

Stricture of the Anterior and Middle Urethra

The importance of the size of the resectoscope sheath as cause of stricture has been overestimated. A thin resectoscope with a small cutting loop does not prevent strictures (see p. 16). After 20 years of experience with cortisone added to the lubricant (ratio 1:1), we have achieved a rate of strictures of the middle and anterior urethra of 1.1 per cent (Table 7). The stricture usually is in the bulbous urethra. This is traumatized more frequently during TUR by extension and compression than are the other parts. So-called "leakage current" also can cause strictures.

Endoscopic Urethrotomy

Endoscopic urethrotomy (see Fig. 122, d) is superior to blind urethrotomy because the stricture can be cut precisely down into sound tissue under direct vision and limited to the diseased section of the urethra. Today, stricture of the bladder neck is treated by endoscopic urethrotomy; in exceptional cases, this is combined with cryosurgery or TUR (see Fig. 182). Stricture at the urethral meatus (0.3 per cent) represents no problem. It is cut and treated with an ointment containing cortisone.

Recently, prevention of urethral strictures has been attempted by instilling 5–10 cc of 10 per cent povidone-iodine cream daily for several weeks. Finally, it should be emphasized that the number of postoperative urethral strictures is an indicator of the quality of TUR. Fast resection with as low a current as possible and with different qualities of current for coagulation and cutting treats the tissue best. Only the pathologic adenomatous tissue is to be resected. Superficially resected capsular and bladder neck tissues (over-resection) tend to indurate, to shrink and to bleed more (see Figs. 88, 97).

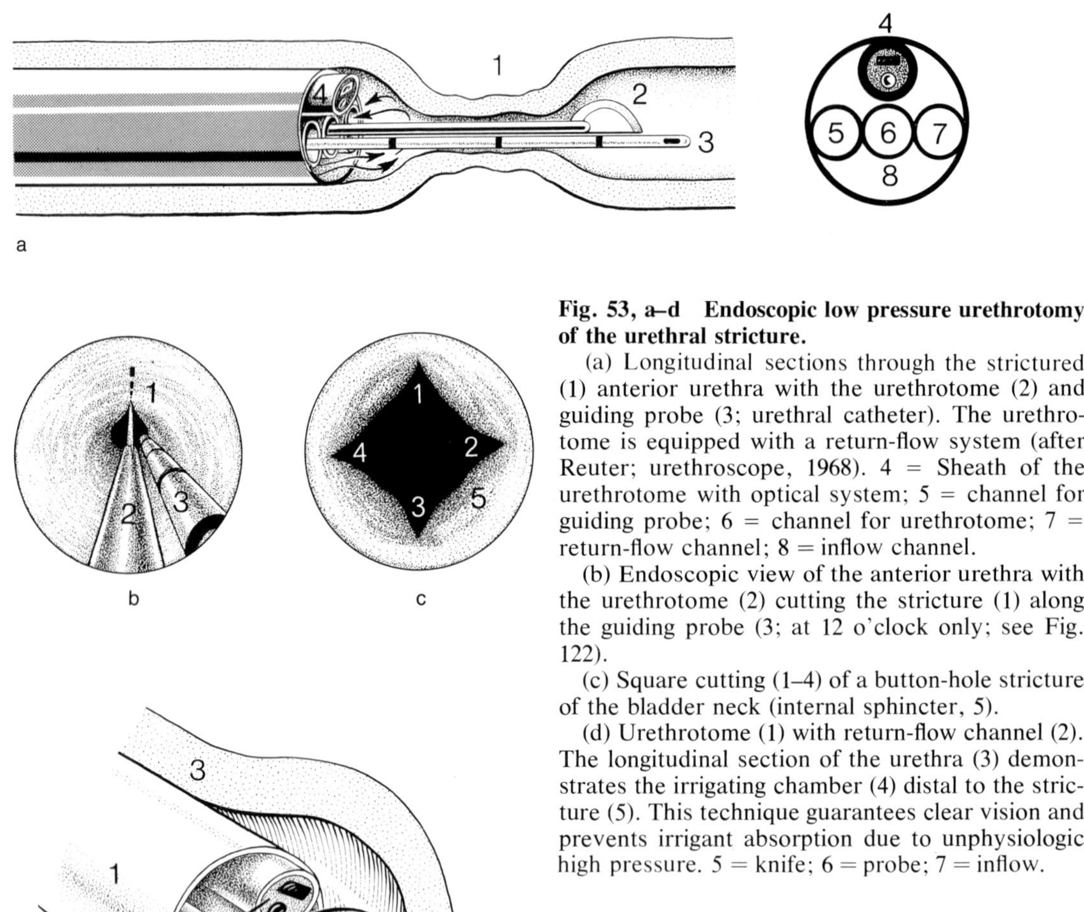

Fig. 53, a–d Endoscopic low pressure urethrotomy of the urethral stricture.

(a) Longitudinal sections through the strictured (1) anterior urethra with the urethrotome (2) and guiding probe (3; urethral catheter). The urethrotome is equipped with a return-flow system (after Reuter; urethroscope, 1968). 4 = Sheath of the urethrotome with optical system; 5 = channel for guiding probe; 6 = channel for urethrotome; 7 = return-flow channel; 8 = inflow channel.

(b) Endoscopic view of the anterior urethra with the urethrotome (2) cutting the stricture (1) along the guiding probe (3; at 12 o'clock only; see Fig. 122).

(c) Square cutting (1–4) of a button-hole stricture of the bladder neck (internal sphincter, 5).

(d) Urethrotome (1) with return-flow channel (2). The longitudinal section of the urethra (3) demonstrates the irrigating chamber (4) distal to the stricture (5). This technique guarantees clear vision and prevents irrigant absorption due to unphysiologic high pressure. 5 = knife; 6 = probe; 7 = inflow.

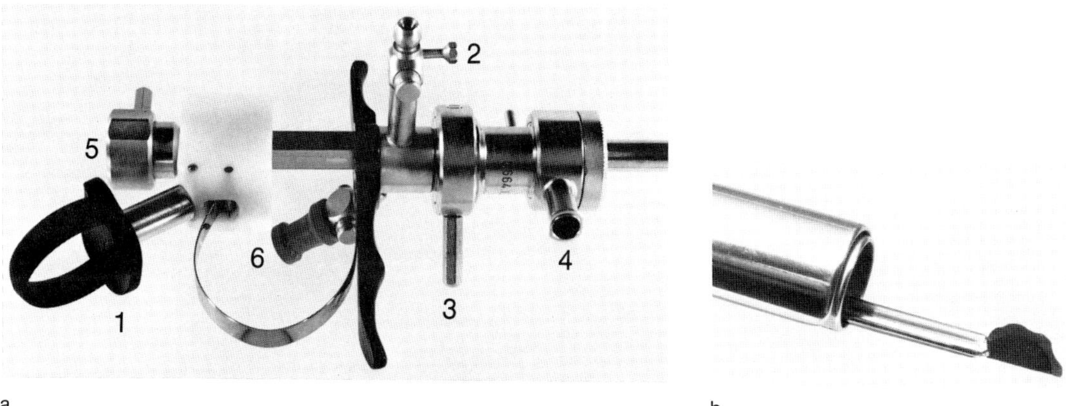

Fig. 54, a–c Endoscopic urethrotome (R. Wolf) with return-flow channel (Reuter) for low pressure urethrotomy.

(a) Insert (1) with return-flow stopcock (2) and sheath lock (3). Revolving cock (4) on the sheath for inflow. The optical system is not installed (5). Channel for probes (6).

(b) Beak with extended knife (sharpened like a saw).

(c) Optical urethrotome (Olympus Winter & Ibe) with scalpel and guiding catheter. The channel for the guiding catheter is inside the scalpel sheath.

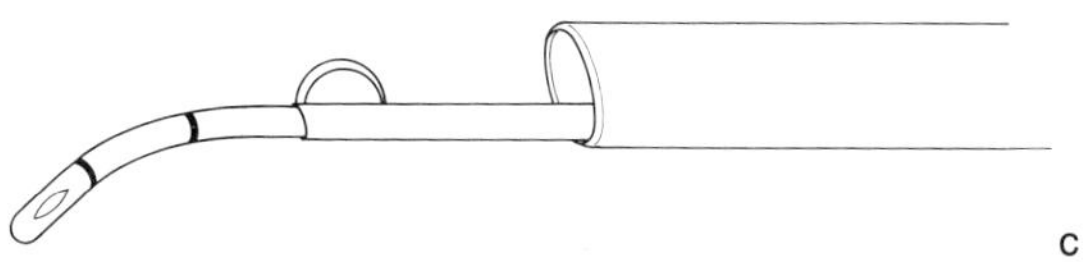

Postoperative Cystogram

This radiographic technique provides an important control by which the surgeon can judge the quality of his TUR. It reveals technical errors and shows the way to improvement. The extension and shape of the prostatic fossa — especially the condition of the apex — are judged. Within a few days, a totally resected fossa contracts to one half or one third its previous size (see Figs. 55–61). A fossa distended during high pressure TUR has no tendency to contract rapidly. This is complicated further by the bladder atony caused by overdistention of the bladder and fossa during high pressure irrigation and use of the compression catheter (cystogram; Fig. 62). Such gross problems as post-TUR ureteral reflux and insufficient partial TUR are easily demonstrated by the cystogram (see Figs. 5, 57, 58). Even small errors can be clearly identified — e.g., a small remnant at the apex at the 12 o'clock position (see Fig. 6). The oblique exposure completes the x-ray examination. When the seminal vesicles are resected they are seen on the cystogram lying adjacent to the bladder (see Fig. 65). After TUR of a subvesical adenoma, a spherical fossa with a clearly distinguishable ring formed by the internal sphincter is seen (see Fig. 58), whereas in the intravesically-developed adenoma, which often overdistends the internal sphincter, the ring is not observed (see Fig. 62). "Sphincter sclerosis" and the "median bar" cannot be treated adequately by making a few cuts; after a correct TUR the cystogram shows a large prostatic fossa (see Fig. 7). The topography of the fossa also depends on the constitution of the patient. This is demonstrated by differences in the relations between symphysis, bladder and fossa (see Fig. 67). For comparison, an atonic prostatic urethra (without TUR) of neurogenic etiology is shown in Figure 68.

(Text continued on page 80)

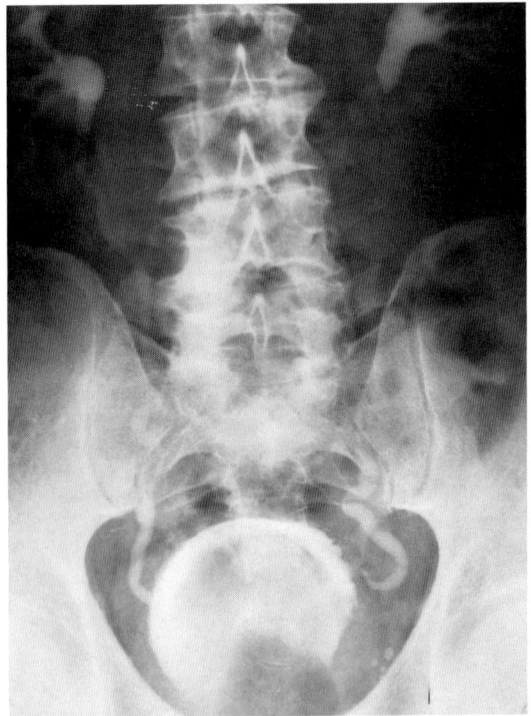

a

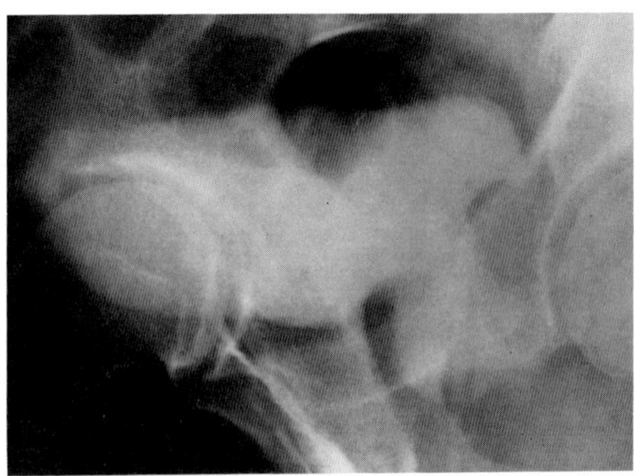

c

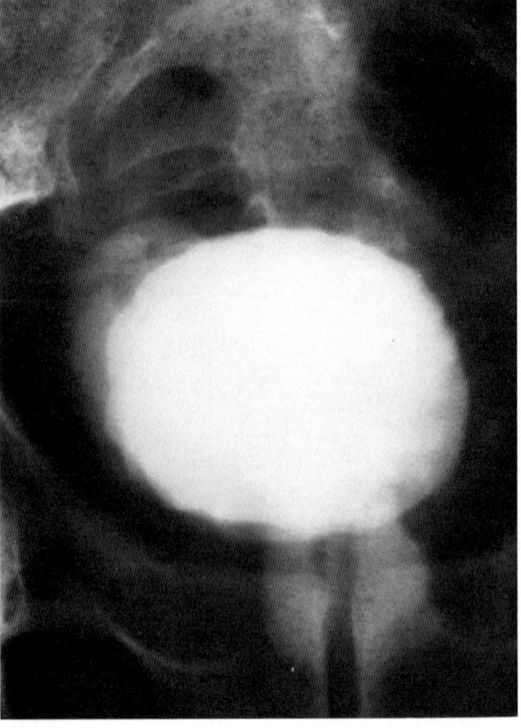

b

Fig. 55, a–c Result of TURP of a giant adenoma (200 gm net weight; about 260 gm gross weight; diameter of 8 × 10 cm) in an 85-year-old patient, risk-degree II.

(a) Preoperative excretory urogram (20 × 30 cm). The bladder is completely filled by the giant adenoma; note the fish-hook-shaped obstructed distal ureters.

(b) Cystogram (AP 10 × 15 cm) six days after TURP. The bladder is filled with 50 cc of contrast medium and is well contracted. Its diameter is 6 × 7 cm. At the left, a small hood is noted (compare Fig. 55, *c*). Below the bladder, there is a remarkably small, spherical prostatic fossa with a diameter of 3 cm. The capsule has shrunken quickly following total resection of the adenoma (low pressure irrigation). Postoperative progress was without complication, and micturition left no residual urine.

(c) Lateral cystogram (13 × 18 cm). The bladder, which is shaped like a sausage, is 14 cm wide and 6 cm high. The posterior part of the prostatic fossa forms a sharp angle with the bladder floor. It is pear-shaped and without adenomatous remnants.

Fig. 56, a–c TURP of a giant adenoma (net weight, 190 gm; 250 gm gross) resected in 110 min in a 69-year-old patient, risk-degree II. Low pressure irrigation with continuous aspiration of irrigant through the suprapubic trocar.

(a) The cystogram (13 × 18 cm) before TURP shows the large intravesical portion of an 8 × 10 cm adenoma. The left ureter is fish-hook-shaped and meets the shadow of the bladder in the upper third near a lucent area that represents the isolated median lobe of the intravesical adenoma (intravenous urography 20 min after injection).

(b) The postoperative cystogram (30 × 40 cm) demonstrates a ball-shaped excavation (5 × 5 cm) that represents the fossa below the bladder five days after TURP. The bladder floor is about 5 cm lower than before TURP (compare Fig. 56, *a*). The internal sphincter is clearly outlined within the bladder shadow. Bladder contraction is reduced; this is made evident by the oval shape of the bladder shadow. The fossa itself has a regular shape. Only at the right is it somewhat enlarged, and there a small capsular lesion may be seen. The bladder was filled with 50 cc of contrast medium through the balloon catheter pictured (20 Fr. catheter with 5-cc balloon in the fossa, providing three means of continuous irrigation).

(c) The postoperative cystogram (13 × 14 cm) in the lateral oblique exposure shows a flat atonic bladder shadow shaped like a cigar (6 × 5 cm). The large spherical prostatic fossa is situated below the posterior part of the bladder. The catheter lies obliquely within the fossa; the apex has been completely resected. The posterior bladder wall is flat and 2 cm high. The bladder roof forms a horizontal plane. The fossa has shrunk to approximately one half to one third of its original size immediately after TUR.

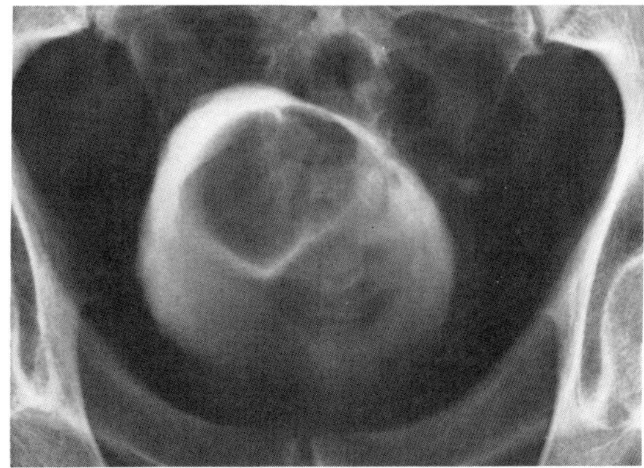

a

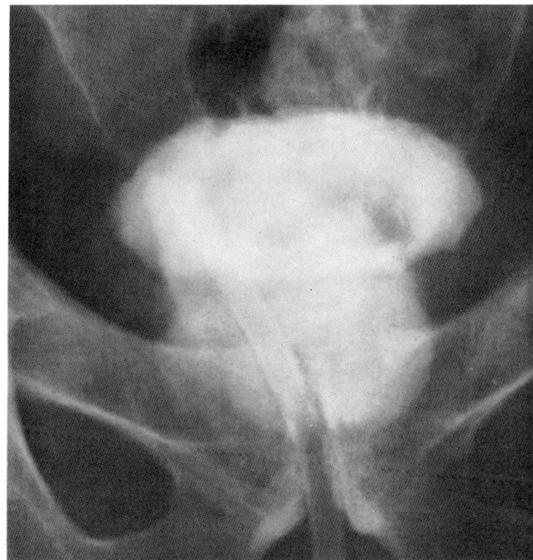

b

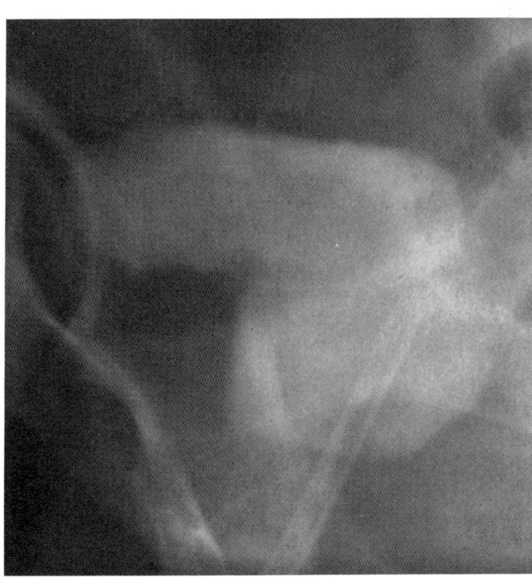

c

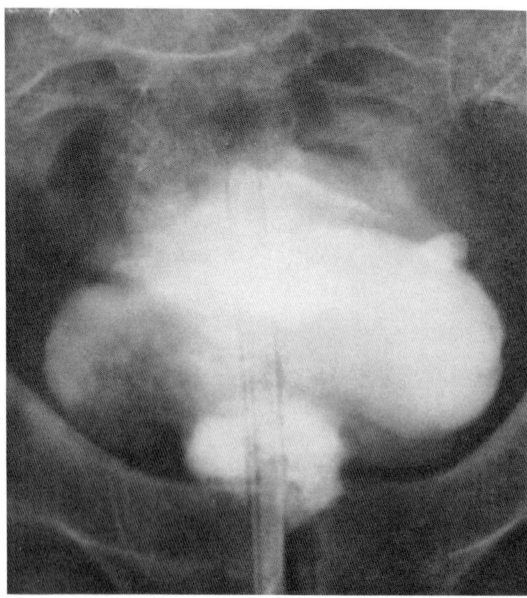

Fig. 57 Partial TUR of a medium large prostatic adenoma (about 40 gm) in a 72-year-old patient (performed by a trainee with experience of about 100 TUR). Low pressure irrigation.

The postoperative cystogram (13 × 18 cm) was obtained three days after TUR. The well contracted shadow of the bladder is partly obscured by intestinal gases at the right and is deformed above by a permanent catheter (20 Fr.) that was introduced too far and extended at the left by a small diverticulum. The internal sphincter separates the bladder neck from the prostatic fossa (3 × 2 cm). The wall of the fossa is irregular at the left. At the lower right a large adenomatous remnant can be seen at the apex. Fifteen gm net of adenomatous tissue were resected in 30 minutes. Six days later, a secondary total resection (TURP) was performed and 15 gm net additional tumor tissue was removed in 25 min.

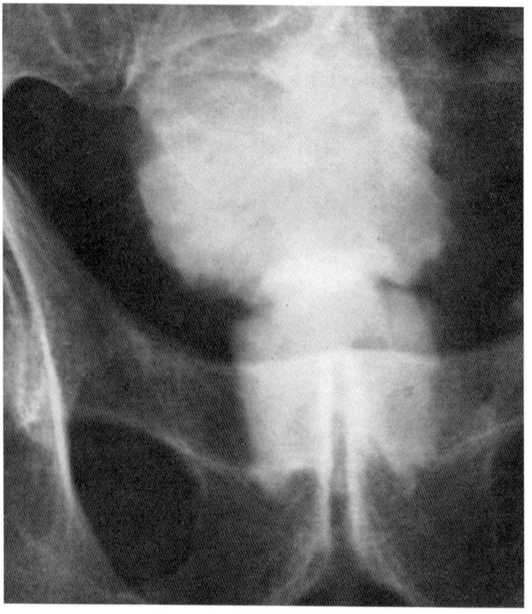

a

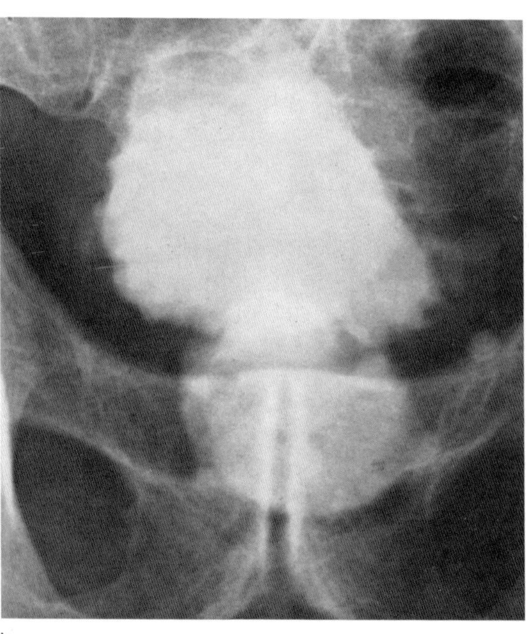

b

Fig. 58, a–b Partial TUR in first session; TURP in second session.

Large prostatic adenoma (about 100 gm) in an 80-year-old patient (risk degree II). Low pressure irrigation with continuous aspiration (trocar).

(a) The cystogram (13 × 18 cm) three days after TUR shows an irregular bladder shadow with a well delineated internal sphincter. Below the bladder, note the cylindric prostatic fossa (4 × 4 cm) with an irregular left lateral wall and the larger adenomatous remnants at the apex. In the first session, 60 gm were removed in 65 min; one week later, 20 gm net were resected in 15 min because 500 cc residual urine had been noted.

(b) The cystogram (13 × 18 cm) after the second session demonstrates a spherical prostatic fossa (4.5 × 4 cm) below the bladder shadow. The lateral walls of the fossa now are concave and the apex is rounded. At the left of the bladder neck, a cuneiform shadow separates the bladder and fossa; probably an overlying intestinal loop is the cause of this shadow.

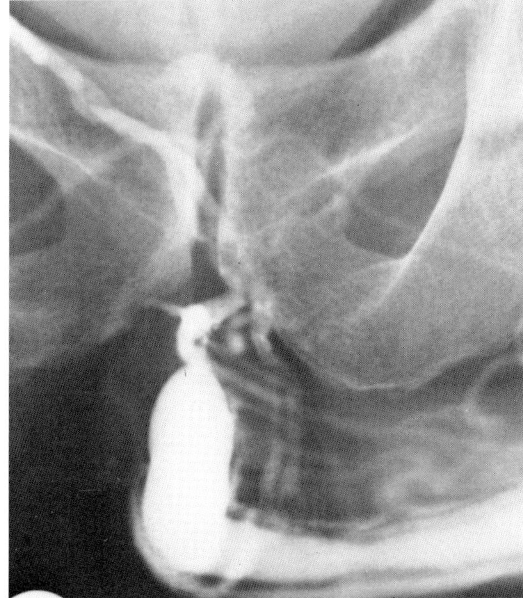

Fig. 59 Urethral stricture four years after TURP. Forty gm net of adenoma were resected in 45 min in this 66-year-old patient. The urethra was filled retrograde with contrast medium, and a stricture in the middle urethra was demonstrated. Extensive reflux into paraurethral veins also was verified. This venous reflux is due to unphysiologic high pressure, which filled the urethra. After treatment with bougies there has been no recurrence (three-year follow-up).

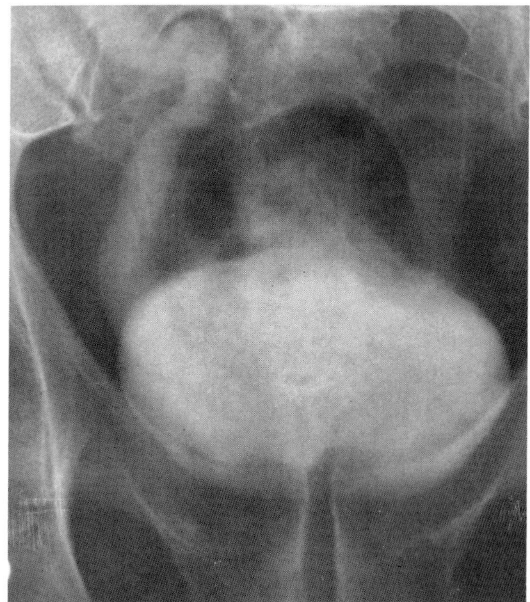

Fig. 60 Partial TUR with stricture of the right ureteral orifice.

One year after TUR (62-year-old patient, risk-degree 0), the bladder has a normal shape and good tension. The bladder floor lies about 1 cm below the upper rim of the symphysis; the straight line is broken by two prominent residual nodes of adenoma. The right ureter is chronically obstructed; the left ureter is delicate. The cystogram (13 × 18 cm) was made one hour after intravenous urography.

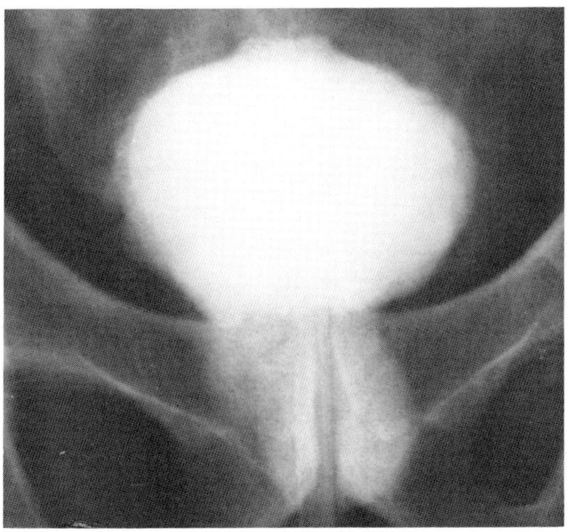

a

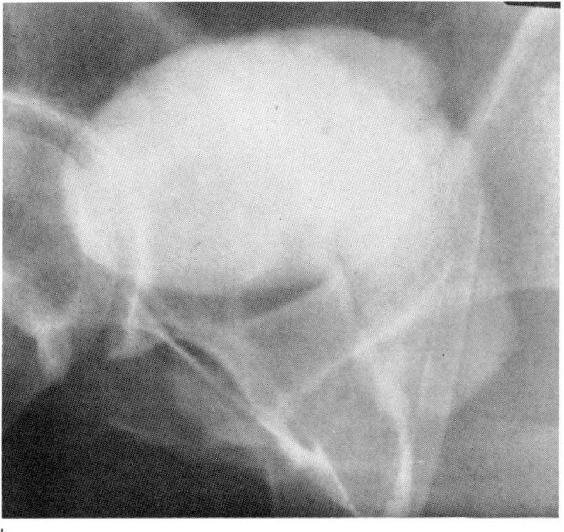

b

Fig. 61, a–b TURP of a giant adenoma (130 gm net in 95 min) in a 55-year-old patient, risk-degree 0.

Five days after operation the prostatic fossa has shrunk to about half its original size.

(a) AP cystogram (13 × 18 cm): the well contracted bladder is separated markedly from the fossa (4 × 3 cm) by the internal sphincter. The right wall of the fossa is distended laterally and has an irregular outline. This indicates over-resection or a lesion of the capsule. The apex is well rounded, and there are no adenomatous remnants. The delicate left ureter can be seen.

(b) The lateral oblique exposure (13 × 18 cm) shows the prostatic fossa (5 × 4 cm) at the dorsal end of the oval bladder. The shape of the fossa is cylindrical and its outline smooth; the apex is convexly formed without adenomatous remnants. The catheter (20 Fr) lies obliquely within the fossa. The posterior wall of the bladder begins about 2 cm above the rim of the trigone.

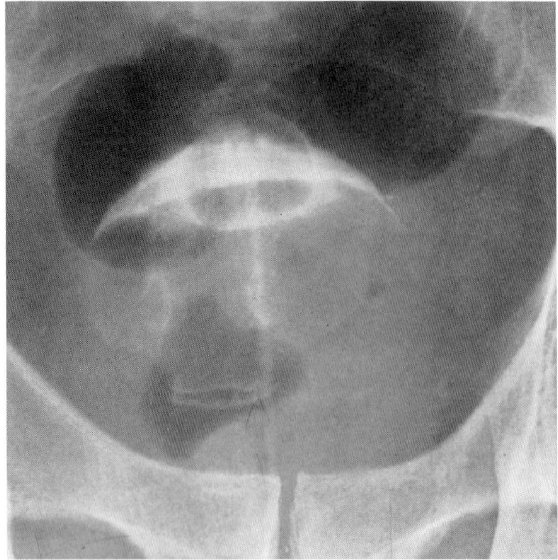

a

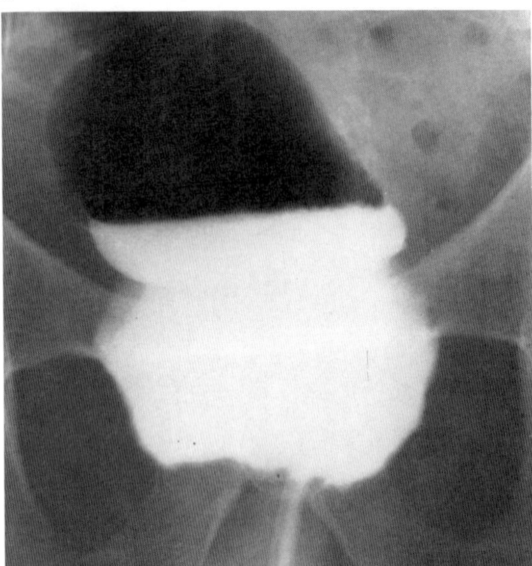

b

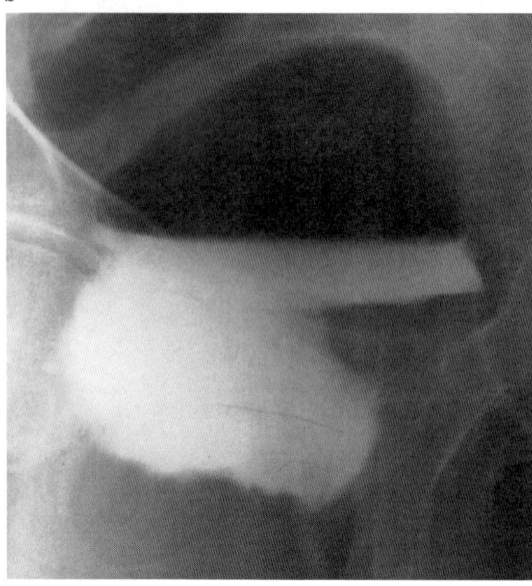

c

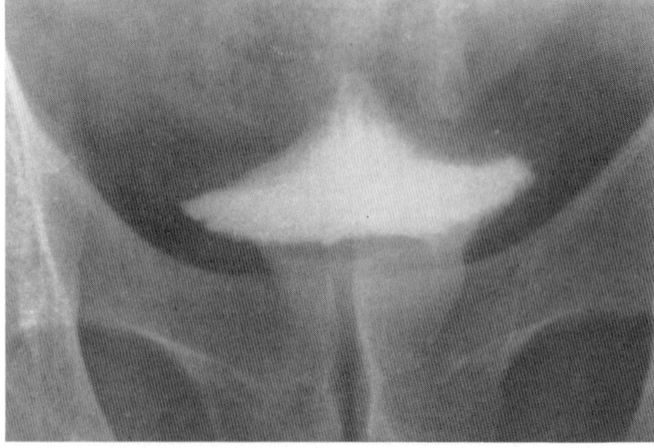

d

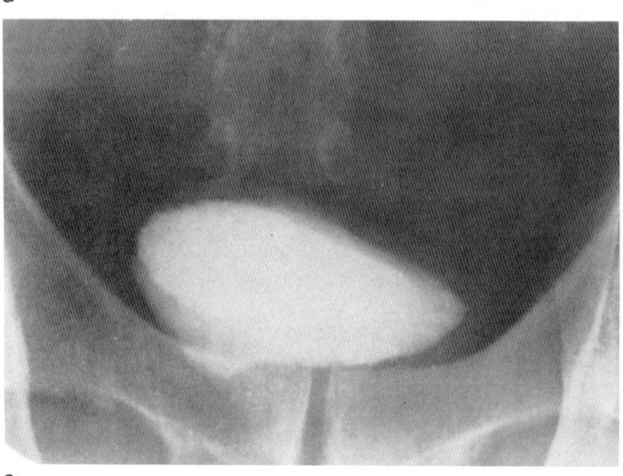

e

Fig. 62, a–e Recovery from an overdistended prostatic fossa due to high pressure irrigation. TURP of an adenoma (9.5 cm long and 240 gm net weight) in two sessions with an interval of 10 days in a 62-year-old patient (risk-degree II).

(a) Preoperative cystogram (13 × 18 cm) with indwelling balloon catheter. The bladder has the shape of a small sickle and lies 6 cm above the symphysis.

(b) Cystogram (13 × 18 cm) three days after the second session. Owing to the high pressure irrigation used, the prostatic fossa is distended to 4 × 8 × 7 cm. The bladder is filled with 50 cc air and the fossa and bladder floor with 100 cc of contrast medium. The apex has an irregular outline; this is not caused by adenomatous remnants (compare Fig. 62, *d*).

Oblique lateral cystogram (13 × 18 cm) shows a fossa 4 × 7.5 cm. The trigone has been completely resected, and the fossa adjoins the posterior bladder wall directly over a small prominence. The anterior wall of the bladder is well set off against the fossa. The anterior fossa extends over all of the inner side of the symphysis.

(d) Cystogram (9 × 12 cm) with 30 cc contrast medium one month after TURP. The fossa is reduced to a ball-shaped excavation 2.5 × 3.5 cm.

(e) Cystogram (9 × 12 cm) three months after TURP. The prostatic fossa has shrunk completely and is no longer seen. Only at the right of the bladder floor is a small recess noted.

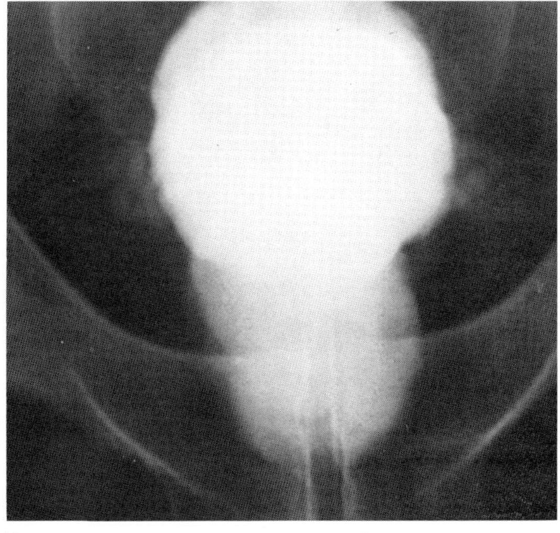

a

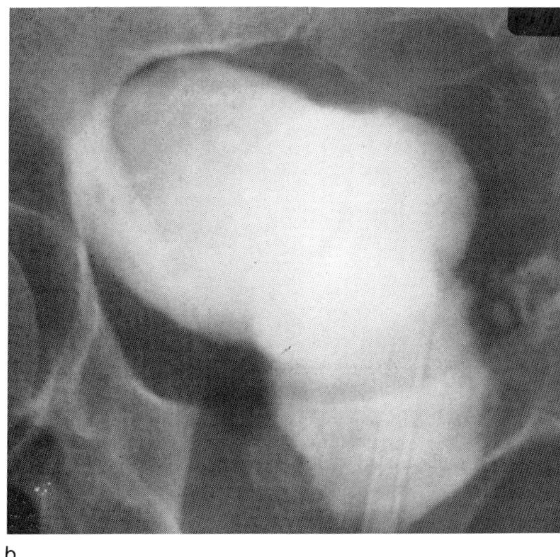

b

Fig. 63, a–b TURP of a large adenoma (75 gm net) in 60 min in a 69-year-old patient, risk-degree II. Low pressure irrigation with continuous trocar aspiration.

(a) The AP cystogram (13 × 18 cm) demonstrates a well contracted bladder with somewhat irregular outlines and a slightly hooded roof (double contour) three days after the operation. The bladder floor (internal sphincter) is well delineated from the prostatic fossa (5 × 4.5 cm); at both sides the seminal vesicles are recognized as worm-shaped shadows. The outlines of the already reduced fossa are somewhat irregular — especially at the right. However, the tumor was well resected and there are no adenomatous remnants.

(b) The oblique lateral exposure (13 × 18 cm) demonstrates a cylindrical fossa (5.5 × 4.5 cm) with a somewhat irregular outline; the apex is cone-shaped. At the posterior wall of the fossa the seminal vesicles are seen to be filled with contrast medium at the rim of the symphysis. The balloon catheter (20 Fr, the 5-cc balloon has been emptied) touches the trigone.

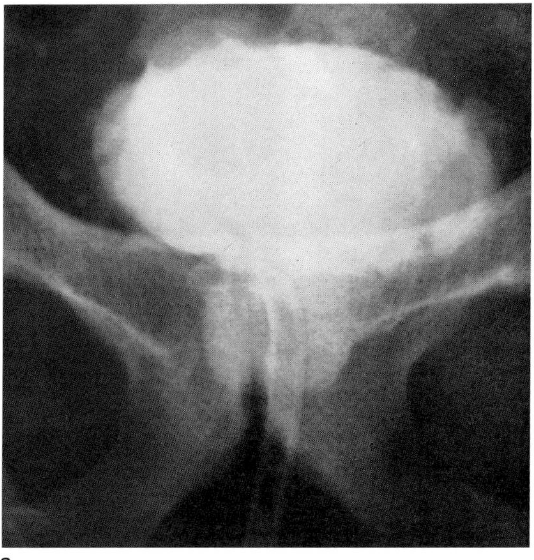

a

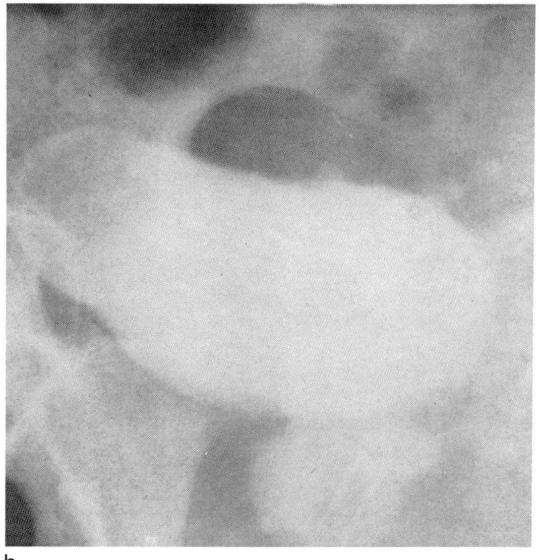

b

Fig. 64, a–b TURP of a subvesical adenoma (35 gm net) in 50 min in a 65-year-old patient, risk-degree I. Low pressure irrigation with continuous trocar aspiration.

(a) The AP cystogram demonstrates a well contracted bladder with somewhat irregular outlines. The prostatic fossa (3 × 3.5 cm) has shrunk well four days after the operation. It is clearly delineated from the bladder floor and has a regular spherical shape. The tip of the catheter (20 Fr) has caught laterally below the trigone and is reversed.

(b) The oblique lateral exposure demonstrates a sausage-shaped bladder shadow. The bladder neck is set off against the fossa (3 × 3 cm) by the annular internal sphincter. The tip of the catheter pushes the wall of the fossa backward.

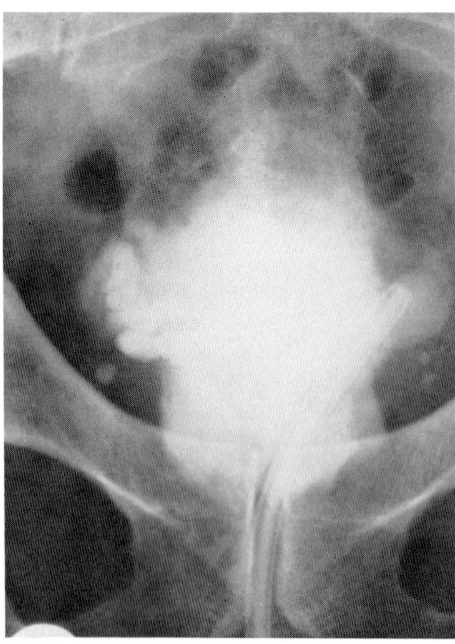

Fig. 65 TURP of a giant adenoma (130 gm net) resected in 105 min in a 74-year-old patient (risk degree II) after prior treatment for uremia due to chronic urinary retention with over 1L residual urine. Continuous low pressure irrigation with suprapubic trocar.

Cystogram (13 × 18 cm): the bladder is loose; its outline is unclear and irregular six days after TURP. At the left, the vermiform outline of a cut seminal vesicle is seen. At the right, the tip of the catheter (20 Fr) is introduced into a cherrystone-sized diverticulum. The internal sphincter forms only a slight waist between the bladder and the broad prostatic fossa (5 × 5.5 cm). It is ball-shaped; only at the left is a small capsular lesion identified as a concavity.

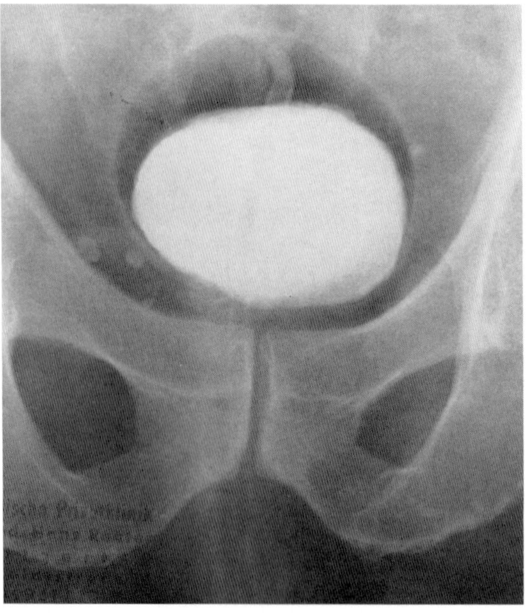

a

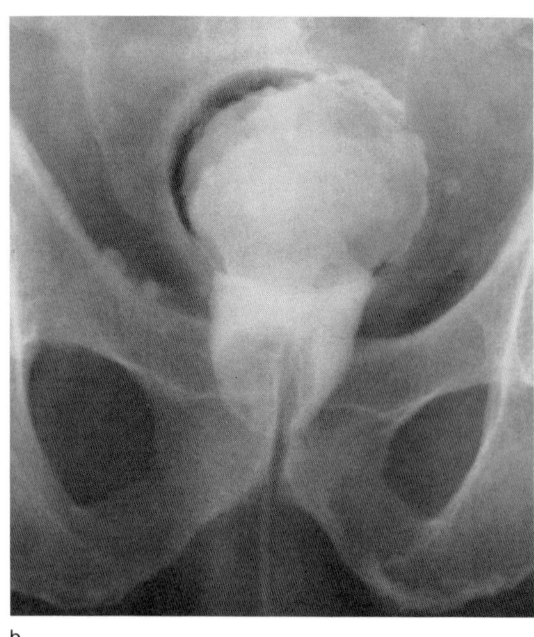

b

Fig. 66, a–b TURP: "sphincter sclerosis" in a 67-year-old patient (risk degree 0). Ten gm net of tissue were resected in 20 min. High pressure irrigation with 80 cm elevation of the irrigating reservoir.

(a) The preoperative cystogram (13 × 18 cm) demonstrates a well contracted bladder of normal shape filled with contrast medium and air. The tip of a Mercier catheter touches the fundus of the bladder. The bladder floor is slightly elevated; a median lobe of adenoma, however, is not recognizable.

(b) The postoperative cystogram (13 × 18 cm) was made three days after the operation. The outlines of the bladder show an inflammatory reaction. The bladder neck passes wide into the prostatic fossa (3.5 × 3.5 cm), delineating clearly the rim of the internal sphincter. The fossa itself is overdistended by high pressure irrigation and has the shape of a thimble; the 5-cc balloon of the catheter is seen at the apex.

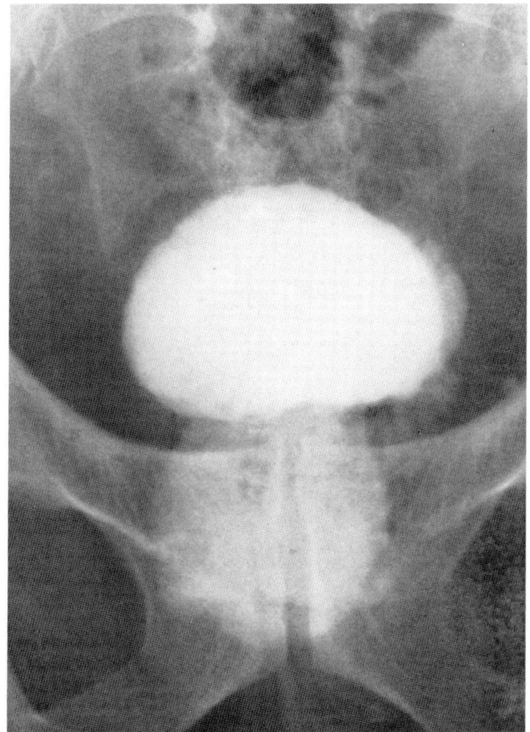

a

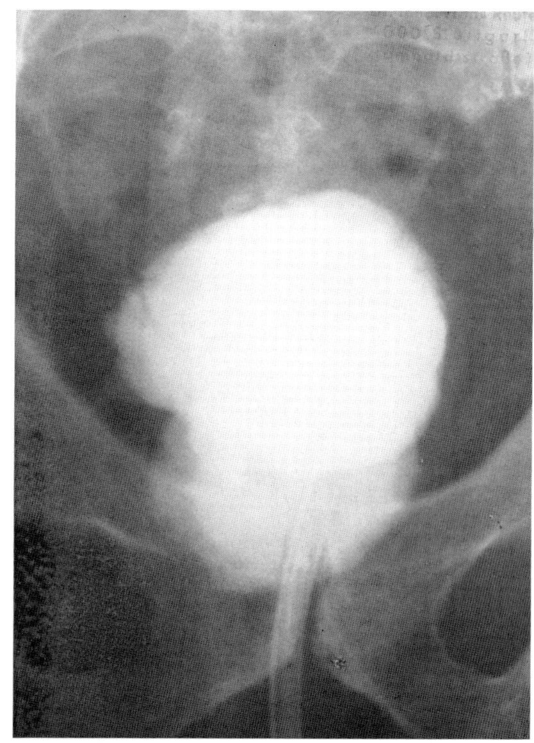

b

Fig. 67, a–c Comparison of the topography of the prostatic fossa after TURP in three different patients (cystograms 13 × 18 cm).

(a) Regular spherical fossa (5 × 4.5 cm) below the bladder after TURP of 35 min (55 gm net). 71-year-old patient, risk-degree I.

(b) Steep angulation between prostatic urethra and bladder, around a somewhat deformed prostatic fossa after TURP of 60 min (80 gm net) in a 78-year-old patient, risk degree II. The spherical fossa (5 × 6 cm) is almost half overlapped by the bladder shadow; the angle between the urethra and bladder is flat.

(c) The large, round fossa (5 × 6 cm) is totally overlapped by the bladder shadow. Eighty gm net of adenoma were resected in 75 min. The patient was 71 years old, risk degree I. In men with pyknic habitus the prostate not infrequently lies higher above the rectum than in men with other builds. This changes, as in this case, the topography of the bladder and fossa; the angle between the urethra and bladder is almost neutralized.

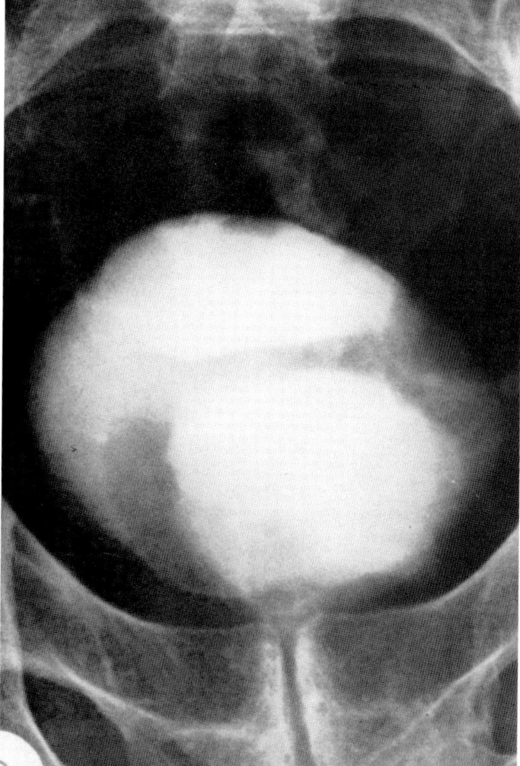

c

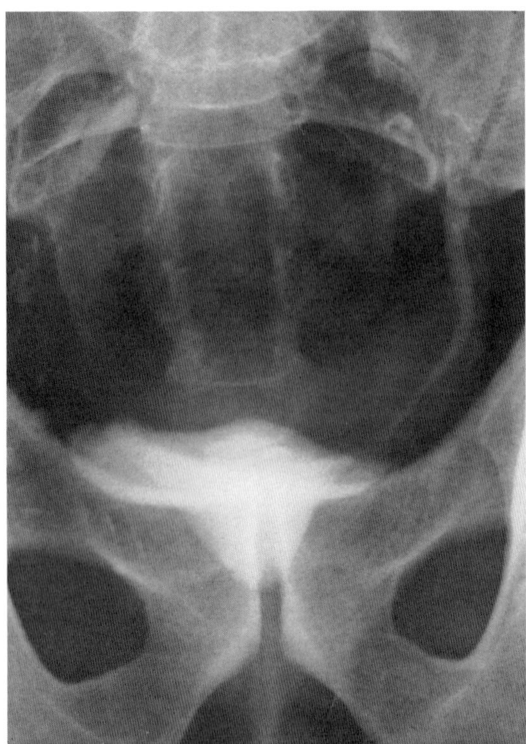

Fig. 68 Neurogenic bladder with atonic bladder neck (no preceding prostatic operation).

The bladder is slightly filled (excretory urogram 15 min after injection; 13 × 18 cm film). An open cone-shaped bladder neck (5 × 3 cm) is demonstrated; the tip of the cone is at the apex. This 60-year-old patient was operated for rectal carcinoma one year previously (at this time, a giant renal cyst was operated).

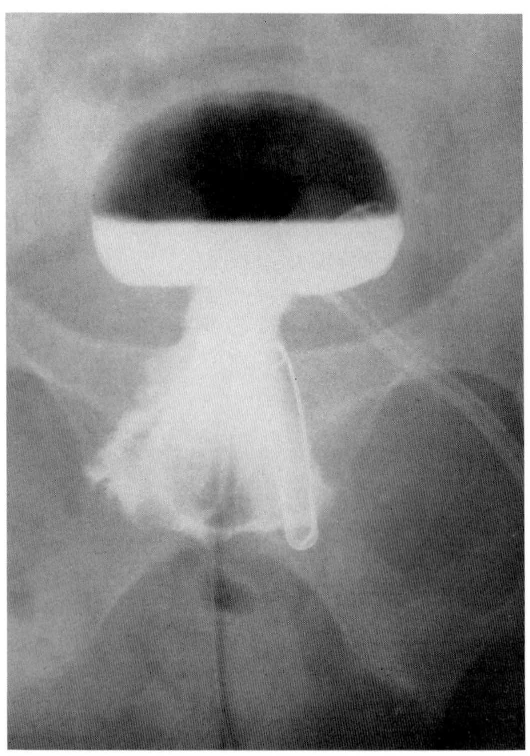

Fig. 69 Suprapubic prostatectomy of a 200-gm (gross) adenoma.

The bladder shows smooth, well contracted outlines three days after the operation. It is half filled with air and half with contrast medium. The bladder neck is narrowed by sutures. The pear-shaped prostatic fossa is 7 cm long and 5 cm wide; the outline of its lateral wall is irregular, especially at the left. A compression catheter is situated in the fossa; its balloon was reduced to a content of 20 cc. At the right, the safety-pin of the wound drainage at the suprapubic fistula catheter is seen. This picture (13 × 18 cm) serves for comparison with results after TUR.

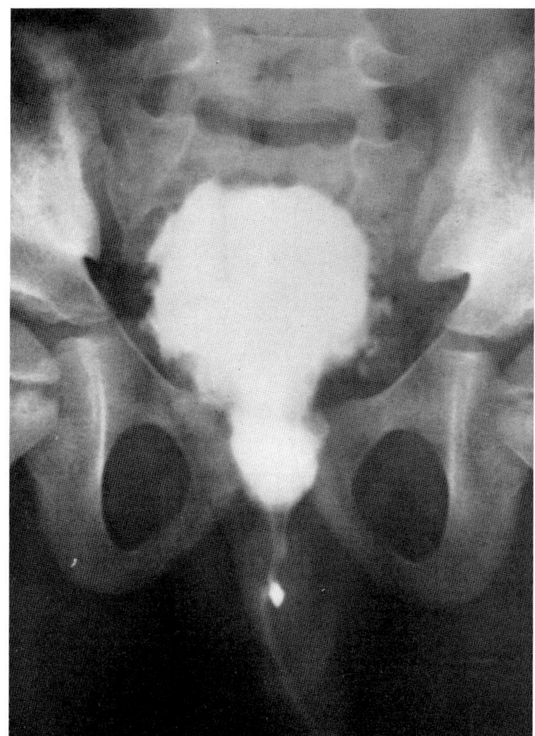

Fig. 70 Cystogram one week after TUR of neurogenic sphincter sclerosis with overflowing bladder and urethral reflux due to dysplasia of the sacral bone in a five-year-old boy (film 13 × 18 cm).

Seventy eight tissue chips were resected in 30 min (see Fig. 3).

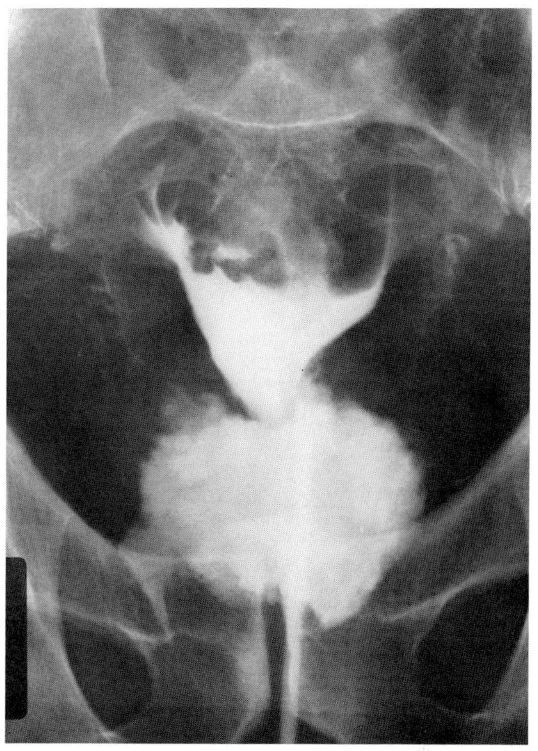

Fig. 71 Retroperitoneal perforation during TUR of 50 gm (net) in 60 min (cystogram 13 × 18 cm).

At the upper rim of the irregular spherical outline of the fossa and bladder, a subvesical cuneiform shadow is visible by contrast medium. Its tip lies within a small perforation below the trigone (cleft formation; see Fig. 93). At the right, beside the tip, the shadow of the catheter is barely visible, even though the contrast medium was passed through it. The prostatic fossa is not clearly distinct from the bladder. At the right, the capsule is defective; here, a small amount of contrast medium has extravasated laterally into the lower periprostatic space. A small adenomatous remnant protrudes at the apex. Postoperative recovery was uneventful; the permanent catheter was left in place for one week (good result).

Cystogram after Radical TUR

In radical TUR, large parts of the capsule are resected, separating the connection between the bladder neck and apex. The excavation leaves periprostatic fatty and connective tissues, which epithelialize to form a new urethra. The resected bladder neck assumes the shape of a bowl; this configuration often remains for life (see Fig. 75).

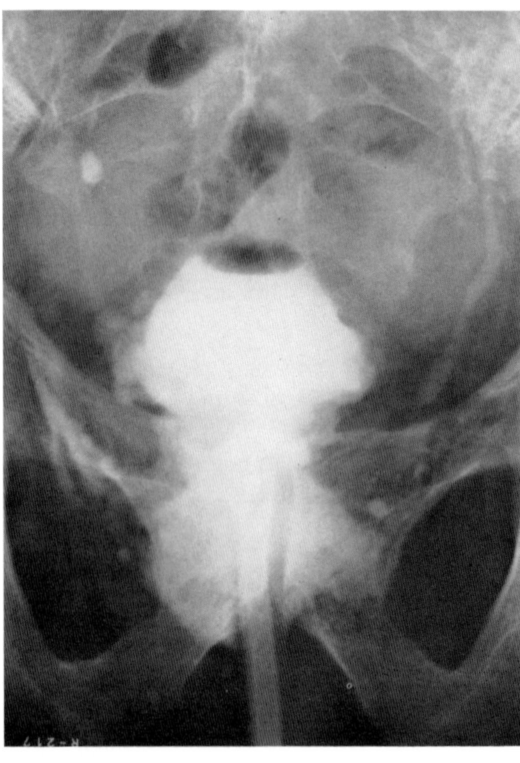

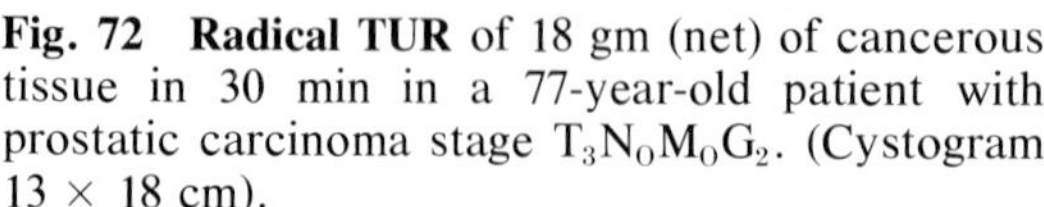

Fig. 72 Radical TUR of 18 gm (net) of cancerous tissue in 30 min in a 77-year-old patient with prostatic carcinoma stage $T_3N_0M_0G_2$. (Cystogram 13 × 18 cm).

The outline of the bladder is irregular; at the left, the seminal vesicles are seen. The prostatic fossa (5 × 5 cm) is spherical, although it has an irregular outline. At the left a large excavation is particularly notable behind the pubic bone. The left ureter (at the right) is made visible by reflux. The patient was without recurrence eight years after TUR.

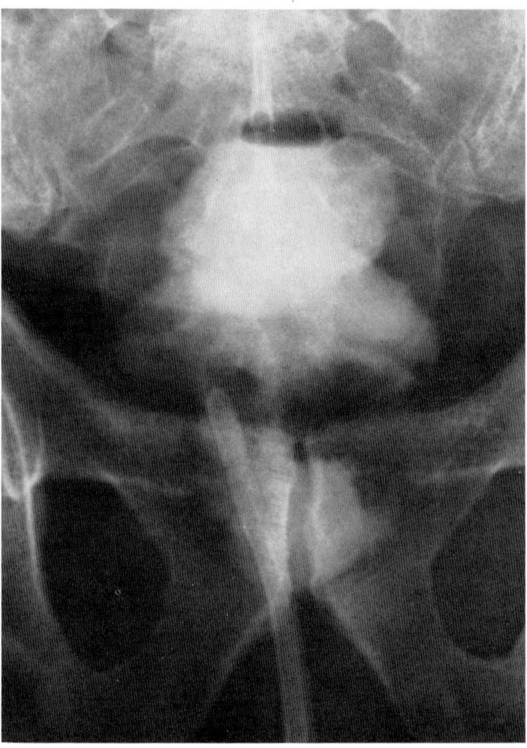

Fig. 73 Radical TUR of 50 gm (net) in 60 min of an undifferentiated prostatic carcinoma (stage $T_3N_xM_0G_3$) with left ureteral obstruction (cystogram 13 × 18 cm). The spherical bladder (which had shrunk after cobalt irradiation) sits above the large prostatic fossa (8 × 7 cm). The fossa itself is deformed; at the left, a larger mass protrudes into the fossa (fatty tissue, coagulate). The carcinoma seemed to be healed in the region of the prostate; however, nine years later bone metastases were confirmed. The patient's physical condition was good following orchiectomy and estrogen therapy.

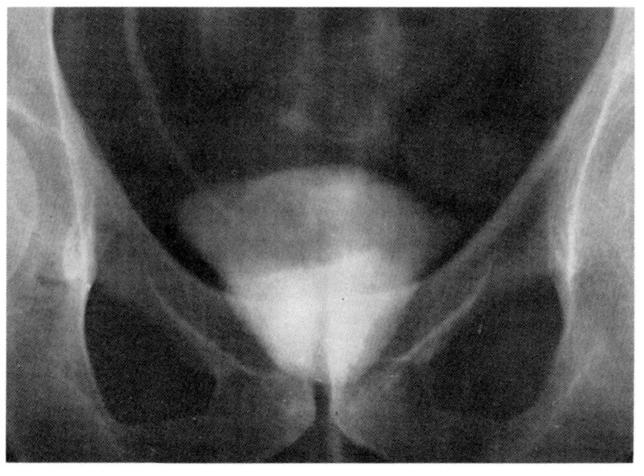

a

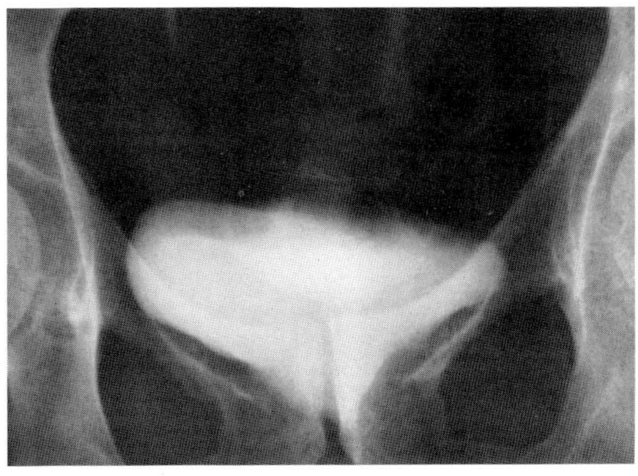

b

Fig. 74, a–b Cystograms (13 × 18 cm) three and ten years after radical TUR of a prostatic carcinoma, stage $T_2M_0N_0G_2$, in a 44-year-old patient.

(a) Three years after TUR, the lower rim of the bladder has a ball-shaped, smooth outline (excretory urogram 20 min after injection). The internal sphincter clearly outlines the fossa (5 × 3 cm).

(b) The excretory urogram ten years after TUR demonstrates a shrunk prostatic fossa (3.5 × 2 cm) with smooth outlines. The patient has had no recurrence. Owing to inadequate erection, a Silastic prosthesis was implanted into the penis (technique after Reuter; lateral cut into the penile crown proximal to the glans with excellent results). No irradiation, no orchiectomy and no estrogens were given.

Fig. 75 Cystogram (13 × 18 cm) three years after radical TUR of 35 gm (net) of a prostatic carcinoma in 50 min (stage $T_3N_0M_0G_2$). There was extended infiltration of the capsule in this 43-year-old patient (cobalt irradiation; castration; estrogen therapy).

Six years after TUR there has been no recurrence. The cystogram demonstrates a bowl-shaped, distended bladder floor with smooth outlines (excretory urogram 20 min after injection).

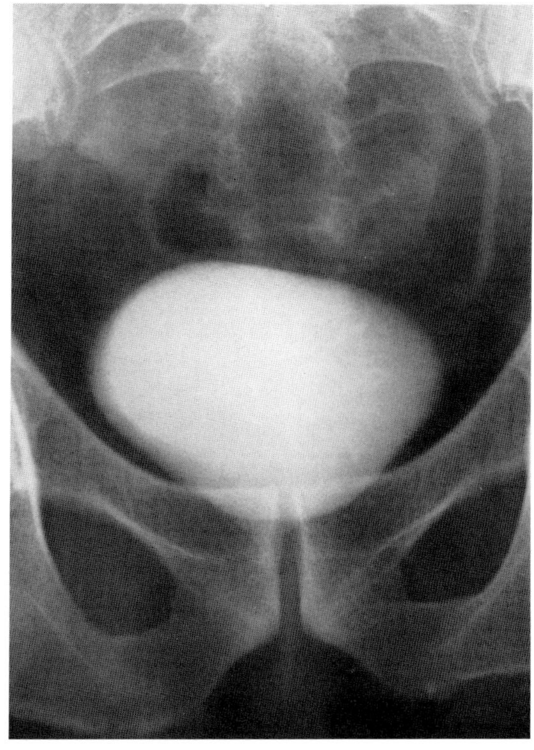

TUR of Bladder Tumors

TUR is today the predominant procedure for treatment of bladder tumors. Open surgical procedures are employed only in malignant tumors. Electrocoagulation is done only for the very small papilloma (see Fig. 129).

TUR is performed:

(1) For all benign papillomas (see Fig. 130).

(2) For papillary carcinomas stage T_1 as radical TUR; it is also used in the upper bladder hemisphere (stages T_2 and T_3 here are treated by open surgery).

(3) For papillary carcinoma (stages T_1 and T_2) of the lower bladder hemisphere — especially in the region of the trigone (radical TUR) (see Fig. 135).

(4) For G_2 and G_3 infiltrating cancer. Here, radical TUR is indicated only in stage T_1. If exploratory excision (performed as total or radical TUR) reveals a histologic pattern corresponding to the clinical appearance, we continue as soon as possible with open surgery, eventually followed by irradiation (see Fig. 132) and chemotherapy (see Fig. 140).

(5) Precancerous lesions (TiS) are treated by TUR, open surgery or cryosurgery (see Fig. 179) as indicated by the findings.

Additive nontoxic chemotherapy is employed to stimulate the immune system (see Fig. 176) as, for example, cryonecroses (Ablin). Cystostatic drugs can be combined with antibodies (immunochemical treatment; Theurer). Also, vitamin B_{17} (amygdalin) has been reported to have a specific effect on malignant cell proliferation and to inhibit formation of neoplasms. Other authors try hyperthermia (Bichler; Harzmann).

Endoscopic cryosurgery either supplements or replaces TUR of the bladder tumor (see Fig. 175). If histologic examination of a seemingly benign bladder tumor shows malignancy, as a rule we freeze the base of the resected tumor. In our experience, this improves the prognosis. We prefer to use trocar cryosurgery in larger tumors because it is more efficient than surface cryosurgery (see Fig. 175).

Technique of TUR of Bladder Tumors

TUR of bladder tumors follows the same rules as TURP. Low pressure irrigation (see p. 25) provides physiologic conditions in the bladder and reduces the risk of complications (perforation, ascending infection of the kidneys, bladder overdistention, irrigant absorption, metastasis). The best instrument for TUR of bladder tumors is the resectoscope

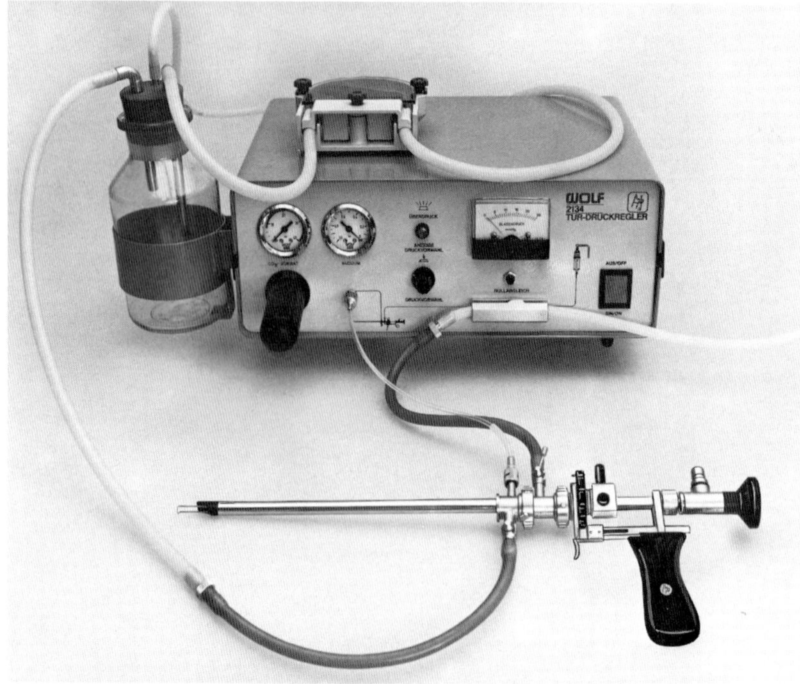

Fig. 76 Low pressure TUR of bladder tumors. TUR pressure gauge unit for automatic regulation of bladder pressure during resection of bladder tumors with the low pressure return-flow resectoscope (with measuring channel; see Fig. 15, c, 6).

with return-flow and continuous irrigation (see Fig. 76). The bladder should not be totally emptied during TUR, because the wall of the empty bladder may be aspirated into the sheath and resected without being noticed. Bladder filling of about 100 cc (to 200 cc at the most) is optimal: the elastic undistended bladder wall can thus escape the cut.

It is recommended that each bleeder be coagulated immediately at the level of bladder wall. This prevents dangerous bleeding from several vessels, where irrigant and vision quickly become clouded. Venous bleeding often is found more easily when the irrigant only flows out (inflow closed), having previously coagulated the arteries.

A tumor on the bladder roof or the posterior wall can be reached by the loop more easily when the bladder is almost empty (20 to 50 cc filling). The bladder roof is pushed with a finger or the whole hand downward toward the loop. A tumor on the bladder floor is lifted by rectal palpation so that it opposes the loop (see Fig. 77).

Superficial TUR at the Level of the Bladder Mucosa (Figs. 129–131)

The aim is to resect the tumor only to the level of the mucosa. The "benign" papilloma (stage T_A) never infiltrates the muscular layer of the bladder; therefore, it is wrong to resect deeper. Deep resection is indicated only when one suspects carcinomatous infiltration (stage T_2; see Figs. 132, 135).

We apply two different techniques: first, the prograde cut; second, the retrograde cut:

(1) *The prograde cut* is performed — as in prostatic adenoma — mostly in the large, broad-based tumor. The cutting loop is inserted behind the mass of the tumor and then retracted distally under current (as in TUR of the prostatic bar; see Fig. 88). The window of the resectoscope sheath is kept as close as possible to the rim of the tumor so that the tissue may be cut with the loop and sheath as with scissors. This prevents semiresected, floating parts of the tumor from hanging at the rim of the resected mucosa. Resection of such remnants can be difficult; risk of perforation is increased (see Fig. 133).

The loop is extended only half way in order to keep the length of the uncontrolled cut as short as possible. During cutting one must not forget to follow the curve of the bladder wall. This is possible only if the entire resectoscope performs an arciform motion. In tumors of the lateral bladder wall, a technique similar to that used for TUR of the adenomatous lateral lobes is employed. We first resect the lower part of the tumor to mark the lower border of the wound in the mucosa. Then the main mass of the tumor is resected from above to below the level of the mucosa until the last remnant falls off (see Nesbit technique for the adenoma, Fig. 38).

The tumor of the posterior bladder wall is resected with a circular movement; like mowing grass. For this technique, special "tennis-racket" loops were developed. However, we use the regular loop (see Fig. 77). The return-flow resectoscope and a nearly empty bladder are helpful.

(2) *The retrograde cut* (see Figs. 78, 130) is more effective than the prograde but also more dangerous. It is always performed at the level of the mucosa in order to separate the tumor from the bladder wall at its base. It is not suitable for morcellation of the tumor layer by layer. This cut must be performed with the entire resectoscope, because it must follow the curvature of the bladder wall. When the course of the cut between tumor and bladder wall cannot be observed perfectly, the cut should be stopped after 0.5 to 1 cm (at the most) to avoid perforating the bladder wall. Only with increasing experience one should believe one's self capable of longer retrograde cuts. Tension of the bladder wall is especially important. The wall can evade the retrograde cut if the bladder is not filled tight (see Fig. 77).

TUR of the Infiltrated Bladder Wall

This procedure is similar to radical TUR of the prostatic capsule (see Fig. 50). Both the bladder wall and the capsule can be divided into three hypothetic layers. The inner layer consists of close-meshed muscle fibers that lie directly under the mucosa. Toward the periphery, these meshes become wider until perivesical connective tissue appears between the fibers (see Fig. 134). The danger of perforation is reduced when these layers are observed. An exception to this rule is a tumor that infiltrates the peritoneum. In this case there is no warning layer in the periphery of the bladder, and the peritoneum is cut without notice (see Fig. 96, c–e).

The TUR of ulcers (irradiation; tuberculous), the sample excision of infiltrates of unknown origin (bilharziasis; cancer in situ; edema; catheter ulcers; inflammation; etc.) or foreign bodies (nylon net immigrated into the bladder after suspension plasty; surgical

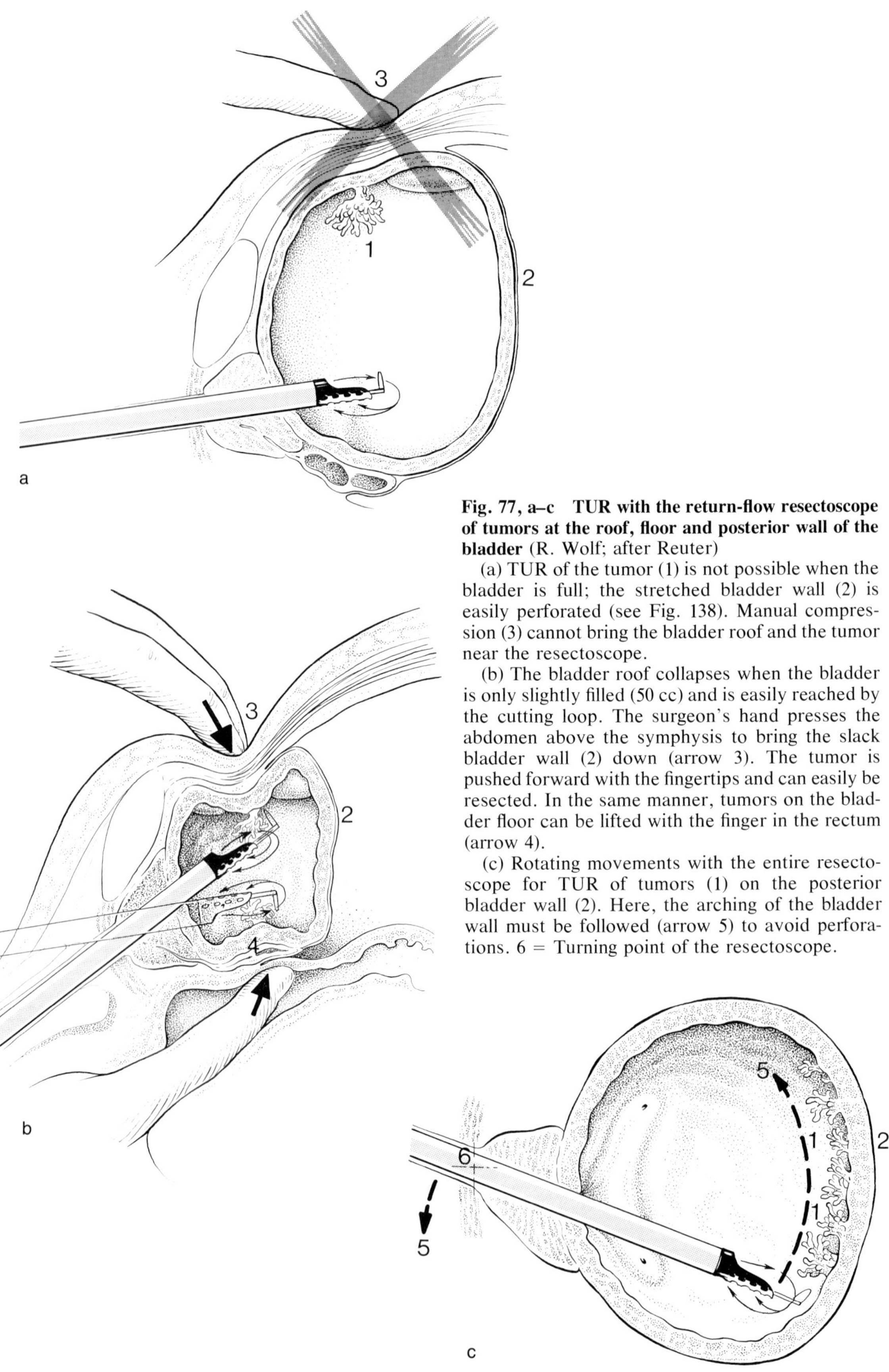

Fig. 77, a–c TUR with the return-flow resectoscope of tumors at the roof, floor and posterior wall of the bladder (R. Wolf; after Reuter)

(a) TUR of the tumor (1) is not possible when the bladder is full; the stretched bladder wall (2) is easily perforated (see Fig. 138). Manual compression (3) cannot bring the bladder roof and the tumor near the resectoscope.

(b) The bladder roof collapses when the bladder is only slightly filled (50 cc) and is easily reached by the cutting loop. The surgeon's hand presses the abdomen above the symphysis to bring the slack bladder wall (2) down (arrow 3). The tumor is pushed forward with the fingertips and can easily be resected. In the same manner, tumors on the bladder floor can be lifted with the finger in the rectum (arrow 4).

(c) Rotating movements with the entire resectoscope for TUR of tumors (1) on the posterior bladder wall (2). Here, the arching of the bladder wall must be followed (arrow 5) to avoid perforations. 6 = Turning point of the resectoscope.

Fig. 78, a–d Retrograde cutting for TUR of bladder tumors with the return-flow resectoscope (after Iglesias; see Fig. 130).

(a) Incorrect cutting guidance. The resectoscope (2) is brought to the base of the tumor (1) at the level of the mucosa with the loop retracted. The loop is then extended for the cut, but the sheath — incorrectly — remains stable. After 1 to 2 cm (arrow 3), the loop perforates the concave bladder wall.

(b) The correct cut is performed with an arched movement (arrow 4) of the entire resectoscope along the surface of the arched bladder wall (3).

(c) When the retrograde cut cannot be controlled by direct vision, the loop is first pushed retrograde, cutting 0.5 to 1 cm into the pedicle (1) of the tumor. Then the cut is stopped and the loop is guided behind the tumor (arrow 2) and cut as usual (d). 4 = Cutting direction of the loop; the sheath now remains immobile.

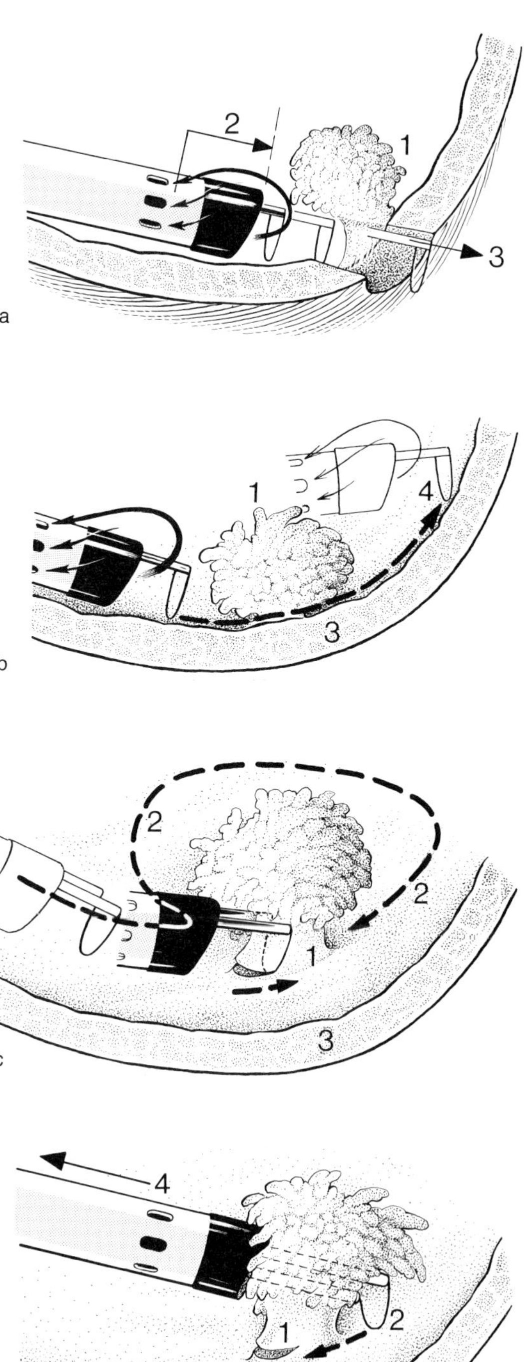

threads) should be treated following the same rules established for TUR of bladder tumors (see Fig. 127).

Postoperative Treatment

If the tumor was resected only to the level of the mucosa, a Foley catheter is not necessary. An exception to this occurs when the bladder is permanently irrigated with cytostatic drugs (not instilled). We follow this procedure in all large recurrent papillary tumors. Outpatients also are treated in this way at intervals of one to four weeks (see Fig. 139). Deeper defects of the muscular layer require urinary drainage by Foley catheter for periods of several days. Total TUR of the bladder wall and perforation into paravesical tissue require urinary drainage for one to two weeks (see Fig. 138).

A special method of postoperative treatment is the permanent intra-arterial infusion of cystostatic drugs — e.g., into the internal iliac artery (see Figs. 79, 140).

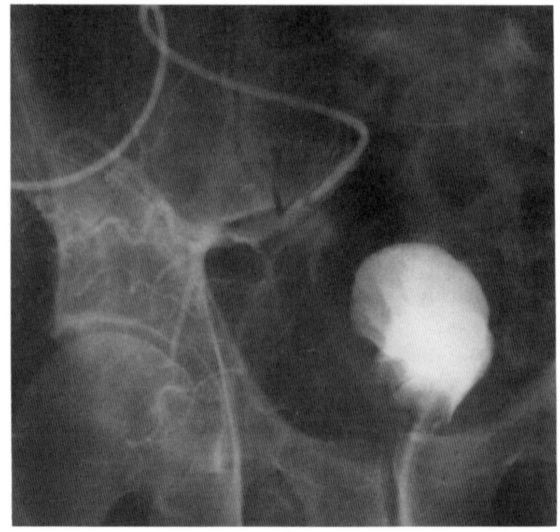

a

Fig. 79, a **Operative angiography** of the internal iliac artery with constant irrigation with cytostatic drugs over two weeks for the treatment of an inoperable bladder carcinoma.

This figure (film 18 × 24 cm) shows the bladder filled with contrast medium through the indwelling catheter; on the left, a tumorous defect is noted. Over the right iliac bone (left side of picture), a plastic tube introduced into the operatively ligated internal artery is seen. Angiography demonstrates the area of circulation of the internal iliac artery, including the external gluteal artery (for necroses on the buttocks, see Fig. 140).

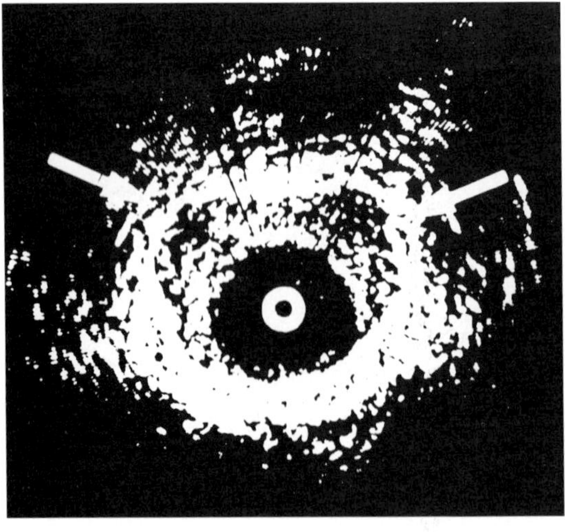

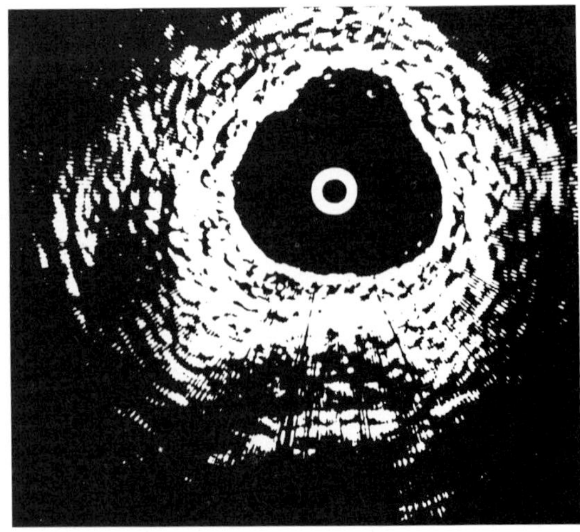

b

Fig. 79, b Transurethral ultrasonic scanning of TURP (Matouschek). Left transurethral scan shows remaining tissue of both lateral lobes (partial TUR) in the prostatic fossa. Right scan shows the result after TURP (no remaining tissue).

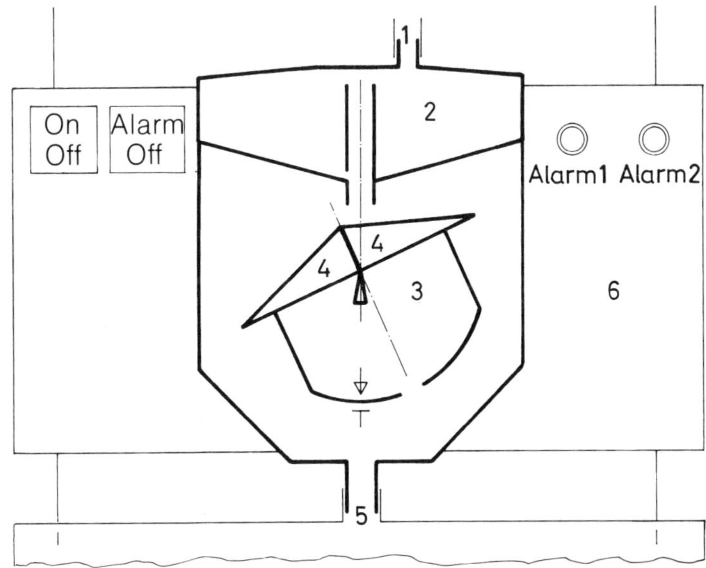

Fig. 80 Electronic catheter control unit (Uromat) (after Reuter; Technovita, Stuttgart, W. Germany).

Disposable measuring chamber with magnetic valve, constructed as disposable part. Its double chambered balance is used for indirect volumetric measurement of flow in a closed system with the aid of an infrared light switch. The wireless alarm sounds when urine flow stops and when the urinal is full.

This unit prevents acute postoperative pyelonephritis and urosepsis (with chills) frequently caused by an obstructed catheter and urinary retention. The Uromat measures 25 × 15 × 6 cm and weighs 2 kg with its batteries.

1 = Inflow; 2 = disposable balanced measuring chamber (3); 4 = urine chambers; 5 = drainage into the urinal; 6 = case with switches; suspension frame (bed).

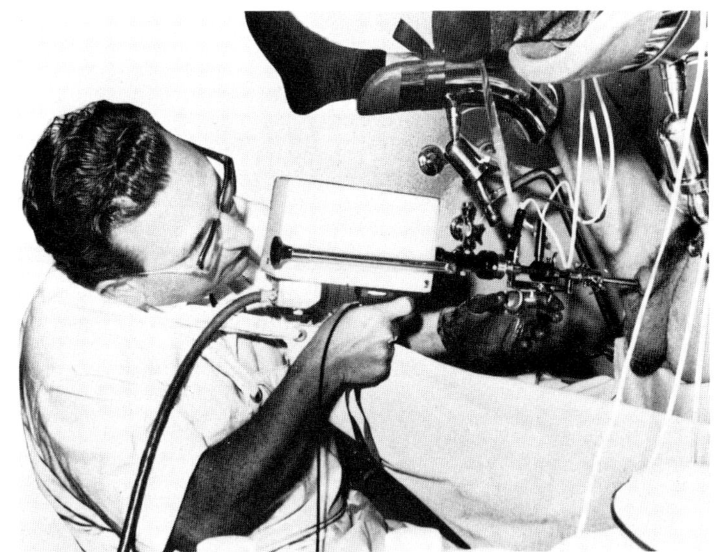

Fig. 81 Live television transmission during TUR (1964) in the Urologic Hospital Prof. Dr. Reuter in Stuttgart (Philips TV camera).

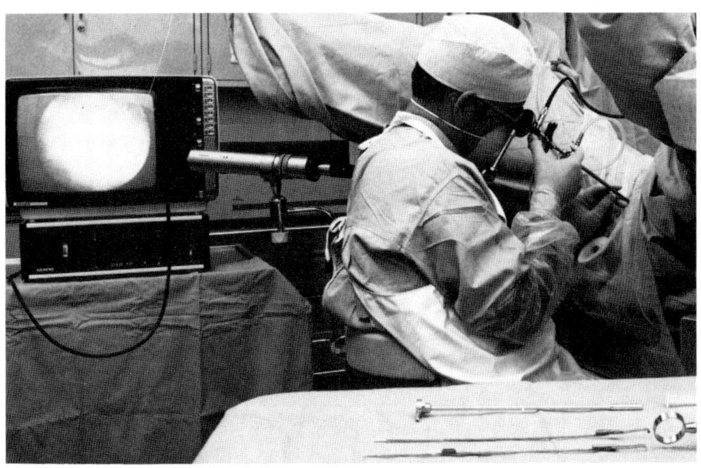

Fig. 82 Videorecording of TUR (1978) by Prof. Dr. Matuscheck in the Urologic Hospital of Karlsruhe through an articulated optical teaching attachment between the resectoscope and TV camera.

83 a–c

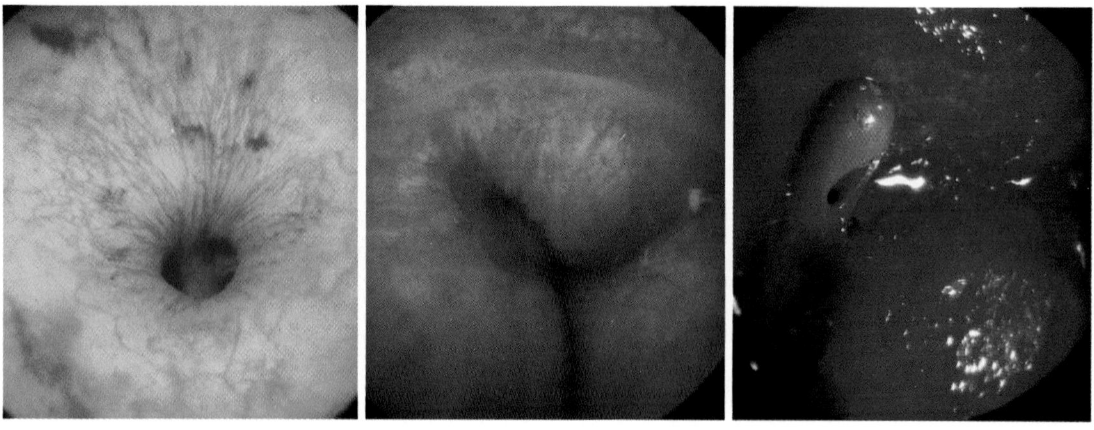

The Bladder Neck as Seen by Suprapubic Trocar Cystoscopy

Fig. 83, a Normal bladder neck of a young man (traumatic disruption of urethra)
The internal sphincter of the bladder is slightly opened; in the lower part of the short prostatic urethra, one can recognize the colliculus seminalis, from which a ridge connects the urethra with the bladder. This can be seen in the path of the vessels, which continue into the trigone with a few inflamed infiltrates. The bladder wall can be seen on the lower circumference of the picture. On the upper part the bladder floor; the interureteral ridge and the ureteral orifices are not visible.

The scar after traumatic urethral disruption is continuously dilated up to 16 Fr. No further stricture was observed over the following 13 years.

Fig. 83, b Prostatic adenoma (see Fig. 107, a)
The adenoma has pushed away the bladder neck and overextended the internal sphincter. It has stretched the prostatic urethra lengthwise and has compressed the lumen. The Y-shaped figure of the internal orifice of the urethra is made up of the three lobes of the adenoma. The median lobe of the adenoma pushes the entire trigone up so that it touches the interureteral ridge. Owing to the compression, the vessels of the mucosa are congested. This picture demonstrates an important phenomenon in TUR. The lateral lobes of the adenoma join in a fold in the urethra at "12 o'clock" (lower margin of the picture) and continue up to the distal end of the adenoma of the external sphincter. It "replaces," so-to-say, the absent colliculus seminalis at 12 o'clock.

Fig. 83, c Giant prostatic adenoma of 180 gm seen before suprapubic prostatectomy.
The mucosa exhibits light reflections caused by the flash camera. The opened and collapsed bladder shows that the veins of the mucosa, which normally are congested, have lost this pattern and have become darker. – The water-filled bladder is under physiologic pressure; therefore, the pattern and color appear more normal. It is now possible to resect these giant adenomas because low pressure irrigation with permanent irrigation used in combination with the new, unusually efficient resectoscope (after Hösel) presents a considerably lower operative risk (0.3 per cent) than does open surgery (3.3 per cent; see Table 8, p. 235).

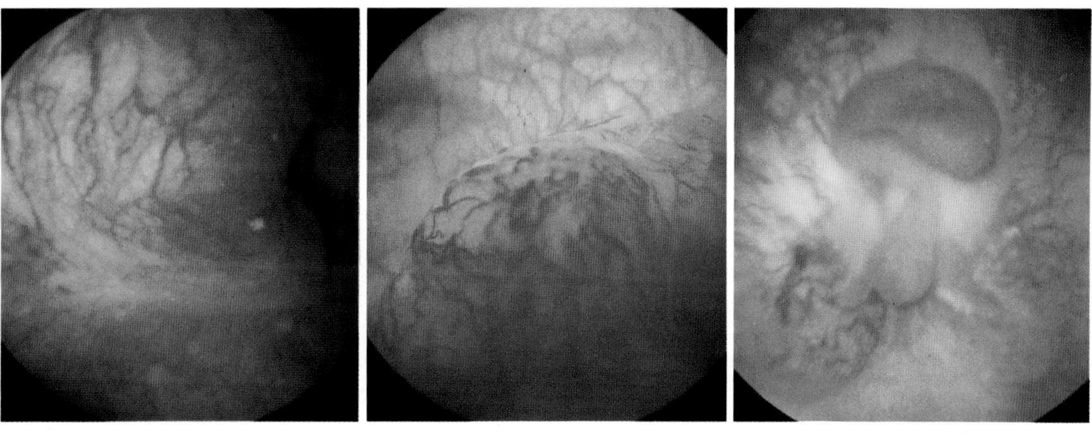

83 d–f

Fig. 83, d Typical right lateral lobe.
The adenoma (see Fig. 83, b) has raised and stretched the mucosa. The blood vessels are congested and bleed easily. Above the interureteric ridge are infiltrates that exhibit inflammation, purulent flakes and granular areas. The lateral lobe continues into the median lobe above at the right. The right ureteral orifice (on the left margin of the picture) and the interureteric ridge are raised from the border of the adenoma (Fig. 107).

Fig. 83, e Prostatic adenoma with carcinomatous infiltration of the lateral lobe (Stage $T_3N_xM_xG_2$).
The cancerous nodule appears as a ball at the left lateral lobe. The blood vessels of the mucosa are deformed and congested. The adenocarcinoma shines white through the mucosa. In the background, the normal bladder wall may be seen (upper part of picture). The left ureteral orifice is hidden by the tumor (see Fig. 133). Subradical TUR (50 gm net). The patient died three years later.

Fig. 83, f Bladder neck with prostatic abscess; bladder neck stricture; prostatic adenoma.
Through the trocar cystoscope one can see that the color of the bladder neck mucosa has changed following medication. The vessels are congested and surround the urethra radially. Pressure from the rectum causes purulent matter to empty from the opening of the urethra into the bladder. This wide angle photograph was taken from a distance and shows almost the entire lower bladder; however, the ostiae and the interureteral ridge are somewhat obscured (see Fig. 122, b). Total cryoprostatectomy with excellent result (see Fig. 167, c).

Urethrocystoscopy of the Prostatic Urethra at the Beginning of TURP

Fig. 84, a Sphincter sclerosis.
The prostatic bar is seen crosswise at the lower margin of the picture. Above the posterior wall of the bladder, trabeculation due to muscle hypertrophy can be seen. The hemorrhagic infiltrates are the result of previous catheterization for acute urinary retention.

Fig. 84, b Prostatic adenoma with urate calculus.
Urethrocystoscopy prior to TUR of the prostate (50 gm net in 55 min with litholapaxy-Bigelow) shows a bar-shaped median lobe above which a lemon-colored calculus is partly obscured by the prostate. The bladder wall can be seen to the left of the calculus; there is slight injection of the mucosa. Hyperuricemia is present. (See Fig. 126; postoperative stricture, see Fig. 122, a, b).

Fig. 84, c Prostatic adenoma with spherical median lobe, trabeculated bladder and chronic cystitis.
On the lower edge of the picture only a small part of the median lobe can be seen. The bladder wall shows trabeculation, and the bladder mucosa demonstrates chronic cystitis. On the bladder floor, several stone remnants are shown. Both ureteral orifices are obscured by the median lobe of the prostate. TURP: 55 gm net in 45 min.

Fig. 84, d Ball-shaped lateral lobe of a prostatic adenoma.
Urethrocystoscopy performed before TURP (45 gm net in 35 min) shows the bladder neck and the intravesical part of the lateral lobe as a ball. Unlike the bladder in previous illustrations, the bladder here is almost empty. Therefore, it appears collapsed. Its wall shows large trabeculations; its mucosa is folded because of the aspiration of bladder irrigation fluid. Since low pressure irrigation (see p. 25) TUR is performed on an almost empty bladder, the volume is only about 20 cc.

Fig. 84, e Ball-shaped lateral lobe.
Urethrocystoscopy was performed in a water-filled bladder before TUR was begun (unlike Fig. 84, d). The posterior wall of the bladder is tense because of the pressure of the bladder irrigant; it shows typical hypertrophic trabeculation. The tension of the tissue in the bladder wall and the fossa caused by high pressure irrigation (see p. 24) increases the danger of perforation because the bladder wall and the prostatic capsule cannot escape a deep cut.

Fig. 84, f Bladder neck with giant prostatic adenoma, collapsed bladder dome and suprapubic trocar needle.
The small median lobe of the adenoma lies in front of the lateral lobes, both of which rise laterally. In the upper part of the picture, the tip of the trocar needle used for suprapubic aspiration of irrigant can be seen. The bladder is filled maximally with 30 cc of irrigant; therefore, the bladder dome is not sufficiently extended, and mucosa is aspirated through the small opening in the trocar needle. The aspiration is made easier if the needle is lowered closer to the bladder floor. Suprapubic aspiration offers so many advantages that we no longer think of TUR without low pressure irrigation (see p. 29). TURP: 190 gm net in 80 min.; 87-year-old poor-risk patient. Blood transfusion: 450 cc.

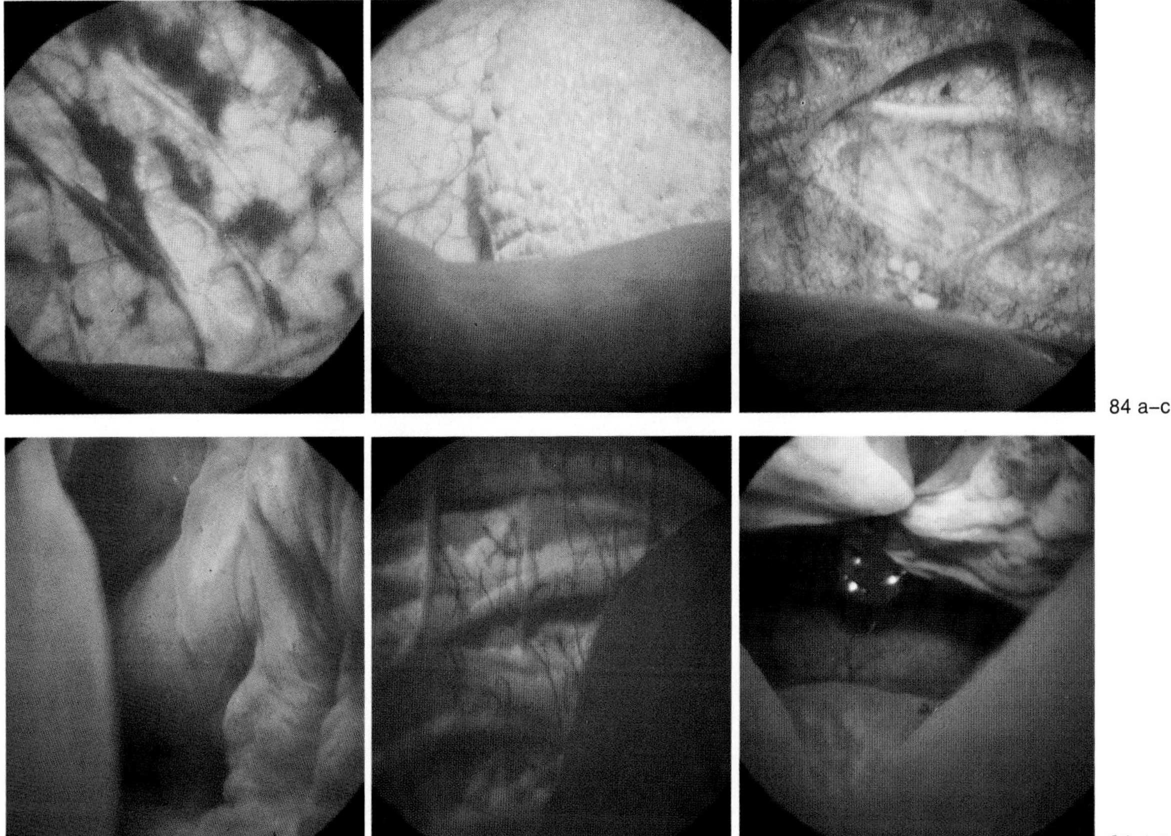

84 a–c

84 d–f

85 a–b

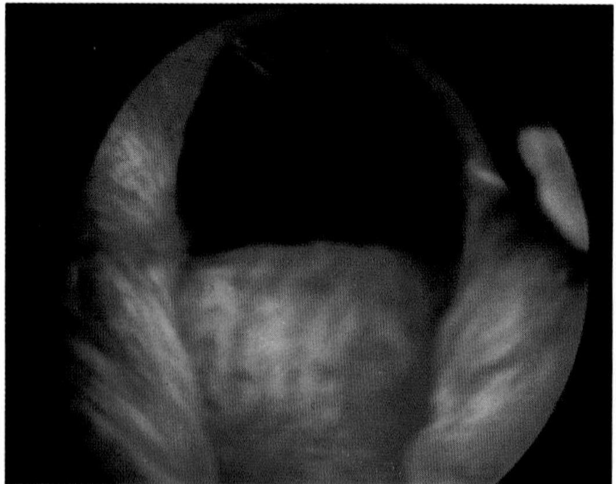

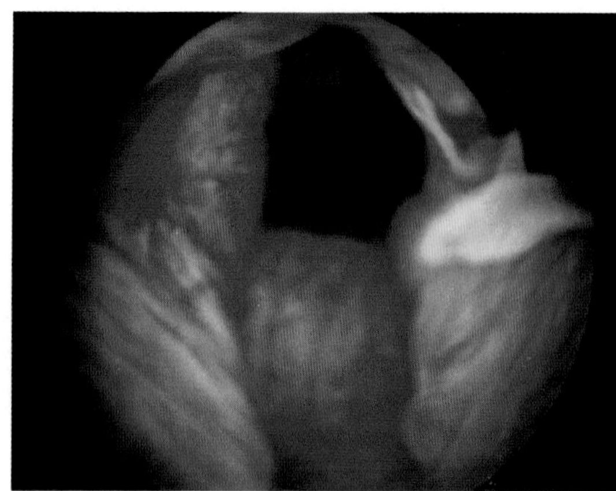

Urethroscopy of the Prostatic Urethra with Resectoscope

before TURP (50 gm net in 60 min) combined with blind litholapaxy of two bladder calculi 4.5 cm in diameter; peridural anesthesia.

Litholapaxy today is performed with suprapubic trocarcystoscopy in air (see Fig. 126).

Fig. 85, a The internal sphincter and the proximal third of the prostatic urethra, which is close to the bladder.
The median lobe protrudes into the bladder. It fills the lower part of the urethra and blocks off half the lumen. The irrigation stream (high pressure irrigation) keeps the urethra open by pressing the lateral lobes outward. The vessels of the mucosa are somewhat congested.

Fig. 85, b The middle part of the prostatic urethra.
The lateral lobes narrow the prostatic bed of the urethra into an oval longitudinal gap. The mucosa of the lateral wall of the urethra is slightly injured by the resectoscope, showing some hemorrhagic changes and some fibrous coating.

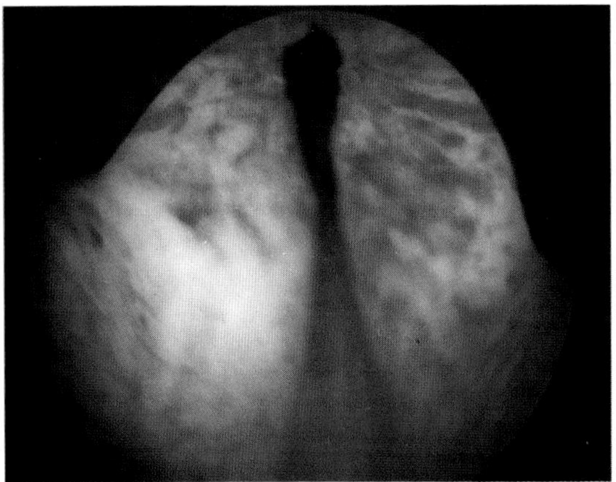

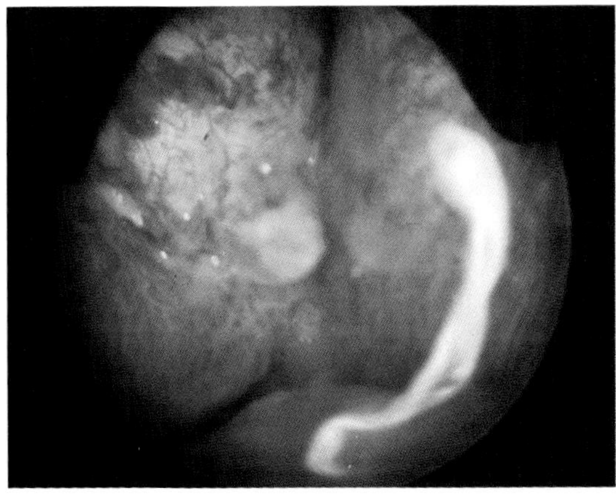

85 c–d

Fig. 85, c Distal prostatic urethra.
The lateral lobes almost touch each other, forming a typical fold at 12 o'clock. In the upper third, one can see the irrigation stream finding its way into the bladder. The mucosa shows congestion of some horizontal vessels due to hemorrhagic inflammation.

Fig. 85, d Distal prostatic urethra with external sphincter.
The lateral lobes have completely occluded the lumen of the urethra. Even with high pressure, the irrigating stream can no longer press them apart. Therefore, we first resect an irrigating channel into the median lobe down to the colliculus seminalis (see Fig. 91, f). The colliculus seminalis lies distally between the lateral lobes. The mucosa reveals inflammatory hemorrhagic alterations with individual small granules. A long fibrin flake is seen in the irrigant in front of the lateral lobes.

86 a–c 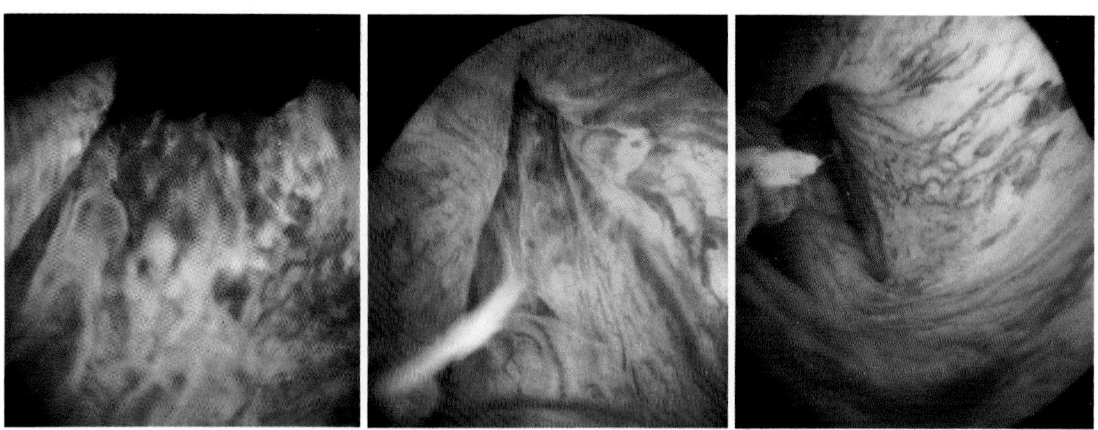

Prostatic Urethra with Internal and External Sphincter. Urethroscopy with resectoscope of a small, soft, glandular adenoma with prostatitis.

Fig. 86, a Bladder neck.
The median lobe of the adenoma is only vaguely visible. The right lateral lobe extends as a marked fold. Two typical ridges stretch horizontally from the median lobe to the hidden colliculus seminalis. The mucosa of the prostatic urethra shows edematous inflammatory changes and hemorrhagic infiltration.

Fig. 86, b Distal prostatic urethra.
At the left, next to the colliculus seminalis, a small part of the right lateral lobe can be seen. Along the urethra this lobe is covered with vessels that show inflammatory reaction. The partially visible internal orifice of the urethra is located in the upper margin of the picture, where the two lateral lobes also converge (see Fig. 85, c). At the right margin of the picture, a fibrin flake can be seen.

Fig. 86, c External sphincter of the prostatic urethra with transition from the posterior to the middle urethra.
At the right margin of the picture, the beginning of the external sphincter can be recognized at 4 o'clock. Its muscle folds in the urogenital diaphragm extend in part as a fan shape to the colliculus seminalis, and partly as a semicircle up to the fibrin flake, which is visible in Figure 86, b. The border between the prostatic and median urethra is sharply defined.

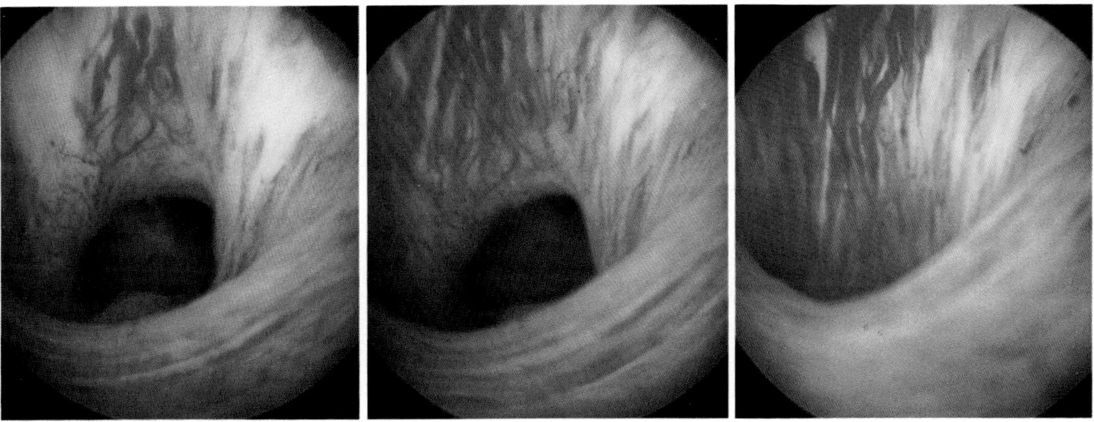

86 d–f

Figs. 86, d–f Urethroscopy of the middle urethra with the external sphincter during TURP (100 gm net in 65 min).

Fig. 86, d Contraction of the external sphincter.
The urethroscopy shows the lower half of the median urethra, which is actually lifted up by the elastic muscle of the external sphincter. The upper half of the urethra remains inactive. The top of the colliculus seminalis can be vaguely seen above the center of the sphincter ridge. The floor of the prostatic urethra and, on its upper margin, the almost closed internal orifice of the bladder can be imagined at the back of the lumen. The lateral lobes disappear behind the external sphincter. The dome of the urethra begins contracting because the horizontal vessels of the mucosa are being pressed together.

Fig. 86, e The resectoscope has been withdrawn 2 cm distally into the median urethra. The irrigating fluid has kept the lumen open, but the contraction of the external sphincter has increased. The shape of the muscle fibers lying under the mucosa can be seen as a traverse fold. The upper circumference of the urethra keeps forming longitudinal folds; the vessels go in the same direction.

Fig. 86, f The resectoscope has been withdrawn farther into the middle urethra. The swell of the external sphincter lifts the tip of the endoscope, and the cystoscopist feels a sudden jerk. The floor of the median urethra is somewhat blurred (lower part of the picture). The external sphincter confines the scope toward the prostatic urethra. The vessels on the upper part of the urethra have moved together even more closely. In this area of the urethral anatomy, there is a bend; therefore it is necessary to use the obturator to facilitate the reinsertion of the sheath into the bladder. (This is a site of predilection for traumatic strictures.)

87 a–c

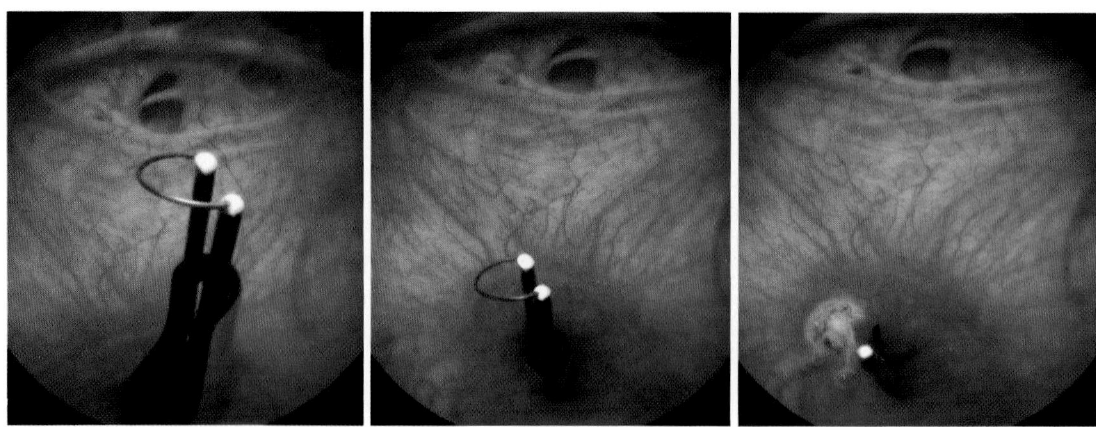

Trocar Cystoscopy in TURP (20 gm net). Bladder neck stricture together with sphincter sclerosis and prostatic adenoma.

Fig. 87, a Bladder neck with resectoscope.
Suprapubic trocar cystoscopy shows a small subvesical adenoma about 1 cm in diameter that displaces the internal sphincter. This is seen clearly as a dark red ring, approximately 5 mm in radius, surrounding the internal orifice of the urethra. Above the orifices the typical vessel pattern of the trigone is visible. The left orifice is closed; the right is dot-shaped. Behind the interureteric ridge there are transverse muscle trabeculae with pseudodiverticula. A 28 Fr resectoscope sheath has been passed, and the overlarge loop protrudes beyond the beak. Resectoscopes with sheaths of 21 to 26 Fr allow passage of only considerably smaller cutting loops, thus lowering the efficiency of TUR. One gram of tissue is resected with 24 Fr by ten cuts; but only four cuts are needed with 28 Fr. The prostatic capsule is particularly sensitive to electric current and reacts to it by shrinking, leading to stricture of the bladder neck and prostatic fossa. In our experience the dilatation of the urethra by the 28 Fr resectoscope plays no important role in the formation of strictures so long as a corticoid lubricant is applied for easy passage of the scope (lubricant with addition of cortisone or povidone-iodine).

TUR was performed in a 77-year-old patient (20 gm net in 25 min) under epidural anesthesia. Histology: 1. Adenoma rich in glandular structures; 2. prostatic tissue deficient in glands; 3, chronic interstitial inflammation.

Two weeks previously, the resectoscope was perforated into the paravesical space (see Fig. 36); about 1 L of isotonic irrigant (5 per cent glucose) was absorbed at that time (high pressure irrigation). A suprapubic bladder stab-fistula was made for urinary drainage.

Fig. 87, b The cutting loop as it begins the first cut of the bladder neck.
The resectoscope is being withdrawn into the prostatic urethra. The loop automatically hooks into the median lobe or the margin of the trigone (see Fig. 87, c). In the urethroscopic view, the loop disappears completely, and the first cut on the bladder neck usually is done blindly (see Fig. 88). If this procedure can be watched, the result is a short superficial cut of 1 to 2 cm, which is typical of a beginner's technique (see p. 50).

Fig. 87, c First cut.
The bladder floor has been photographed from a distance (bird's eye view from about 10 cm). The semicircular slough of the first cut can be seen in the mucosa of the bladder neck at 7 to 8 o'clock; the cutting loop already has disappeared. The first cut is made slowly without interruption from the bladder neck toward the verumontanum; thus faulty cutting of the adenoma margin of the bladder neck is avoided.

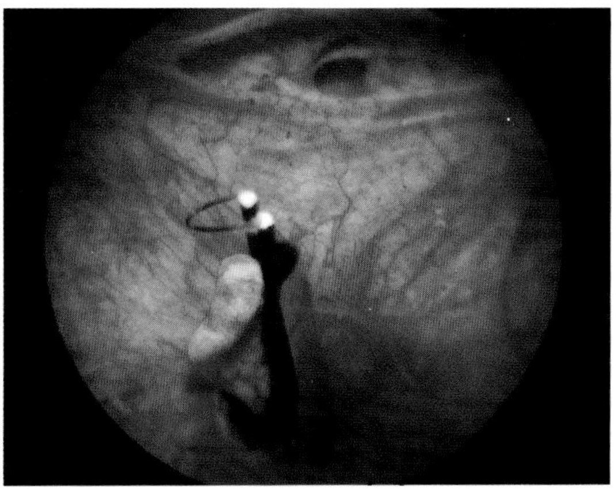
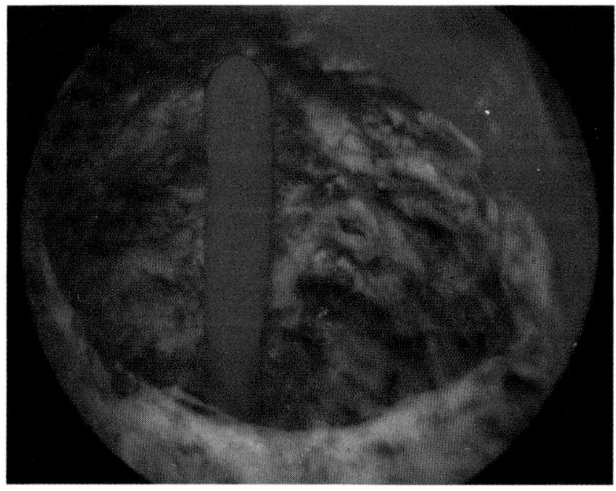
87 d–e

Therefore, it is important to control the position of the resectoscope sheath of the verumontanum. The resectoscope is held horizontally or parallel to the longitudinal axis of the patient's body. Any deviation from this position may result in faulty cuts (Fig. 88, a). In each case we control the course of the cut with the finger in the rectum. A rectal shield and a special apron to collect irrigant assure asepsis and keep the operating room clean and dry. Low pressure irrigation simplifies these problems (see p. 25) because, thanks to permanent aspiration, the irrigant need not be collected further.

Fig. 87, d Ejecting the first tissue chip.
The beak of the resectoscope protrudes from the prostatic urethra. The first tissue piece has been caught in the cutting loop. The resectoscope is pushed into the bladder; at the same time, the loop is fully extended so that the thick tissue piece can be carried by the irrigating fluid into the bladder. Following this, the cut fossa is checked and, if necessary, bleeding vessels are coagulated. The ring muscle fibers of the internal sphincter often can be seen in the margin of the trigone. These muscles no longer belong to the prostatic capsule but stem from the bladder wall. To protect the internal sphincter, the cutting loop is now positioned for the next cut 1 to 2 cm distal in the prostatic urethra or fossa (see Fig. 91).

Fig. 87, e Bladder neck with prostatic fossa.
One week after TURP the bladder neck is completely resected and the prostatic fossa has a diameter of more than 5 cm. It is shaped like a regular semi-round cavity. Its wall consists primarily of circularly structured prostatic capsule fibers covered with thin necrotic tissue. There is a 20 Fr rubber catheter in the fossa. The mucosa is cut off exactly on the bladder floor; below, a slight over-resection in the anterior bladder wall is noted.

The size of the fossa after TURP depends on two factors:

1. The kind of irrigation and/or the irrigation pressure.
2. The compression of the fossa postoperatively with the balloon catheter used.

In high pressure irrigation (ca. 100 cm H_2O = ca. 10 k Pa), the dynamic pressure of the irrigating stream dilates the elastic fossa during TUR and infiltrates the tissue with irrigant. In addition, the compression catheter with its 30- to 50-cc balloon prevents the desired active contraction of the fossa and its vessels. Therefore, principally for these reasons, we use only physiologic low pressure irrigation and a 5-cc balloon catheter, 20 Fr, with an irrigant canal (closed system with three-way-catheter for permanent irrigation; see p. 59).

88 a–c
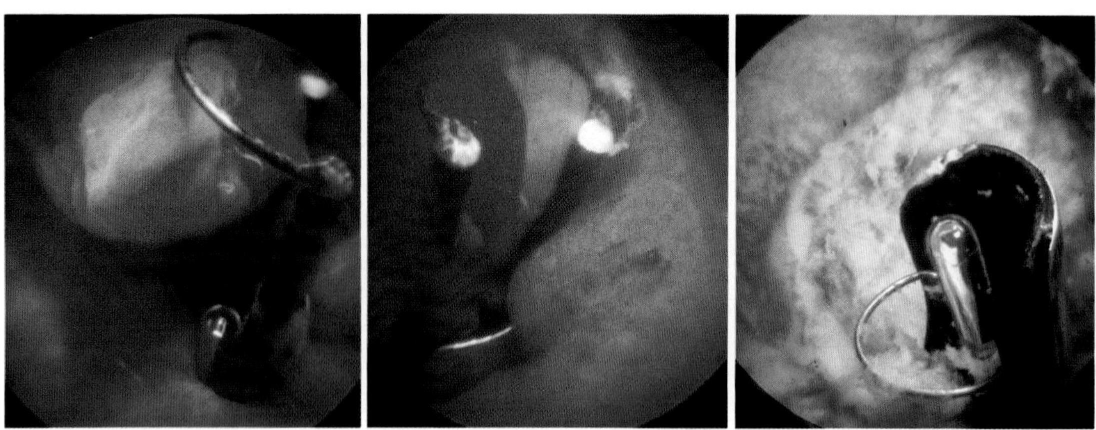

TURP of a Medium-sized Recurrent Adenoma 6 cm Long and 40 gm. Net Weight After Suprapubic Prostatectomy. Trocar Cystoscopy.

Fig. 88, a Incorrect initial position of the cutting loop.
For the first cut, the loop is placed sideways on the overlapping median lobe. The next cut is more difficult because a moving piece of tissue has formed that interferes with the cutting loop. The cutting loop is completely extended. The eyepiece of the optical system has disappeared in the prostatic fossa; i.e., the loop is placed blindly in the correct position on the bladder neck. Still visible is the top of the electric bulb, which is seen on the left next to the insulated wire of the cutting loop. The resectoscope sheath is bent sideways; therefore, the cutting loop is not in the correct position. The sheath always should be held along the horizontal axis of the body (Fig. 41).

Fig. 88, b Corrected position of the cutting loop.
In trocar cystoscopy, the sheath of the resectoscope lies along the horizontal axis of the body. The loop is now positioned at the center of the median lobe. The metal margin of the beak of the resectoscope can be vaguely seen in the orifice of the urethra. The position of the loop explains why the cutting process cannot be observed if the loop is fully extended. If we make a film of the TUR procedure, and if we want a clear picture, we must not press the loop completely into the tissue.

This technique is basically incorrect, but it does enable us to demonstrate the cut through the tissue on film. In actual practice, we cut blindly (as already mentioned); in addition, we press the tissue toward the loop with the finger in the rectum while simultaneously covering the eyepiece of the optical system.

Fig. 88, c Partial TUR.
The resection loop is extended only half way; therefore, the effective motion of the cutting loop has been shortened considerably. The loop starts at the bladder neck and resects only the first third of the prostatic fossa. A funnel develops in the adenoma; its base is on the bladder neck and its top is in the middle of the prostatic urethra (see Fig. 4).

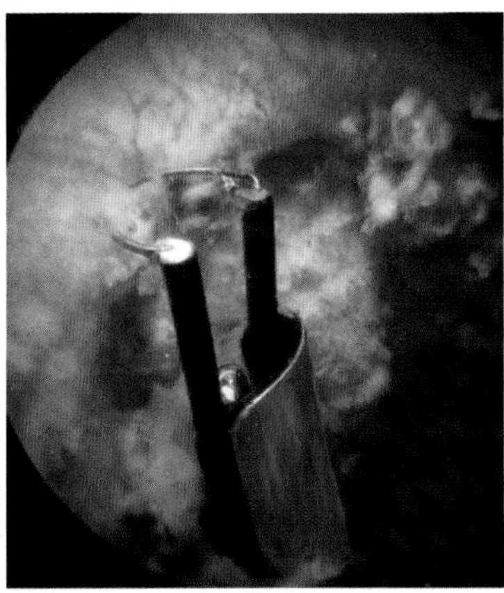
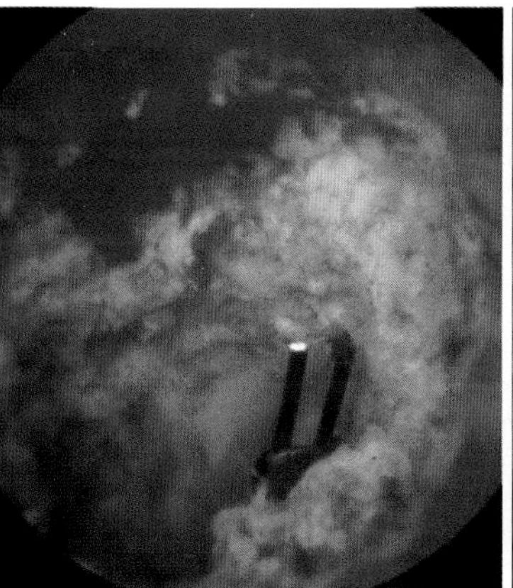
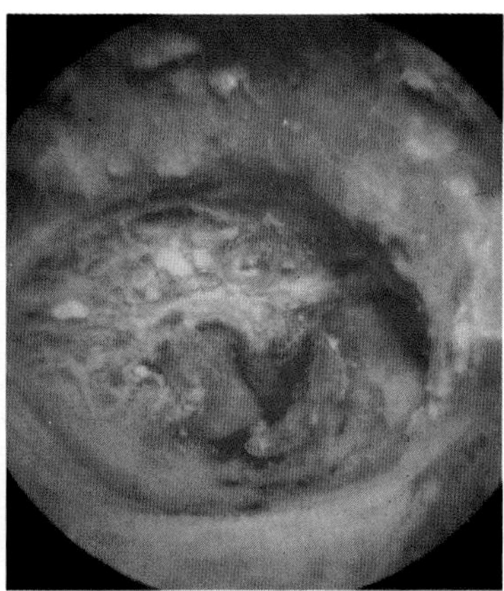

88 d–f

Fig. 88, d Incorrect position of the cutting loop on the bladder neck.
Trocar cystoscopy shows an irregular cut and rough adenomatous tissue covered with necrosis — due to overly rapid cutting. Placing the cutting loop at the mucosa of the insufficiently resected bladder neck has resulted in unnecessary over-resection of the bladder wall (Fig. 97, b), and the loop is now lost in healthy tissue. In this case the bladder wall, internal sphincter and ureteral ridge were resected by mistake. In an extreme case, the ureteral orifice also can be resected. To avoid over-resection in TUR, it is important to keep the cutting loop fully extended out of the resectoscope sheath and to hold the resectoscope horizontally. It is incorrect to position the resectoscope on the bladder neck at a sharp angle to the axis of the body. Owing to the pressure on the adenoma lying underneath, the bladder neck arches out, thus producing an over-resection. This position is correct only in the distal fossa in order to resect tissue remaining at the apex. An additional advantage is that one can use the finger in the rectum. If possible, the resectoscope should be placed near the verumontanum to obtain the full benefit of the loop (see Fig. 13).

Fig. 88, e Correction of a partial TUR during a second session.
Trocar cystoscopy shows the prostatic fossa as a large funnel in the bladder neck. The fossa extends too far into the bladder wall (over-resection). This surgical error frequently leads to pathologic scar formation and stricture of the bladder neck (see Figs. 120–122). The fully extended loop cuts the adenomatous tissue blindly 2 cm off the edge of the bladder neck, thereby enlarging the funnel (Fig. 88, c). In blind cutting only the position of the resectoscope in its relation to the verumontanum can be controlled. It should be horizontal to the body axis. To judge the enlargement of the funnel, the size of the already resected fossa can be compared with the diameter of the loop (8 mm).

On the right margin of the picture, an over-resected area can be seen on a large border of the wound on the bladder floor. In the deep fossa some convex protruding adenomatous remnants are still present. We should point out again that the prostatic capsule (true prostatic tissue) is always concave, whereas adenomatous remnants protrude in a convex fashion. Consequently, all convex tissue portions in the prostatic capsule can be resected as long as the capsule has not been perforated (see Figs. 91, a; 95, b, e).

Fig. 88, f Complete view of the prostatic fossa as a result of TURP (40 gm in two sessions).
Trocar cystoscopy shows a round, regular semi-spherical cavity in the prostatic area of the bladder neck. After 10 days, almost all of the necrosis has been shed from the wound. The wall of the prostatic fossa therefore is smooth, and only in the deepest portions (to the right of the ureteral orifices) can the fibrous structure of the capsule be recognized. The fossa has already shrunk considerably and is divided into two layers:

(a) The first flat resection funnel (compare Fig. 88, c) with over-resection toward the trigone (upper margin of picture), which is still covered with a small amount of necrosis.

(b) The corrected floor of the fossa in the distal part of the apex, which was not resected until the second session of TUR.

In the center, the cut lumen of the urethra can be seen. The verumontanum divides the lumen into a V-shaped gap. On the right, the wall of the urethra slightly overlaps the fossa (note pieces of mucosa to the left of the center of the picture). No more adenomatous tissue can be seen, the prostate having been fully resected. It is easy to understand that the x-ray of a fully resected fossa always shows a typical round shape (Fig. 6). The contour of the semi-spherical lobe extends to the center of the symphysis; thus, the quality of the TURP can be controlled at any time by viewing the x-ray film.

TURP of a Giant Adenoma After Palliative Partial Cryoprostatectomy, Second Session (TURP: 65 gm in 40 min)

Three months previously, total trocar cryosurgery of a bladder tumor (angiomyofibroma 4 cm in diameter) and partial cryoprostatectomy of a 6 cm long adenoma were performed. *Indication:* A 73-year-old high-risk patient with renal insufficiency. TURP was performed when renal function had been restored. Postoperatively the patient was incontinent for a short time while sludge impaired the external sphincter. Two months later the patient was symptom-free. At age 77, all urologic findings were normal.

Fig. 89, a Placing the loop for TUR.
An adenomatous nodule of the left lobe remains after cryosurgery. This nodule is covered with a yellowed, scarred mucosa. In the background, the underexposed posterior wall of the water-filled bladder is visible.

In Figure 89, c the right wall of the prostatic bed can be seen: it is concave, which means that the larger part of the adenoma was shed after freezing. The cutting loop was completely extended from the sheath and then positioned at the center of the left lobe. Its wire is no longer visible. Therefore, the surgeon must adjust the window of the resectoscope correctly at the verumontanum. The novice finds it difficult to fix the resectoscope because when he places the loop prior to cutting he moves it in an uncontrolled fashion. He should remember the rule: "control-knob at the apex." The cutting process itself can only be controlled by palpation from the rectum.

Fig. 89, b Incorrect starting position of the cutting loop.
The picture shows an epithelialized channel in the lower half of the prostatic urethra after partial cryoprostatectomy. The scarred, infected mucosa shows edema and spreads irregularly across the remaining adenomatous tissue. The cutting loop is placed only superficially. Therefore, only the mucosa is injured. Only when the loop is deeply hooked behind the nodule or bar does it cut with full capacity. A retrograde cut through this remaining adenomatous tissue is possible but dangerous.

Fig. 89, c Correction of the starting position of the cutting loop.
The sheath window of the resectoscope is adjusted above the verumontanum. Both the control knob on the sheath and rectal palpation of the apex may help one to place the loop in the correct position. Next, the handle of the resectoscope is lowered and the loop is fully extended toward the bladder. The loop is turned slightly to the left because the middle lobe of the adenoma is not visible. Then the loop is placed behind the lateral lobe (see Figs. 89, a, d). In the background, the tip of the suprapubic trocar used for low pressure irrigation is visible. The trocar aspirates the irrigant directly in front of the prostatic bed so that the bladder volume never exceeds 20 to 50 cc. The water pressure in the fossa is lower than the venous pressure, thus avoiding all the problems of the TUR water syndrome.

Fig. 89, d Insertion of the cutting loop at the bladder neck.
An air bubble above reflects the picture of the mucosa, thus simulating overhanging tissue. The floor of the fossa is divided by a longitudinal fold into the remaining right and left lateral lobes. The cutting loop is set onto the trigone and hooked at the rim of the adenoma. Then it is turned to the right to achieve optimal utilization of its capacity. The cutting motion is controlled by the finger in the rectum. The cut ends directly at the verumontanum. The air bubble disappears when the sheath is turned.

Fig. 90 Prostatic fossa in TURP (85 gm in 45 min).
The first cut exposes the circular muscle fibers of the internal sphincter on the bladder neck and the pink-colored superficial capsule. The resected tissue piece is covered with mucosa. It drops backward into the bladder when the loop is again extended. The boundary between the internal sphincter and the prostatic capsule can be recognized as a gap. The deeper the cut, the more different the tissue appears, making the difference between the ring muscle and the capsule more distinct. Finally, the bladder wall separates from the prostatic capsule, and a gap develops as a first step to perforation (see Fig. 93, a–d).

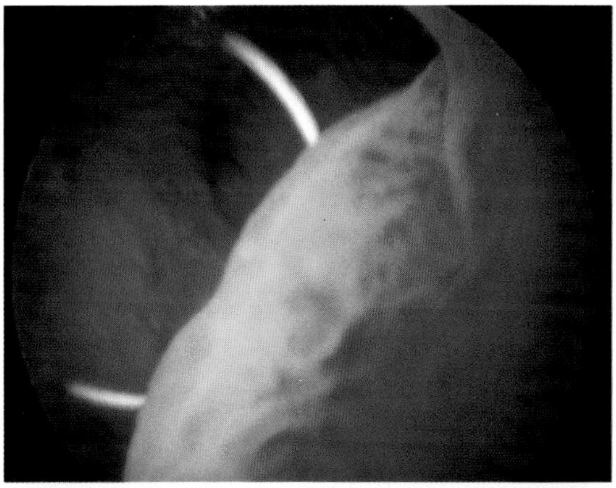

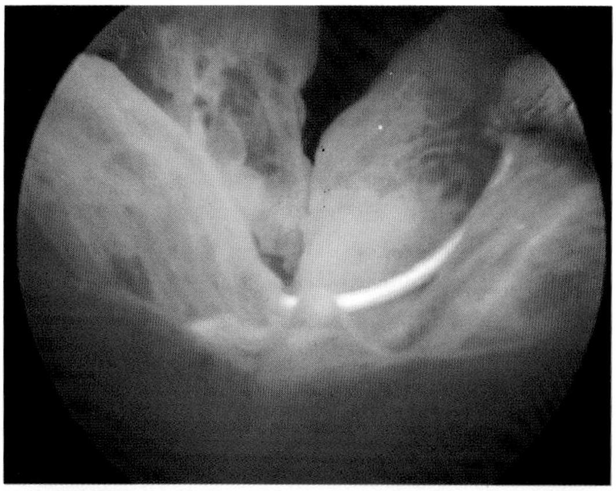

89 a–b

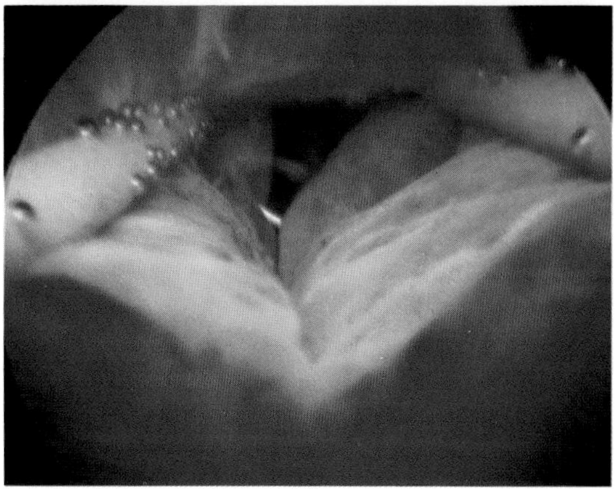

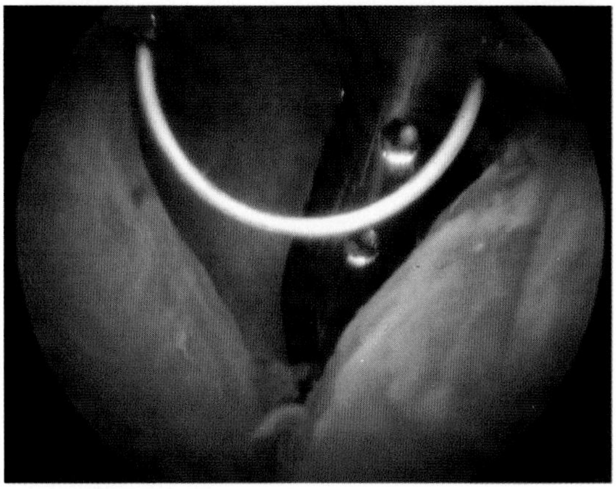

89 c–d

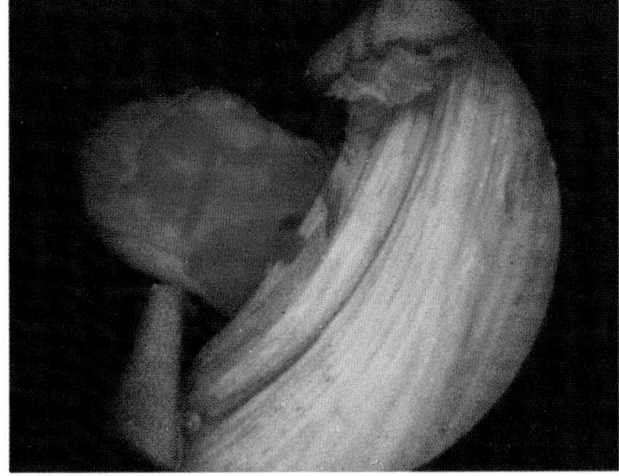

90

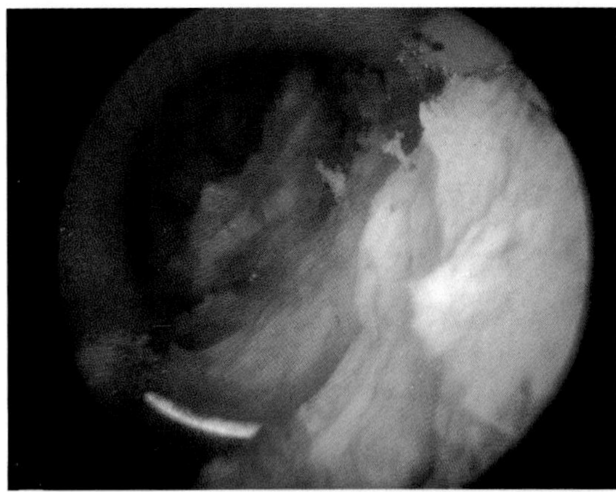
91 a

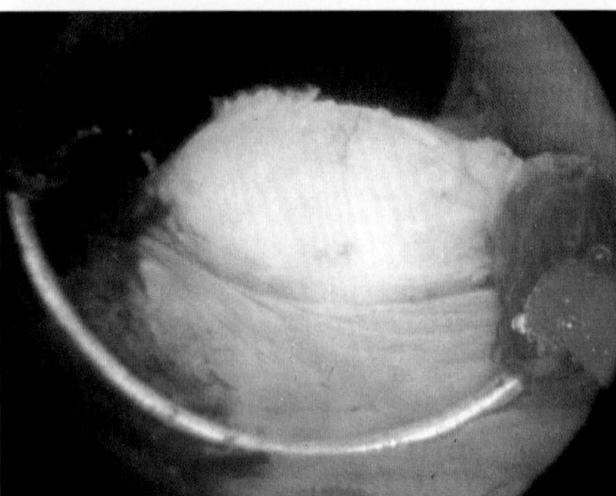
91 b

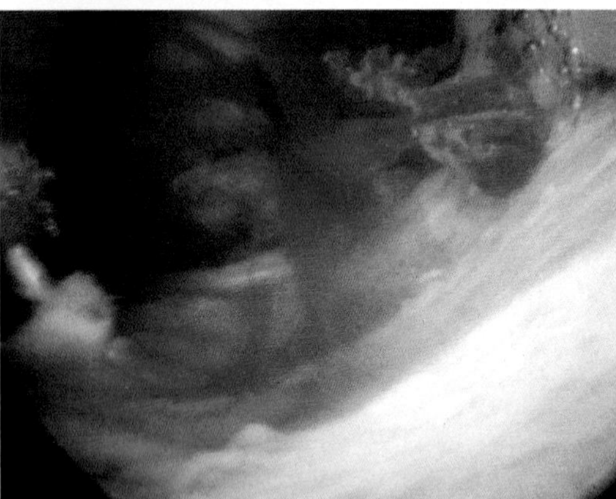
91 c

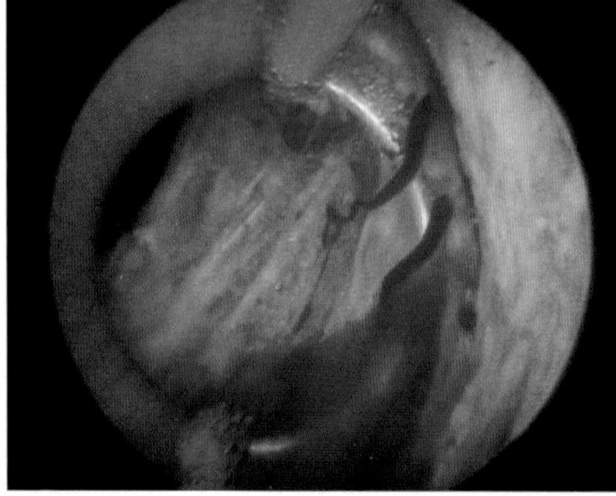
91 d

Prostatic Capsule During TURP

Cryosurgery and TUR in one session. In this 75-year-old patient, the adenoma first was frozen for 3 minutes and then resected immediately afterward (25 gm net in 20 min). A late complication was the shedding of deep cryonecroses after seven weeks. At 82 years, the patient was well and symptom-free. Cryosurgery before TUR (first tested in 1967 by me) subsequently was given up, because continuous low pressure irrigation proved superior.

Fig. 91, a Prostatic fossa with tissue of capsule and adenoma.

Because several cuts were made, the surface of the wound at the apex is irregular. Proximal to the bladder, the superficial capsule is already exposed to the loop and can be recognized by its typical structure, its concave surface and its reddish color. Distal to the loop (at the right), the white adenoma tissue can be seen. The cut surface of the adenoma is rough, owing to rapid cutting or poor current quality. Its surface can be compared to wet snow. It also protrudes convexly (*Rule*: Convex tissue can be resected; see Fig. 88, e). In front, in the lower part of the photo, blue-shaded capsule tissue shines through.

Fig. 91, b Prostatic fossa with superficial capsule infiltrated with blue dye.

After resection of the whitish adenomatous layer (Fig. 91, a), the so-called "false capsule" (hypothetic layer between capsule and adenoma) is exposed. The tissue of the capsule is blue, because indigo dye was injected through the rectum. In the background, a chip of adenoma floats in the irrigating stream toward the bladder.

We divide the true prostatic tissue into three hypothetic layers to help orientation during TURP:

(a) Superficial capsule. Its fibers are very narrow-meshed (Fig. 91, d).

(b) Middle capsule. Here the fibers are coarse and less plaited (Fig. 91, e, j).

(c) Deep capsule. The distances between the fibers are wide. In the gaps between, one can see the true, fibrous capsule as well as periprostatic connective or fatty tissues (Figs. 91, k; 94, a).

Fig. 91, c Smooth cut in the pale blue-coloured capsule on the left lateral wall of the prostatic fossa.

The middle capsule in the foreground (on the right) is overexposed by too strong a light. The loop is used to coagulate a diffuse venous hemorrhage. Continuous suprapubic aspiration (low pressure irrigation) of the bloody irrigant facilitates coagulation and makes interruptions to empty the bladder unnecessary.

The foreground is lighted too well, because modern fiberoptics provide too strong a light source. Thus, the details in the tissue structure are lost.

Therefore, we use gray filters in front of the projector lamp to reduce the light.

Fig. 91, d Superficial capsule.
Two streams of blood appear on the left lateral wall of the fossa. These are freshly cut veins. The stream of blood falls almost vertically down the wall of the fossa and is then opened to resemble a fan by the stream of water and is drawn toward the bladder. Distal to the loop, part of the superficial capsule appears; proximally (toward the bladder), part of the middle capsule with its loose fibers can be seen. The left margin of the picture is formed by the beak of the resectoscope. At 9 o'clock, one can recognize the opening of the urethra toward the bladder and the ring of muscle fibers of the internal sphincter.

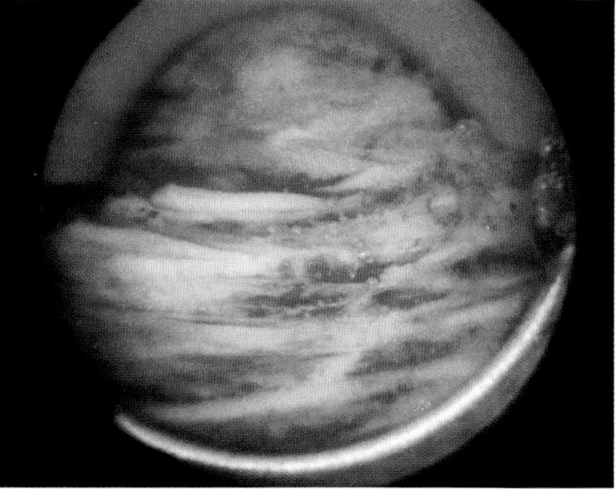
91 e

Fig. 91, e Structure of the middle capsule.
In the middle part on the floor of the fossa, the cut has penetrated the capsule slightly deeper than in Figure 91, d (superficial capsule). We call this layer the middle capsule, because from here on the fibers become coarser. In this patient the structure somewhat resembles that of the bladder mucosa. Unfortunately, a light inflammatory infiltration is sufficient to conceal the structure of the capsule, which increasingly resembles adenomatous tissue. Rarely, this resemblance to adenomatous tissue can lead to unwanted capsule perforation. It is therefore necessary to pay attention to any symptoms that may indicate such capsular perforation:

(a) Thickness of the bladder wall (rectal palpation).

(b) Mobility of the wall (floating of the capsule).

(c) Concave surface of the fossa.

(d) Diffuse hemorrhage (parenchyma).

(e) Fissures in the tissue in the deeper peripheral capsule.

(f) Smooth, metallically gleaming layer of the true capsule (fibrous capsule).

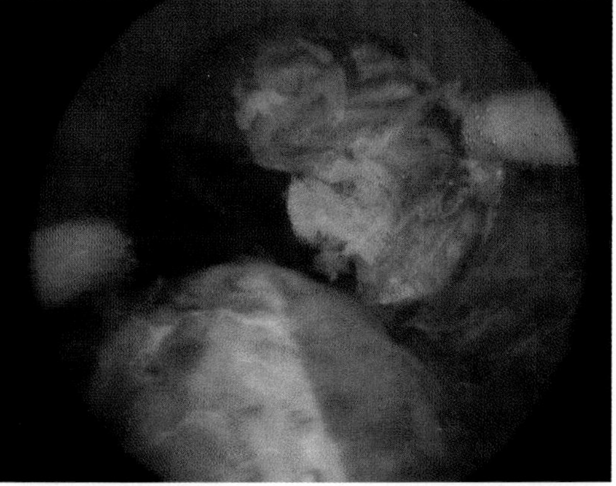
91 f

Fig. 91, f The fossa at the apex.
The cut ends at the colliculus seminalis. The resectoscope has been withdrawn into the median urethra to control the external sphincter. Since it is close to the optics, the colliculus seminalis is greatly enlarged. The cutting loop outlines the border of the fossa. In the right half of the illustration, the left part of the lateral lobe rises vertically. The margin of the mucosa is irregular.

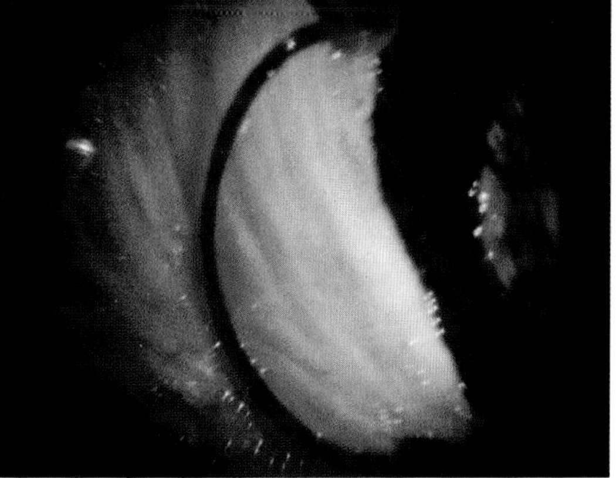
91 g

Fig. 91, g Superficial capsule.
This marked structure of the capsule on the lateral wall of the prostatic bed at 8 o'clock is typical of the third of the fossa that lies close to the bladder. The fibers of the capsule are closely connected, blending to the right into the pink, pale fibers of the internal sphincter. In the left margin of the picture they are bluish-colored and are arranged in a circle. The cutting surface is smooth and without any changes due to inflammation, infiltra-

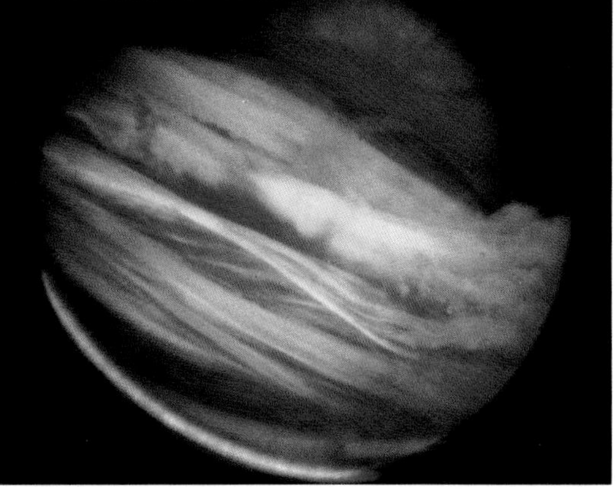
91 h

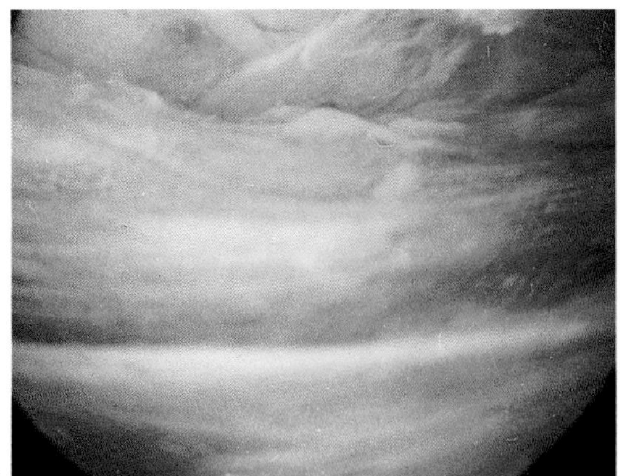
91 i

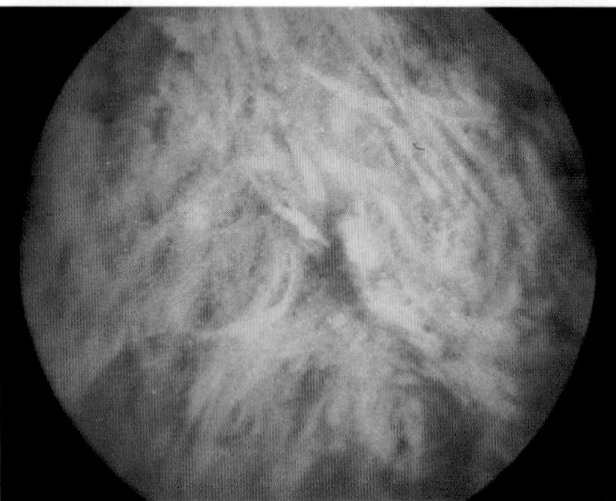
91 j

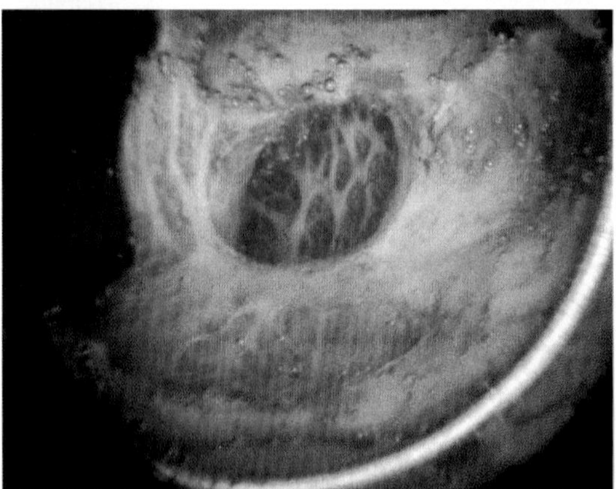
91 k

tion or hemorrhage. The superficial capsule corresponds to the so-called "false capsule," in which, in open surgery, the adenoma is enucleated by the finger. Unfortunately this layer is not recognized in a fissure during TUR.

Fig. 91, h Internal sphincter.
The circular muscle fibers of the internal sphincter are part of the bladder wall. They surround the adenoma on the bladder neck. Owing to the cryosurgery of the tissue, the fibers are slightly separated and thus can be readily recognized. In the lower margin of the photo, the cutting loop is just appearing in the sheath window of the resectoscope. The mucosa of the bladder can be seen at the margin of the wound. It is recommended that the first cuts of TUR be used to expose most of the sphincter and to demonstrate these fibers exactly before extending the procedure to the next section in order to confine precisely the fossa from the bladder neck (see Fig. 121, d).

Fig. 91, i Medium capsule.
The longitudinal fibers of the middle capsule layer are exposed on the floor of the fossa at 7 o'clock. The cutting surface is smooth. In the upper third of the picture, the fiber structure above a longitudinal fissure is irregular and coarse. Here the subvesical, deeper section of the prostate begins to cover the seminal vesicles. The light is too bright; therefore, the details of tissue structure and color are lost.

Fig. 91, j A typical superficial capsule near the apex.
The capsule fibers are closely connected; the cutting surface is somewhat irregular and has a fresh pink color. In contrast to the third of the prostatic bed closest to the bladder, the fibers in this illustration converge concentrically in the direction of the colliculus seminalis, which begins in the lower margin of the picture.
In this 83-year-old poor-risk patient, an adenoma of 125 gm net was resected totally in 75 min (peridural anesthesia; continuous low pressure irrigation with suprapubic trocar). At age 87, all urologic findings remained normal.

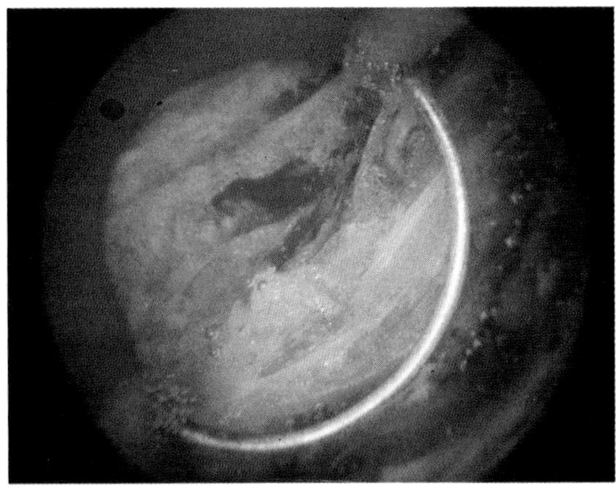

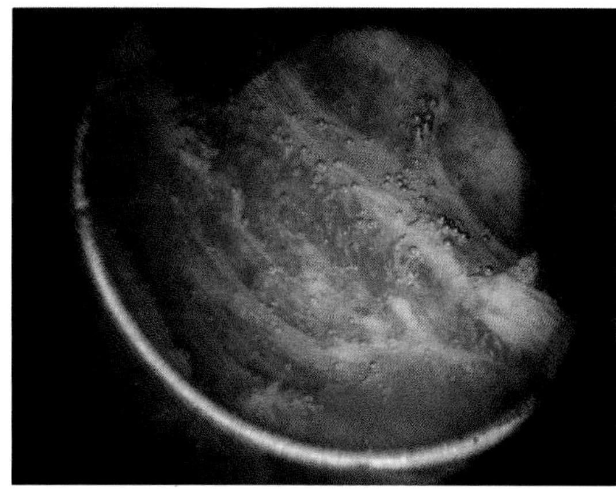

91 l–m

Fig. 91, k Medium and deep capsule.
The cutting loop is about to appear at the sheath window. In the lower half of the picture, the loose fibers of the middle capsule can be seen in the center of the fossa (artificial blue coloring). Above, there is an oval opening whose depth is filled by the fiber net of the deep capsule. This defect was caused by incorrect cutting technique. The finger was bent in a semicircle, and the prostate was mainly lifted with the tip of the finger so that only a certain area of capsular tissue was compressed. Instead, the palm should be held vertically and the prostate lifted with the stretched-out finger during the entire cutting process. The picture covers an area with a diameter of 1 to 2 cm — which is revealed by comparing it with the cutting loop (8 mm diameter).

Fig. 91, l Deep capsule and peripheral capsule (true, fibrous, metallic).
At 5 o'clock there is a deep cut in the prostatic capsule at the center of the prostatic urethra. The tissue fibers have a coarse structure. To the right of the loop there is semicircular coagulation tissue necrosis, because the coagulation was done, in error, with a fully extended loop. At 1 o'clock an almost white cord of tissue appears a few millimeters beneath the blue insulated wire of the loop. It is as smooth as plastic, and a metallic light is reflected on its top. This is a small gap in the surrounding deep capsule that allows one to see the fibrous capsule. Inflammatory infiltrations that had largely changed its typical structure were the reason why the resection was mistakenly performed. These fibers are loosely connected and edematous. To the left of the picture center a vein is visible that spreads fanlike across the floor of the fossa.

Fig. 91, m Fibrous capsule.
A small white ribbon crosses the upper third of the picture (between the sides of the resectoscope beak). It is a remnant of the fibrous capsule. The true prostatic tissue is entirely resected. Below this ribbon, the bloody, gelatinous connective tissue of the periprostatic area can be seen with single, thin fibers in between. A ramified trunk is visible in the right half of the picture between the loop and the fibrous ribbon. Such an exact illustration is possible only if the tissue is under physiologic pressure (low pressure irrigation). A high dynamic pressure due to a high-hanging irrigating reservoir pushes irrigating fluid into the loose tissue (Extravasation; see Fig. 93, e).

Bleeders

Fig. 92, a Hemorrhage from a sinus.

Deep capsule with venous sinus in radical TUR of an immature prostatic carcinoma (stage $T_2N_xM_0G_3$). In the center of the picture, the distance between the fibers becomes ever larger, so that they finally form a gap. A thick stream of blood that stems from a cut venous sinus gushes from the lower part of this gap. The picture shows several characteristic features:

(1) The venous sinus is preferably located in the deep peripheral capsule layer, often in the upper distal lateral wall of the fossa.

(2) The blood stream is aspirated in the direction of the bladder (low pressure irrigation) so that the operative field is irrigated by clear water.

(3) If there is physiologic pressure in the bladder (below 10 to 15 cm of water; 1 to 1.5 kPa), the blood can leave the vessel. As soon as the pressure is increased (over 15 cm of water; 1.5 kPa) it pushes the irrigant into the vessel so that it is forced directly into the circulation, thereby temporarily stopping the bleeding (see Fig. 98, a). This — rather dangerous — effect can be used for speedy coagulation.

Generally speaking, it may be said that almost any sinus bleeding can be coagulated. Therefore, we do not use a compression catheter but only a 20 Fr three way 5-cc irrigation catheter that causes the prostatic capsule to contract relatively fast — a desired effect. Continuous irrigation prevents the formation of coagulate, whose fateful role in bladder tamponade is well known. Radical TUR is a difficult procedure and puts extraordinary stress on the patient, which explains the long resection period (1 hour for 35 gm). The carcinomatous infiltrate into the capsule is completely resected, including the infiltrated trigone. The extensive bleeding made a transfusion necessary. Estrogen therapy was declined by the patient; orchiectomy was performed. Five years later, all findings were normal (79 years).

Fig. 92, b Hemorrhage in the blue-colored peripheral capsule (fibrous; true; metallic).

The net of coarse fibers is visible in the center of the fossa. In the lower two thirds of the picture, the contours, which are tinted with indigo-carmine, are blurred. Above, two untinted periprostatic fibers can be recognized. From above on the right, blood from an artery gushes to the left lower margin of the picture. At the right bottom of the picture, thick, slow bleeding from a vein can be seen. Between, there is a filamentous blood stream.

To better identify the capsule we color it by injecting indigo-carmine transrectally. When proper technique is used (Fig. 91, a, b), the adenoma remains uncolored. TURP of 30 gm net was performed in 35 min. Epidural anesthesia; after 11 years findings were normal (75 years).

Fig. 92, c Arterial hemorrhage from periprostatic tissue.

The prostatic capsule is completely resected on the right lateral margin of the fossa. Erroneously, an infiltrated inflammation in the capsule was diagnosed as a carcinoma infiltrate and was resected up to the healthy tissue (low pressure irrigation). Only three gray-blue fibers of the fibrous capsule meeting in the lower margin of the picture remain. An arterial hemorrhage appears in the lower half of the picture; its pressure gives the appearance of a red fountain splashing to the left margin of the picture. Blurred venous bleeding can be seen above. It is aspirated by the suprapubic trocar needle and crosses the floor of the fossa in serpentine fashion in the direction of the bladder, just as the arterial stream is turned toward the bladder (Fig. 91, d).

TURP (20 gm net); 10 years later the 66-year-old patient had no complaints. Prostatic fossa still evident on x-ray.

Fig. 92, d Vein in the periprostatic tissue (TUR of a sphincter sclerosis).

The center of the picture shows the vascular tube of a vein cut from above. There are fibers of the fibrous peripheral true metallic capsule in the right and left margin of the picture. In between, there is a reddish loose tissue covered with small air bubbles. Low pressure irrigation makes possible the total resection of the capsule and the natural presentation of the extraprostatic region without the tissue being traumatized, nor does the irrigant distort the extraprostatic area, as often occurs in high pressure irrigation.

From a surgical viewpoint this is a covered perforation, because — unlike open perforation — no cavity has been opened in the body and no artificial cavity in the periprostatic region has developed. Therefore, no acute complications can be expected. Consequently, it is best not to speak of "perforation" but rather of total capsule resection. The visible periprostatic tissue hardens within a few hours — thus consolidating the defect.

Deep capsular resection augments the tendency for scar and stricture formation as does over-resection of the bladder. After one year, a bladder neck stricture had to be resected in this 62-year-old patient (Fig. 122, c). *Histology:* Capsule with transverse striped muscle; chronic inflammation. At age 75 all findings were normal.

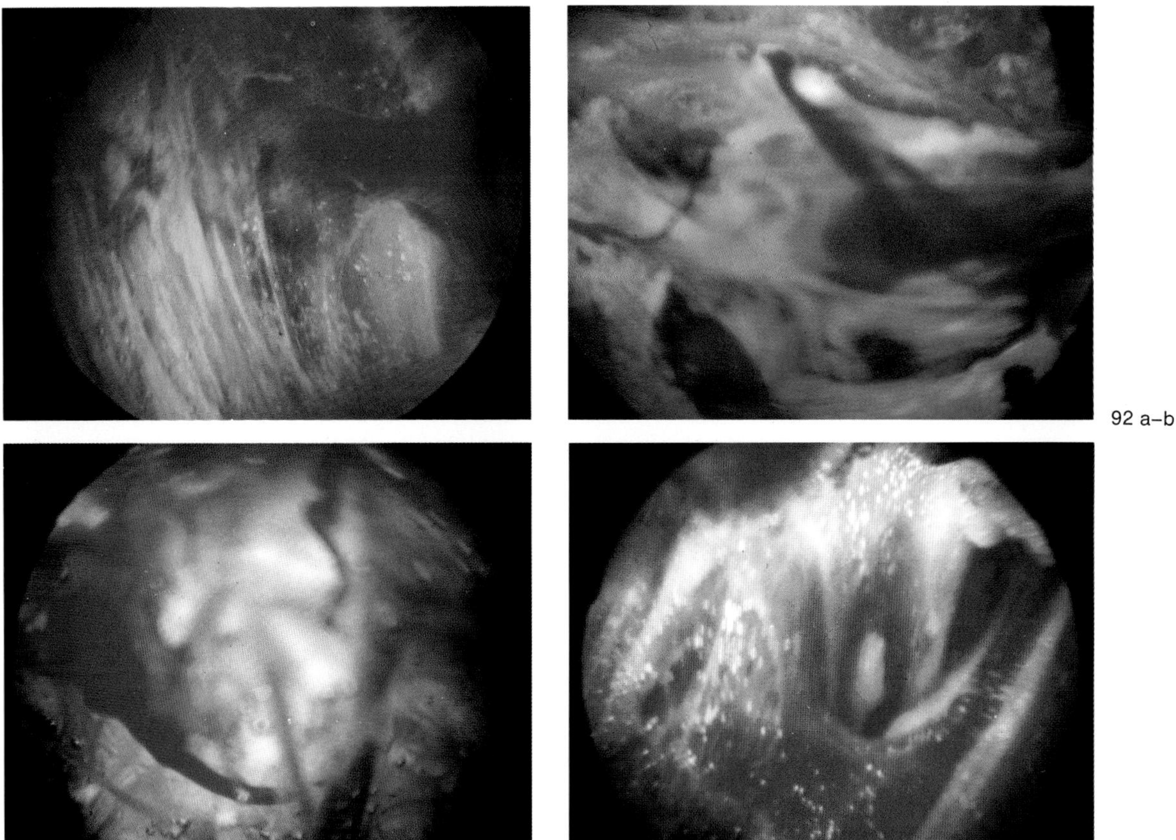

92 a–b

92 c–d

93 a–c
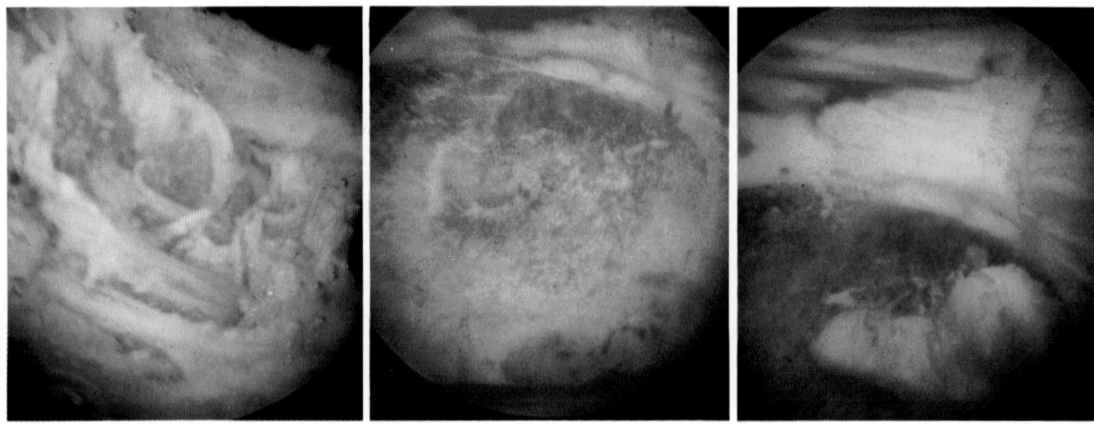

Junction Between Bladder and Prostatic Fossa

Fig. 93, a TURP (20 gm in 30 min).
The junction between the muscle fibers of the internal sphincter belonging to the bladder wall and the prostatic capsule (true prostatic tissue) is relatively thin. If the tissue is resected too deep at this point, a gap develops. In the center of the picture such a gap can be seen, from which emerge torn capsular fibers and subvesical tissue. Above the defect is the internal sphincter, which, owing to over-resection, is atypically narrow. Below the gap, coarse fibers of the deep and middle capsule (see Figs. 39, 91) are visible.

This condition is not dangerous and does not present any complications. However, under unphysiologically high dynamic irrigation pressure the gap may be torn open (Fig. 93, d).

Fig. 93, b Gap between bladder and prostatic fossa.
The continuity of the subvesical connective tissue between bladder wall and prostatic capsule is not interrupted. The cut bladder wall is seen above; a small tissue chip is at the right, below the margin of the prostatic capsule. This condition is the initial stage of disruption and perforation. It does not involve any serious consequences if the urine is drained continuously by an indwelling catheter for four to six days with a small balloon (5-cc)

Fig. 93, c Disruption of the bladder and the prostatic fossa (TURP of a sphincter sclerosis; 10 gm net in 20 min).
In the area of the trigone the connection between the bladder wall and the prostatic capsule was completely severed at 5 to 7 o'clock. Above the trigone, the circular muscle fibers of the internal sphincter can be recognized. Underneath, connective tissue of the subvesical region is noted; it is partially covered by a resected tissue chip. The dynamic pressure of the irrigation has opened the gap below the bladder and has lifted the trigone. The higher the dynamic pressure, the more the bladder neck and trigone retract and the more the fossa is distended. The final result is subvesical perforation.

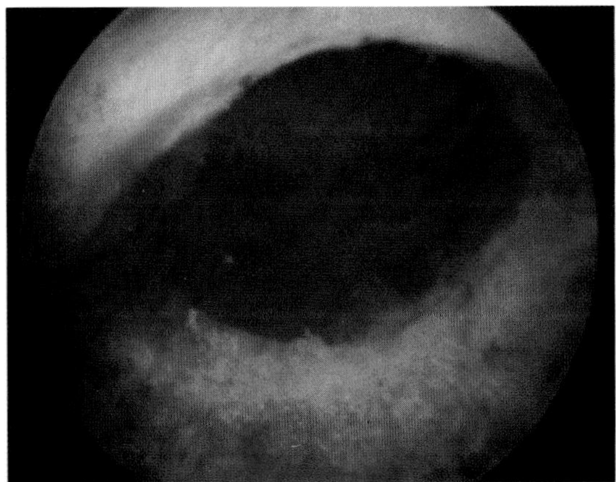

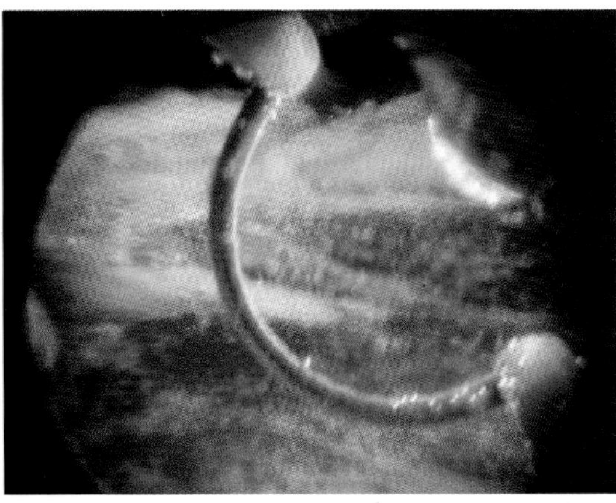

93 d–e

Fig. 93, d Subvesical perforation.
Illumination of the gap shows that a water deposit has developed. Unphysiologic dynamic pressure (high pressure irrigation) has torn open the tissue gap between the bladder and prostate and has undermined the bladder. The severed retracted bladder wall can be seen in the upper margin of the picture. Underneath, there is a perforating cavity filled with irrigant and loose perivesical connective tissue. This irrigant extravasation, which may have a volume of several liters, can extend through the retroperitoneal area to the renal bed. In some cases, this extravasation can be expelled by pressing the abdomen; the water flows out through the indwelling catheter (5-cc balloon in the big fossa, not in the bladder). This ensures an uncomplicated postoperative course. A compression catheter should not be used, as it might shift the perforation hole. Only with continuous low pressure irrigation in TUR can such complications be safely avoided.

Fig. 93, e Water infiltrated prostatic tissue.
In the foreground, the resection loop and its red insulated wires can be recognized. Above, the margin of the resected trigone and the muscle fibers of the internal sphincter cross the picture. Below, the connection of the coarse wide fibers of the deep prostatic capsule is still intact (unlike Figs. 93, c,d). Here, the irrigant was forced through its fibers (irrigant absorption). High pressure irrigation causes a watery extravasation into the periprostatic tissue that may develop into the so-called "water intoxication syndrome." TURP with high pressure irrigation; 110 gm net in 65 min (see Fig. 94, b). Postoperatively, no complications occurred in this 63-year-old man, since 30 cc of 10 per cent NaCl and furosemide were administered IV immediately.

Total TUR of the Prostatic Capsule and Consequences of Water Pressure Caused by Irrigation and Bladder Filling

Any attempt at complete resection of the prostatic capsule under high pressure irrigation (p. 23) is bound to fail a priori, because serious complications — such as water intoxication, perforation and total alteration of the topography of the fossa — will compel the surgeon to discontinue the operation. TUR (TURP, radical TUR) with minimal risk is achieved with the following:

1. Secure knowledge and differentiation of tissues through optical aids.
2. Palpation by rectum for evaluation of consistency and quality of the tissue and for topographic orientation.
3. Prevention of distention of the fossa by keeping the bladder empty with continuous aspiration of irrigant through the suprapubic trocar or the return-flow resectoscope.
4. Physiologic low static and dynamic water pressure in the fossa (p. 21; low pressure irrigation, p. 25) which enables the surgeon to excise larger portions of the prostatic capsule.

Fig. 94, a Total TUR of the prostatic capsule with low pressure irrigation.
Above the stump of the fibrous capsule (lower margin of the picture) reddish periprostatic tissue without water infiltration can be observed (compare Fig. 92, b–d), still covered with a few thin fibers of the capsule. During TUR, physiologic low pressure irrigation avoids extravasation of irrigant into the tissue (compare Fig. 93, e) or veins (compare Fig. 92, a): it also avoids lifting of the bladder mucosa (Fig. 93, d). This technique makes possible TUR of more parts of the true prostate (subtotal, total, radical TUR).

Fig. 94, b Watery infiltration of the prostatic capsule during TURP with high pressure irrigation.
Between the longitudinal fibers of the levator ani, which are pictured vertically at the left, and the margin of the prostatic capsule (right), a gap exposes watery infiltrated periprostatic tissue. The difference between physiologic, tissue preserving, low pressure irrigation and unphysiologic, traumatic, high pressure irrigation is clearly visible when Figures 92, a–94, c are compared. Thus, it is easy to understand how important irrigation is for TURP and how many complications can be avoided if the resection is performed under physiologic conditions — e.g., with an empty bladder and a low irrigating reservoir. The novice will be able to watch the clearly visible operative field without interruption, and he can improve his technique without being disturbed.

Fig. 94, c Radical TUR of carcinomatous prostatic capsule (stage T_3G_3) with low pressure irrigation (see Fig. 113).
The prostatic wall, together with the carcinomatous infiltrate, is completely excised. The traverse muscles of the pelvic floor and the long fibers (levator ani) on the right wall of the fossa are exposed at 8 o'clock. The muscle fibers are partly torn off and lie vertically in the gap of the capsular wall. In the right margin of the picture, periprostatic fat with a glittering surface is seen. This is not a perforation of the prostate but a specific excision of the carcinomatous prostate into the sound periprostatic tissue. In this 75-year-old poor-risk patient (two cardiac infarctions), 50 gm net were resected in 40 min; 10 months later, the patient died following a third cardiac infarction.

Fig. 94, d Perforation of the prostatic capsule. TURP with high pressure irrigation.
The total excision of a suspicious deep nodule in the prostatic capsule has caused a perforation in the periprostatic tissue. In the upper margin of the picture, only a white, sail-like remnant of the fibrous capsule is left. A cavity filled with irrigant has formed that is crossed by the muscle fibers of the levator ani. The wire of the cutting loop has been deformed by heavy use. On the right, in the lower margin of the picture, the red cloud of hemorrhage can be seen in the irrigant. The harmful consequences of high pressure irrigation (p. 23) compared with physiologic low pressure irrigation are obvious (see Fig. 94, e). TURP of 80 gm net in 55 min; peridural anesthesia; blood transfusion. Histology; adenoma.

Fig. 94, e Total TUR of the trigone.
In the upper margin of the picture the bow-shaped stump of bladder floor can be recognized. The trigone has been totally resected because subvesical carcinomatous infiltration was suspected in the area of the seminal vesicles, whose oblong lumina were thus exposed.
Underneath, the blue-colored prostatic capsule (true capsule) is visible. A few bloody threads spread across the field of vision. In all infiltrating processes, resection into the seminal vesicle is necessary, the pathologic tissue being, if possible, resected into healthy tissue. The resection of the seminal vesicles does not involve any complications if, as is usual, vasectomy is performed along with the TUR.

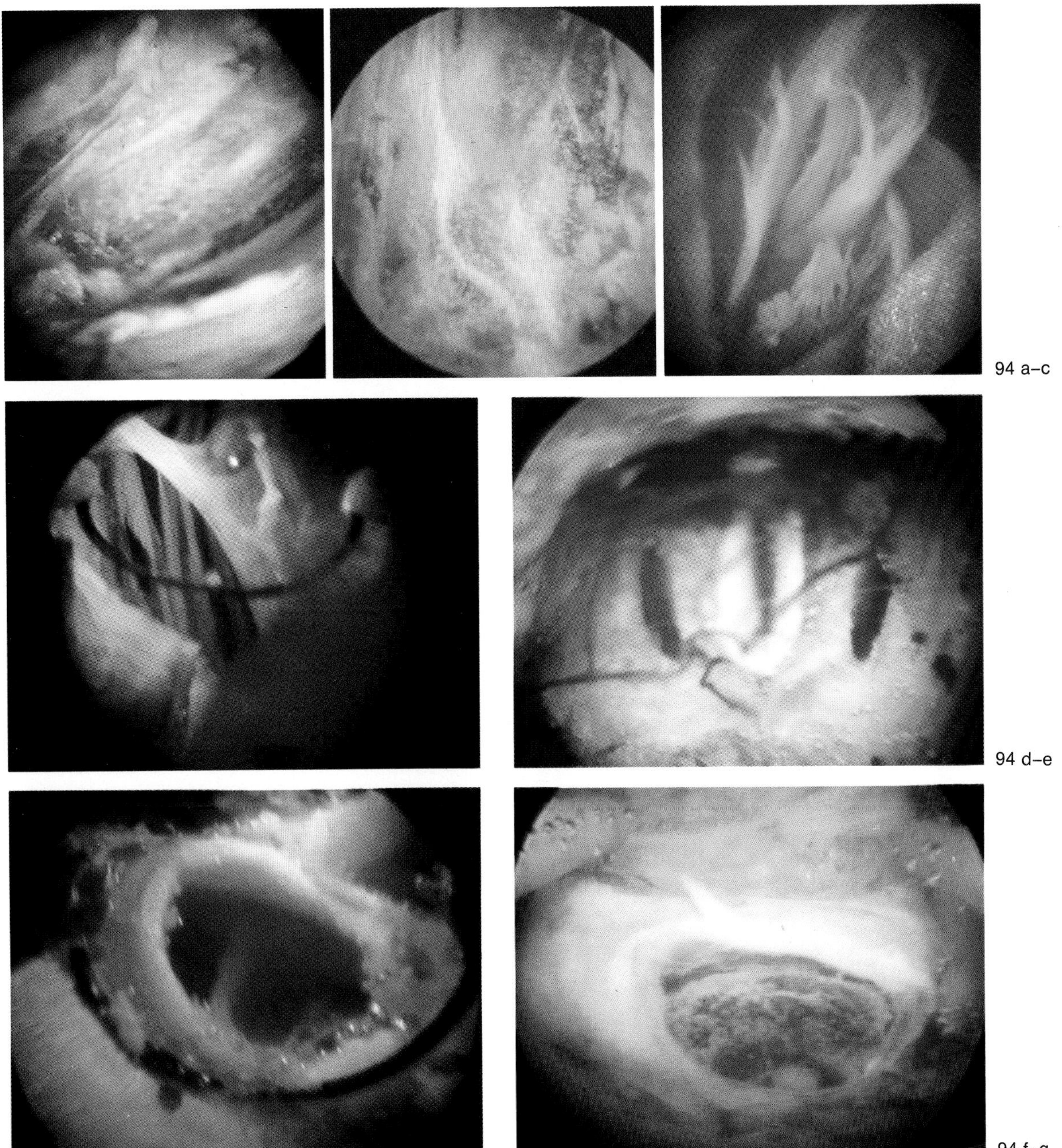

94 a–c

94 d–e

94 f–g

Fig. 94, f Partial TUR of seminal vesicles in prostatic carcinoma (stage $T_2N_0M_0G_2$; low pressure irrigation).
The firm, irregular seminal vesicles were cut above the palpating finger in the rectum. Except for a slight hypertrophy of the wall, the seminal vesicles are not infiltrated by cancer. Note the way they are clustered and the characteristic subdivision of their lumina by segments. Radical TUR in a 75-year-old patient (35 gm net in 30 min). After three years, TUR of a bladder neck stricture was performed. At 80, the patient died following an aortic rupture. No further carcinoma could be found.

Fig. 94, g "Table-cloth perforation" of the prostatic capsule (high pressure irrigation).
In the lower half of the picture a hole in the fibrous capsule almost as round as a circle can be recognized between the fossa and the rectum. It can be compared to a hole burnt into a tablecloth by a cigarette. Not infrequently, this typical covered perforation occurs when the prostate is lifted from the rectum with the tip of the index finger (compare Fig. 91, k). The perforating defect is filled with loose connective tissue. The two gray lateral wires of the cutting loop are visible. TUR of a 58-year-old high-risk patient was disrupted after 35 min (40 gm net) because of a water-intoxication syndrome due to high pressure irrigation. The second session (40 gm in 45 min) was performed two weeks later. Histology: adenoma; connective tissue; smooth muscle; fatty tissue. Two years later the patient died of MS (no urologic symptoms).

Radical TUR of the Prostatic Capsule with Carcinoma Under Low Pressure Irrigation

Fig. 95, a Muscles of the rectum.

The capsule above the outer longitudinal muscles of the rectum is totally resected. In the upper margin of the picture, a transverse portion of the remaining capsule (below the trigone) can be seen in the fossa. Underneath, the smooth longitudinal muscles of the rectum cross the picture vertically. If TUR is performed carefully there is little risk of perforation into the intestinal lumen, because the layer of connective tissue between the prostate and rectum is sufficiently elastic to keep from being cut by the loop. (Photograph taken from the movie, "TUR of the Prostatic Carcinoma," which was shown at the AUA meeting in San Francisco in 1969).

When the bladder is filled under high pressure irrigation, the fossa stretches like the side of a balloon. This is readily palpated by the finger in the rectum and is an important sign of an overfilled bladder in TUR. If the sheath — or, later, the catheter — is pushed forward somewhat forcefully under the trigone, its tip perforates into the thin rectum. We have seen this occur twice, one week after TUR, when the residual urine was controlled. Radical TUR (115 gm net in 80 min; stage T_3G_2). Six years later this 75-year-old patient is without symptoms or carcinoma (Figs. 110, e, 116 a–c).

Fig. 95, b A cluster of adipose tissue.

At 1 o'clock, periprostatic fat is seen pushing into the cavity. Fat droplets glisten in the light; the base of the hanging fat cluster is about 2 cm in diameter. This fat must not be confused with adenomatous tissue and therefore resected, because it closes the gaps in the capsule like a plug and indurates in a short time by leukocyte infiltration. Fat tissue has varying colors and structures. Smaller fat particles also occur in the capsule as accompanying tissue of vessels. It loses its typical appearance in infiltrations, but still can be readily distinguished from the capsule or an adenoma (see Fig. 95, c).

Fig. 95, c Muscles of the levator ani.

On the right lateral wall of the fossa (*left*) pale, bloodless, slack transverse muscles of the pelvic floor are exposed. Above and below there is still a remnant of the capsular wall. In the right margin of the picture, some fat can be seen floating out. The use of low pressure irrigation has made the tissue clearly visible (Figs. 94, c; 95, d–f).

Fig. 95, d Muscles of the levator ani.

The left wall of the prostatic capsule has been completely resected (see Fig. 69). The tense muscles of the pelvis are seen in the right half of the picture: they are well supplied with blood, which spreads from above downward. In the left half of the picture, reddish-colored portions of fat tissue can be seen next to the sail-shaped edge of the muscles. Since the fat tissue is indurated it does not flow out (compare Fig. 95, b).

Fig. 95, e Spherical fat plug.

A loose, pale yellow fat ball flows below the stump of the prostatic capsule into the lumen of the urethra after complete resection of the prostatic capsule at 1 and 2 o'clock. Low pressure irrigation prevents the irrigant from penetrating through tissue defect in the capsule and into the periprostatic capsule area.

Fig. 95, f Spherical fat plug.

The irregular bow-shaped stump of the totally resected distal capsule of the prostate can be seen at the upper and right margins of the picture. Behind it, the spherical plug of fat flows into the fossa. This fat ball is deformed by the irrigation stream because the irrigating reservoir is elevated more than 50 cm above the bladder. If it is raised farther, the fat ball is pushed farther into the prostatic region by dynamic pressure, thereby causing considerable extravasation of the irrigant into the connective tissue in this area (high pressure irrigation).

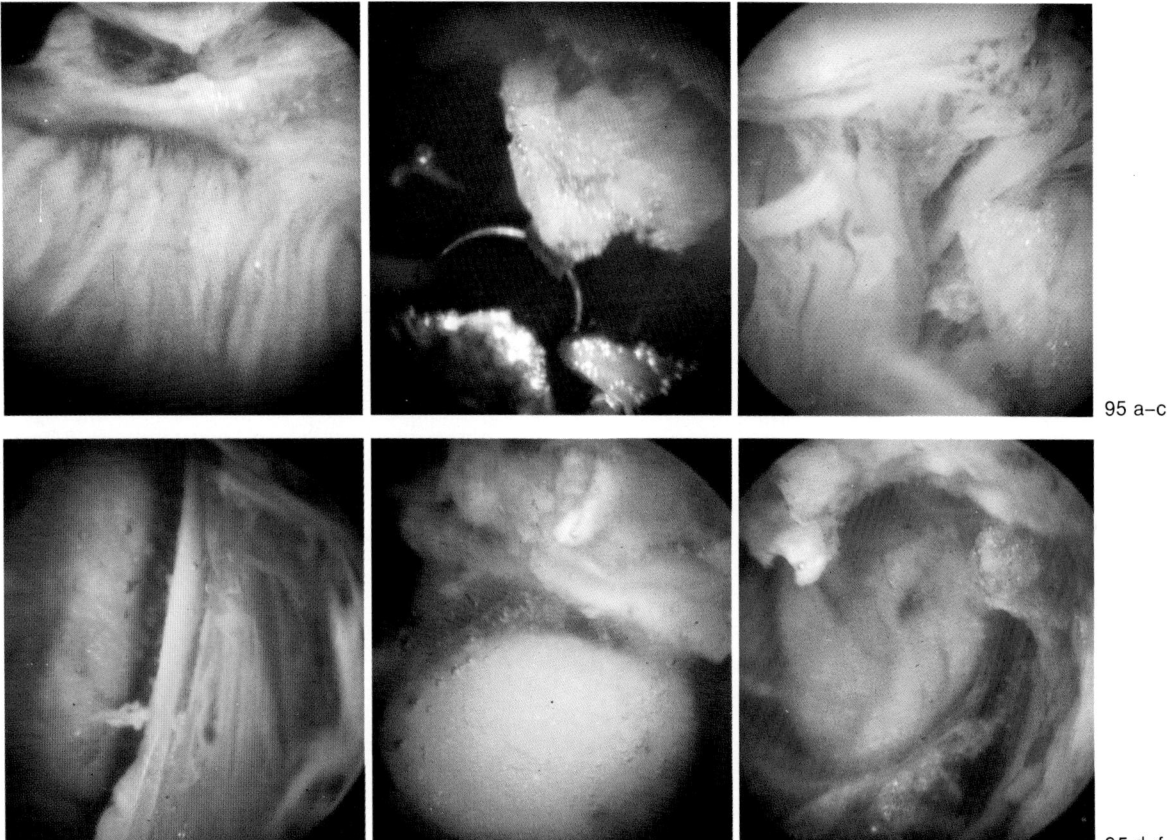

95 a–c

95 d–f

Perforation of the Prostatic Capsule and Peritoneum

Fig. 96, a Accidental perforation.
An oval tissue defect has been created because one specific cut penetrated accidentally through all the layers of the prostatic capsule. In the background, periprostatic connective tissue can be recognized. At the right margin of the picture, the lumen of a blood vessel in the capsule has been severed; however, owing to irrigation pressure, there is no hemorrhage. This unintended perforation of the capsular wall can be distinguished from an intentional one by its shape. By comparing Figures 92, b–d, one can recognize that here a deep isolated channel was resected. The division of the capsule into a deep and a medium layer is clearly recognizable, whereas, in the intended resection, a wide area is removed cut by cut. (TURP 100 gm net in 60 min.)

Fig. 96, b Perforation and resected tissue.
The defect in the capsule was blocked by a chip of resected tissue. This piece could be extravasated into the perforation area outside the capsule, provoking inflammatory complications. It is obligatory to examine any perforation with the illuminated endoscope to establish the extent and kind of perforation (see Figs. 93, d; 94, d). With low pressure irrigation this can be done without risk. When in doubt, a ureteral catheter can be inserted into the perforation and the perforation area filled with contrast media and x-rayed. A cystogram also can prove the diagnosis.

Fig. 96, c Perforation into the peritoneum (radical TUR of a bladder carcinoma infiltrating into the prostate; stage $T_4N_2M_0G_2$).
The infiltrating carcinoma of the bladder (*right*) has grown into the prostatic capsule. Here, the carcinomatous tissue lies directly on the peritoneum; the so-called "warning tissue" is missing. Moreover, in this case, the peritoneum goes more caudad, thereby covering the dorsal outer wall of the prostate. During TUR of the carcinoma, the peritoneum was opened. In the center of the picture the peritoneal defect is bent outward like a sail. At the right margin, a cloudy venous hemorrhage covers the border of the peritoneum. The distal bright stump of the scarred prostatic capsule crosses the lower margin of the picture. Open surgical control is mandatory (see Fig. 180).

Fig. 96, d Perforation into the peritoneum.
The perforation is illuminated. The irrigating stream presses an intestinal loop downward. On the rounded intestinal wall, typical thin blood vessels can be seen. Above this, the posterior wall of the abdomen is obscured by yellow peritoneum. The defect is confined above by the white peritoneum and on the right margin of the picture by the stump of the capsule.

Fig. 96, e Perforation into the peritoneum.
The beak of the resectoscope has been inserted through the perforation into the abdomen. Several intestinal loops are seen floating in the irrigant. At the left a deformed, slightly used cutting loop can be seen.

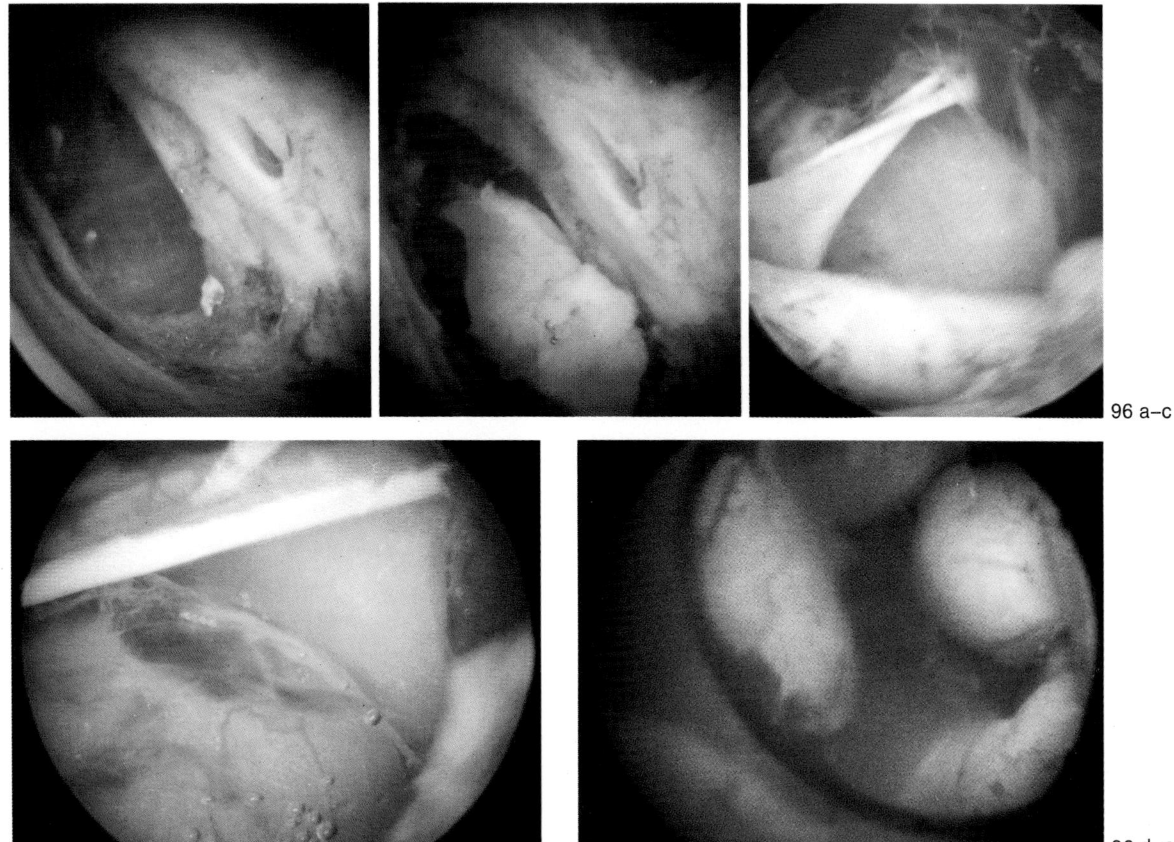

96 a–c

96 d–e

Over-resection into the Bladder (Fig. 97)
Venous Sinus with Thrombus (Fig. 98)
Atrophic Prostatic Capsule (Fig. 99)
Prostatic Stones (Fig. 100)

Fig. 97, a Resected ureteral orifice in the prostatic bed.
The oval opening of the ureteral stump lies in the center of the transverse fibers of the bladder floor and the trigone. The injected mucosa has become edematous owing to the inflammation. To the front and on the right a coagulation slough can be seen. (Over-resection during TURP of 100 gm net in 65 min.) Resection of the orifice is usually well tolerated. Follow-up complications are due to the development of scarring, although this is not frequent. We lost one patient, however, when a tamponade catheter was inserted on the 16th postoperative day to treat a hemorrhage. This resulted in acute pyelonephritis due to compression of the orifice in the prostatic bed. (Publication on TUR of 73 pathologic ureteral orifices. Z Urol *59*:633, 1966.)

Fig. 97, b Over-resection.
In the lower half of the picture, the resected bladder neck can be recognized. Part of the surface of the mucosa has been removed a few centimeters beyond the edge of the internal sphincter. Therefore, the muscular bladder wall is exposed below the irregular edge of the wound. This is a result of poor technique, whereby short cuts were made on the bladder neck and the sheath of the resectoscope was bent excessively. (TUR of a subvesical adenoma of 30 gm net in 25 min; see Fig. 119, h.)

Fig. 97, c Bladder neck after partial TUR (trocar cystoscopy).
The prostatic fossa can be recognized as a flat funnel on the bladder neck. The tissue of the prostate (adenoma and scar tissue) was resected only superficially, whereas the bladder neck was resected all around about 1 cm too deep into the tissue. In the upper margin of the picture, wound necroses adhering to the mucosa are still present. These developed during the first TUR, performed three weeks earlier. In the prostatic bed, freshly resected adenomatous nodules can be seen with chronically inflamed injected areas. The patient had had two previous resections. Several times the remnant of the adenoma caused bladder stones when necrotic tissue shed. Thanks to the subsequent TURP, the patient has healed and has lived 11 more years without recurrence.

Fig. 98, a Venous sinus; radical TUR.
The left lateral wall of the fossa was resected into the pericapsular fatty tissue (right). In the upper center of the picture an oval gap opens. The lumen of the vessel has retreated. Only granular yellow-gold fat can be seen. The venous hemorrhage is minimal because of the increased dynamic irrigation pressure; only at the lower left can a cloud of blood be recognized (see Fig. 92, a). A venous sinus hemorrhage almost always can be coagulated, but sometimes great patience is necessary, as the coagulated vessel repeatedly resumes bleeding. Coagulation with an empty bladder is important in order to relax the tissue of the capsule.

Fig. 98, b Venous blood vessel with thrombus.
Not infrequently, thrombosed blood vessels are resected in the outer capsule. In this illustration, the tubelike vessel is cut open transversally and is surrounded by the deep capsular fibers. There is a thick clot in its lumen. Frequently blood escapes from the vessel next to the thrombus and must be coagulated.

Fig. 98, c Extraction of a thrombus from the vein with a cold resectoscope loop.

Fig. 98, d Thrombotic remnant in front of a smoothly cut vein.
If the irrigation is now reduced there will be massive hemorrhage from this vessel. Coagulation is relatively easy if the current is turned on only after pressing the vessel walls together with the cutting loop or after pushing the loop deep into the lumen.

Fig. 99 Prostatic fossa with sievelike structure.
A small adenomatous remnant can be recognized at the top of the illustration. Below, a relatively smooth membrane is extended; it has numerous small perforating holes. This sievelike structure developed when the true prostatic capsule was atrophied by the pressure of the adenoma and the glandular tubes of the prostate became over-extended.

Fig. 100 Prostatic calculi.
There are numerous round or angular calculi up to the size of a pea in the deep capsule (*Transurethral Prostatectomy of Prostatic Calculi*. Urol Int (Basel) *20*:336, 1965.) Prostatic calculi are always present in the capsule, the true prostatic tissue. Calculi in the area surrounding the verumontanum are always excised in retrograde fashion to protect the external sphincter. Small calculi normally drop from the capsule into the prostatic fossa and are passed spontaneously.

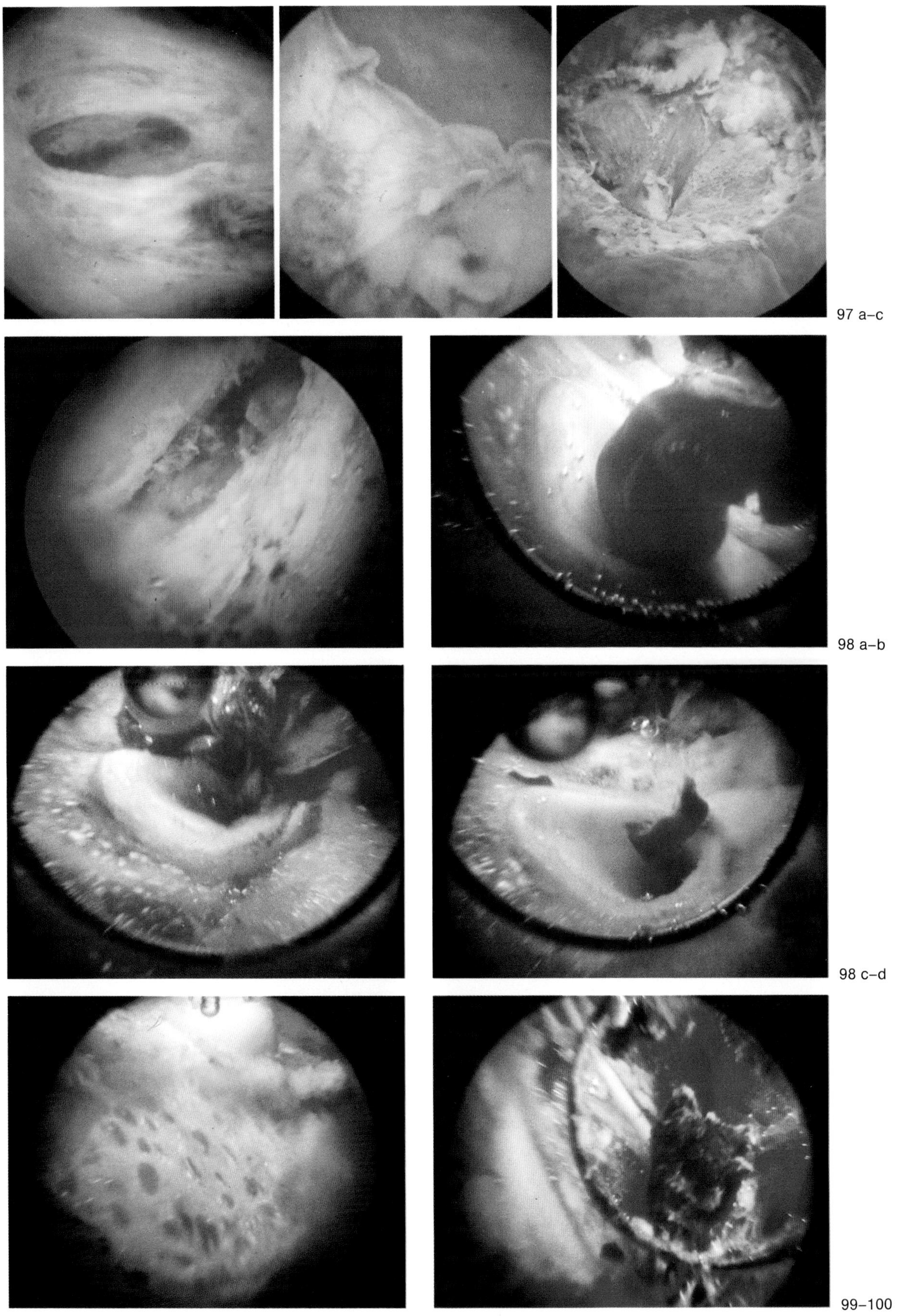

97 a–c

98 a–b

98 c–d

99–100

Distal Limitation of the Prostatic Fossa and Transition into the Middle Urethra (External Sphincter)

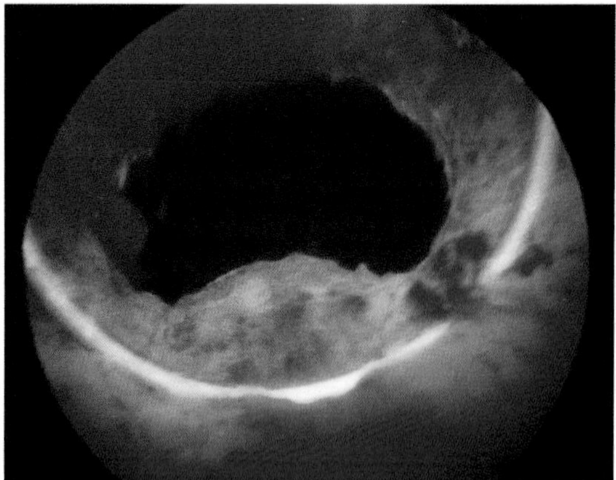
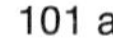

Fig. 101, a External sphincter after TURP.
At the end of TUR, the beak of the resectoscope was pulled back slightly into the median urethra to control the shape of the external sphincter in relation to the verumontanum below. To demonstrate the proportions in the picture, the cutting loop has been extended (diameter, 7 mm). The irrigation pressure has indirectly caused the external sphincter to open. The pillar of the right lateral lobe (*left*) shows slightly irregular indentations and a small cloud-shaped hemorrhage. Here, the median urethra begins.

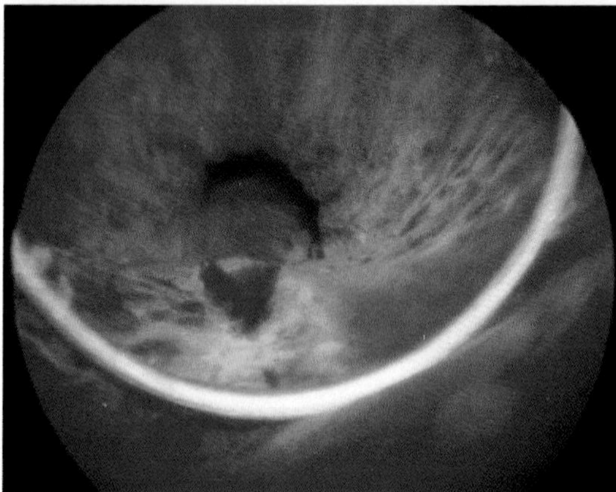
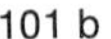

Fig. 101, b Contraction of the external sphincter.
The resectoscope is pulled farther back into the median urethra. The sphincter lumen contracts over the verumontanum like a half-moon while small longitudinal folds are formed in the mucosa. Monitoring the shape and function of the external sphincter is indispensable to control of the distal extension of the fossa during TUR.

The mucosa of the median urethra is irritated by trauma during TUR. Above the cutting loop, the fibers of the external sphincter can be seen.

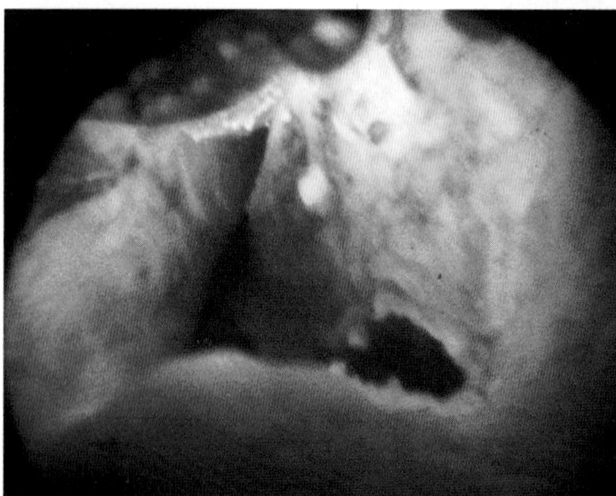
101 c

Fig. 101, c Deformed external sphincter in partial TUR (25 gm net in 45 min).
At the level of the external sphincter, the contours of the lumen of the urethra are triangular. Below, the verumontanum rises. On the right side, at the margin of the picture, the left stump of the lateral lobe protrudes into the lumen, having been undermined from below and resected above up to the sphincter. There is a large adenomatous remnant between the upper and lower resections. On the left, the pillar of the right lateral lobe remains. Also, the adenoma has not been resected up to the edge of the median urethra or the external sphincter. There is a risk of polyp formation on the left. Such a polyp, if lodged in the sphincter, can lead to mechanical incontinence. TUR must be continued to achieve a round tube that demonstrates complete resection of the adenoma (Fig. 103, c).

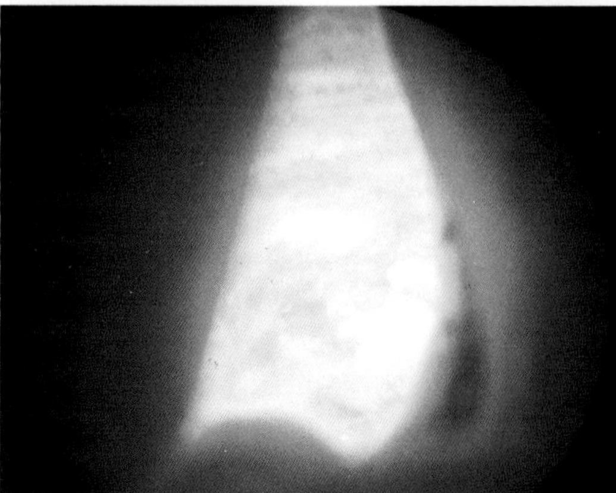
101 d

Fig. 101, d External sphincter and colliculus seminalis after partial TUR (25 gm net in 40 min).
The transition from the median to the healed prostatic urethra (fossa) is seen as a silhouette. This effect occurs because the scarred mucosa of the prostatic urethra is brightly lit by the distal light source while the half-closed external sphincter lies

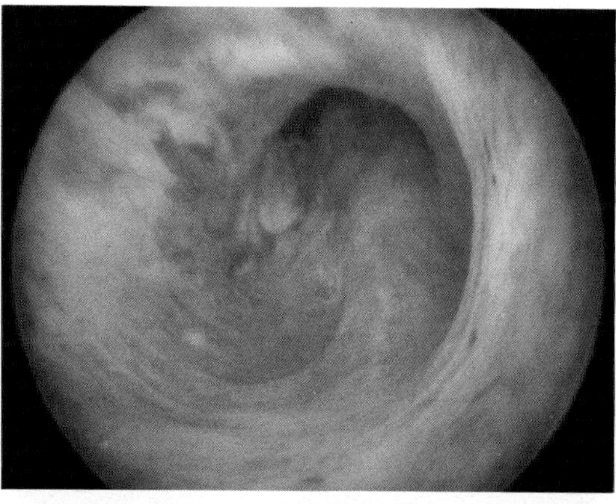
101 e

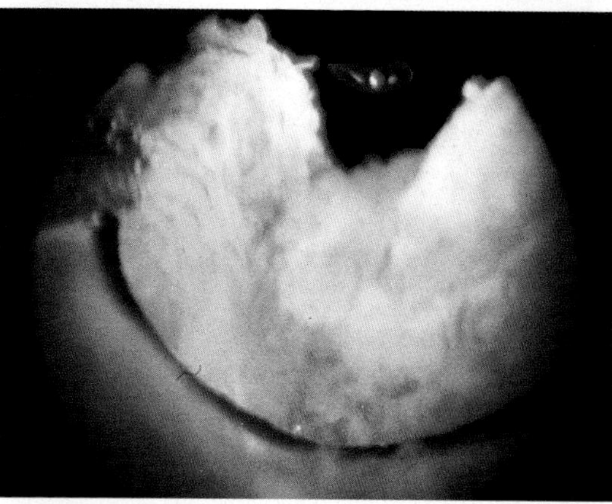
101 f

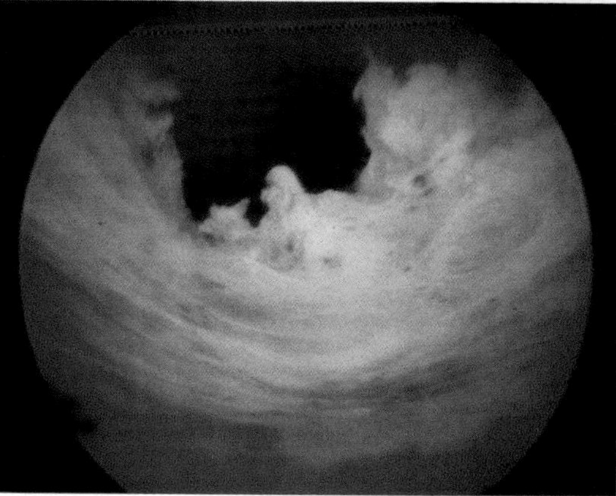
101 g

in shadow. The verumontanum protrudes from below into the vertical oval lumen of the external sphincter. On the left, the silhouette of the stretched pillar of the right lateral lobe protrudes farther into the cavity than on the other side. On the right, a small adenomatous remnant is seen at the apex (see Figs. 87, 88). In the center, the brightly lit mucosa of the healed fossa can be recognized. This adenomatous remnant is enough to cause a continuing chronic *E. coli* infection that causes pain on urination. Only after completion of the TUR do these complaints vanish (Figs. 102, a; 103, c).

Fig. 101, e Median urethra with external sphincter.
The round lumen of the median urethra surrounds the center of the colliculus seminalis, which itself already has been lifted by the urogenital ligament. The median urethra is distended by irrigation pressure, whereas the crescent-shaped lumen of the prostatic urethra is almost closed. The verumontanum continues into the median urethra as a long stretched ridge whose distal end dissolves in the muscle fibers of the external sphincter, which stretch sideways under the mucosa. The utriculus no longer can be seen, having already retreated into the prostatic urethra. The mucosa of the pillar of the right lateral lobe is slightly injured.

Fig. 101, f Over-resection into the median urethra.
Typical superficial lesion in the region of the external sphincter. The mucosa of the median urethra is resected in the corner between the verumontanum and the right lateral lobe. The cutting loop has cut a tongue-shaped defect by penetrating distally about 1 cm too far into the median urethra. The external sphincter usually tolerates this well — and even deeper lesions; therefore, no incontinence occurred after this TUR. In the right margin of the picture, half of the resected verumontanum can be seen. Medially and distally to it, the mucosa of the median urethra is excised; left to the center of the picture is the intact pillar of the right lateral lobe; distal to it, the cutting loop is visible.

Fig. 101, g External sphincter after radical TUR of a prostatic carcinoma.
In the lower half of the picture, typical muscle fibers of the external mucosa cross the urethra and lift the mucosa, which is shown in dramatic relief. Above, the cut-off lumen of the median urethra extends into the resected prostatic bed. The mucosa is lacerated and the verumontanum is largely resected. Although here, too, the carcinoma was resected a few millimeters too far distally, there is no incontinence. Resecting the carcinoma up to the external sphincter involves extreme risk (Figs. 92, a; 98, a; 113, e).

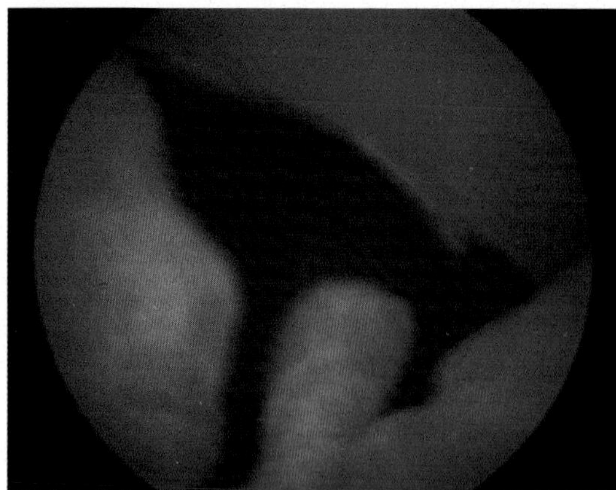
101 h

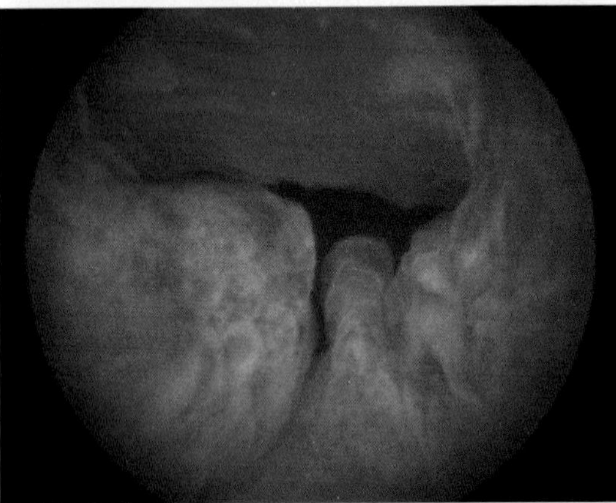
101 i

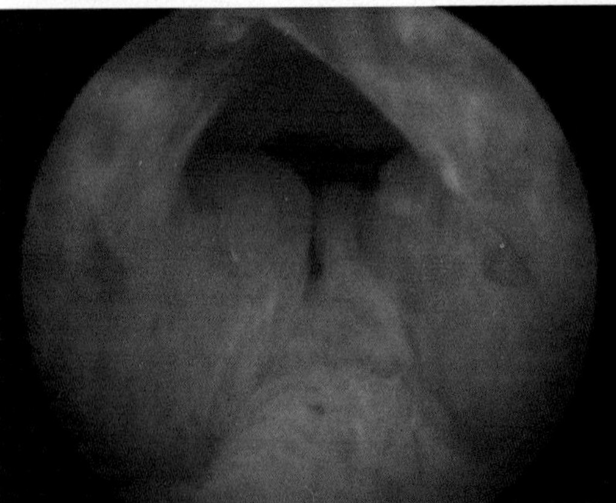
101 j

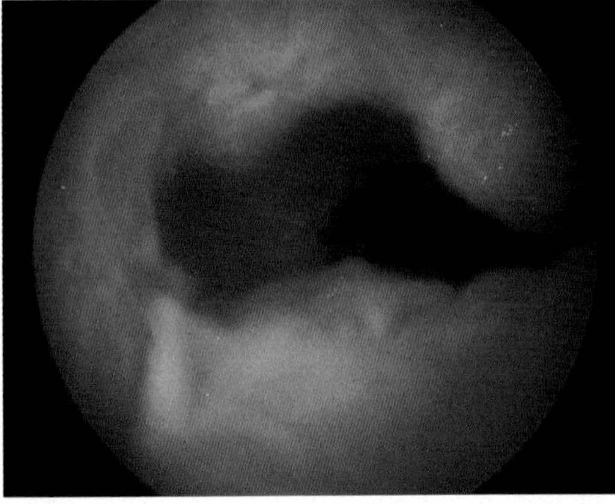
101 k

Fig. 101, h Lesion of the external sphincter with temporary incontinence.
The irregular black figure in the center of the picture is the stump of a median urethra. At 6 o'clock, the verumontanum protrudes like a cone into the unilluminated (and therefore black) fossa; on either side, deep channels have been resected into the median urethra. These defects are more marked than in the preceding Figure because the contours of the urethral stump show. This 73-year-old patient had been partially resected 17 years before. TURP (20 gm net) was performed because of chronic urinary retention (600 cc). The relative incontinence disappeared spontaneously after one year.

Fig. 101, i Lesion of the external sphincter.
The star-shaped deformed lumen of the urethra contracts when the irrigating stream is reduced; the urethra does not close completely, however. The defects (compare Fig. 101, h) continue far into the median urethra. The dome of the urethra is flat; underneath, the median urethra forms a horizontally contracted gap. Here, too, it is noticeable that the lower half of the urethra is actively lifted when closed. The upper half remains mostly passive. The mucosa shows edematous inflammatory changes.

Fig. 101, j Median urethra and view of injured external sphincter.
The resectoscope has been pulled back as far as the transition from the median to the anterior urethra. The ridge of the verumontanum continues to the lower margin of the picture. Even now, the external sphincter does not completely close. The deformed star-shaped lumen of the urethra remains unchanged. At 12 o'clock, the two pillars of the lateral lobes converge approximately at a right angle.

Fig. 101, k Defective external sphincter with incontinence.
The deformed lumen of the urethra is opened by the irrigating stream. The transition from the median to the prostatic urethra can be seen. On both sides, defects from the previous resection are recognizable in the scarred regenerated mucosa. The injured verumontanum is only vaguely visible. The mucosa is edematous and inflamed. The earlier resection, performed by a different surgeon, was only partial and most of the left lateral lobe was not resected. The right lateral lobe was too extensively resected.

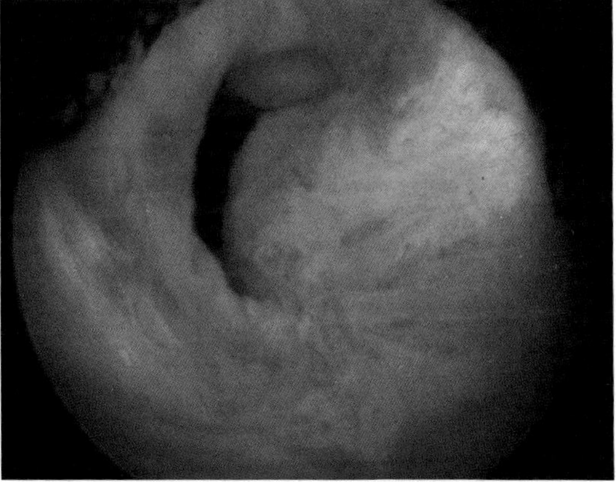
101 l

Fig. 101, l Defective external sphincter with incontinence.
A sickle-shaped defect in the right wall of the median urethra is revealed if the urethroscope is pulled a few centimeters distally toward the median urethra, thus causing the external sphincter to contract. The stump of the median urethra (Fig. 101, k) protrudes like a polyp in the upper angle of the sickle. In the area of the lesion there is chronic inflammation of the mucosa. The Berry surgical procedure failed. The patient won several law suits after three unsuccessful surgical procedures for incontinence.

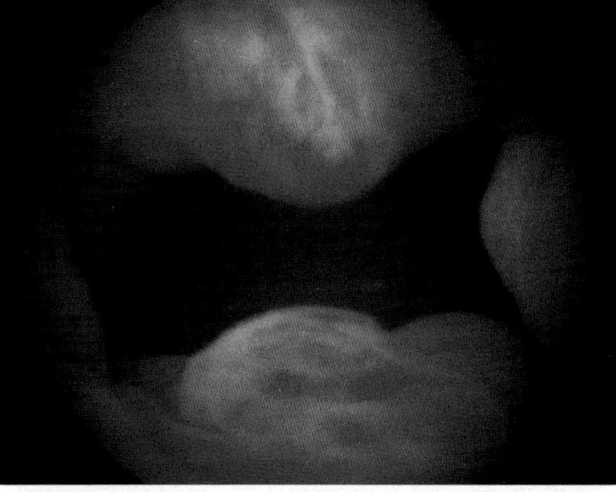
101 m

Fig. 101, m Deformed external sphincter without incontinence.
Urethroscopy shows the situation in the area of the apex of the prostate about one year after TUR. The irrigation opens a transverse lumen of the urethra that is narrowed from above and below. On either side, defects in the area of the sphincter are recognized. The verumontanum is mostly resected. Surprisingly, no incontinence occurred — apparently because the irregular remnants fit into the defects (partial TUR of 35 gm).

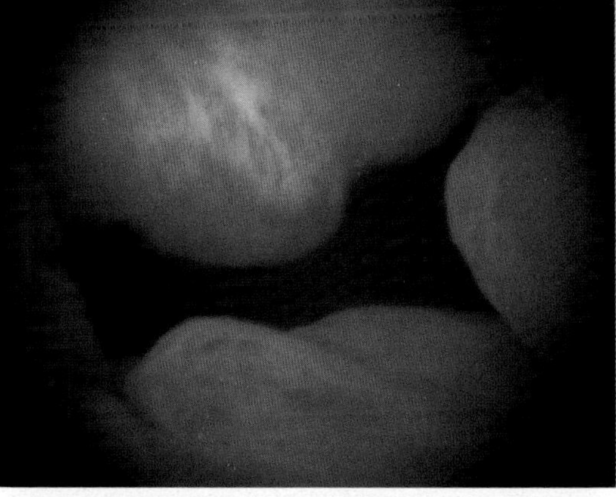
101 n

Fig. 101, n Deformed external sphincter.
At the transition from the median to the prostatic urethra, urethroscopy with a reduced irrigation stream shows a lumen half contracted by the external sphincter at the level of the urogenital diaphragm. The remaining adenomatous nodules on the apex cover the defects in the lumen, thus forming an "H" in the urethra.

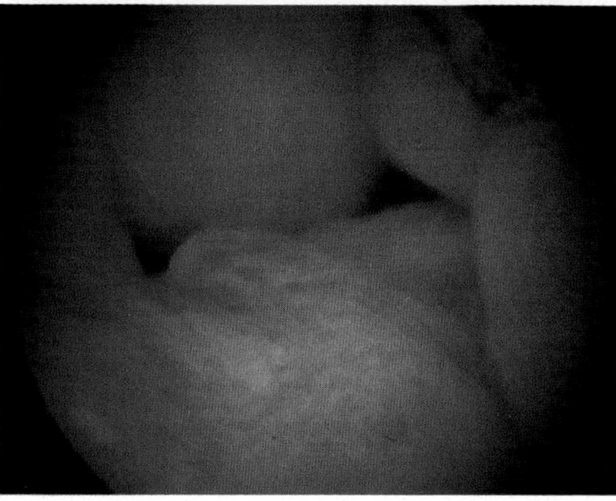
101 o

Fig. 101, o Median urethra with closed deformed internal sphincter.
The cushion-sphaped ridges of the urethra wall contract when the external sphincter closes. Therefore, the channel-shaped defects in the urethral wall fold together. The largely resected verumontanum is irregularly deformed by an adenomatous remnant at the apex and is lifted upward by the contraction of the urogenital diaphragm. Continence is not affected by the channels because these are filled by nodules.

Function of the External Sphincter

Fig. 102, a Column of the lateral lobe four years after TURP (20 gm net in 25 min).
The transition from the middle urethra into the healed prostatic fossa is wide open. The flat, scarcely illuminated bottom of the completely resected fossa is visible behind the opening. The black spot over the rim of the trigone is the entrance to the bladder. In the center, the verumontanum protrudes into the lumen of the urethra. It becomes wider toward the middle urethra, where its fibers continue within the external sphincter to both sides of the middle urethra. A complete TURP always results in a completely rounded urethral lumen (compare Fig. 103,c). Here, columns of the lateral lobes remained. For surgical trainees and in patients with cerebral disease, sparing of columns of the lateral lobes is a necessary measure against incontinence (Fig. 102, b; c).

Fig. 102, b Contraction of the external sphincter.
The urethroscope has now been retracted distally into the middle urethra, and the irrigation has been reduced. Contraction of the sphincter and the urogenital diaphragm lifts the bottom of the middle urethra and pushes the verumontanum up toward the prostatic urethra. This is well demonstrated here. The lumen of the urethra is rounded by the contraction.

Fig. 102, c Sphincter almost closed.
When the urethroscope is retracted farther, the lumen of the fossa forms a sickle over the verumontanum. Both remnants of the lateral lobes meet in a fold at the margin of the picture at 12 o'clock. Here, the prostatic urethra (or fossa, respectively) ends (compare Fig. 85, c). The typical foldings of the middle urethra due to contraction of the urogenital diaphragm are seen:

(1) The lower dorsal half of the tube is lifted actively and the verumontanum with its wedge-shaped process is pushed upward.

(2) The upper ventral part of the urethra is more or less passively compressed from below and is folded longitudinally. The contraction of the loop of muscle and the formation of a cushion are clearly visible.

Fig. 102, d Defect in the right column of the lateral lobe after freezing and radical TUR; no incontinence.
Below, the oblique fibers of the external sphincter meet the verumontanum. The left lateral lobe column (*right*) is well resected. In the right column, however, a large defect like the point of a star is cut at 11 o'clock. To compensate for this fault, a small part of the adenoma has been left beside the verumontanum (*left*).

This 60-year-old uremic patient was first treated with a permanent catheter for seven weeks. Then his prostatic carcinoma ($T_2N_0M_0G_2$) was frozen (4 min) and resected immediately afterward (40 gm net in 40 min). There was no incontinence. Six years later, several carcinomatous nodules had grown in the fossa and at the apex (T_3): cryosurgery with the trocar cryoprobe was repeated four times, freezing for 1 min; then the cryoprobe Special was used three times for 1 min. Orchiectomy, radiation therapy with cobalt (5000 R) followed. Fourteen years later, at the age of 74, the patient had had no recurrence.

Fig. 102, e Compensation of the defect by adenomatous remnant.
The lumen of the urethra is contracted by the external sphincter. The defect (Fig. 102,d) is reduced to a small indentation at 11 o'clock. The gap is closed by the adenomatous remainder (compare Figs. 101–103).

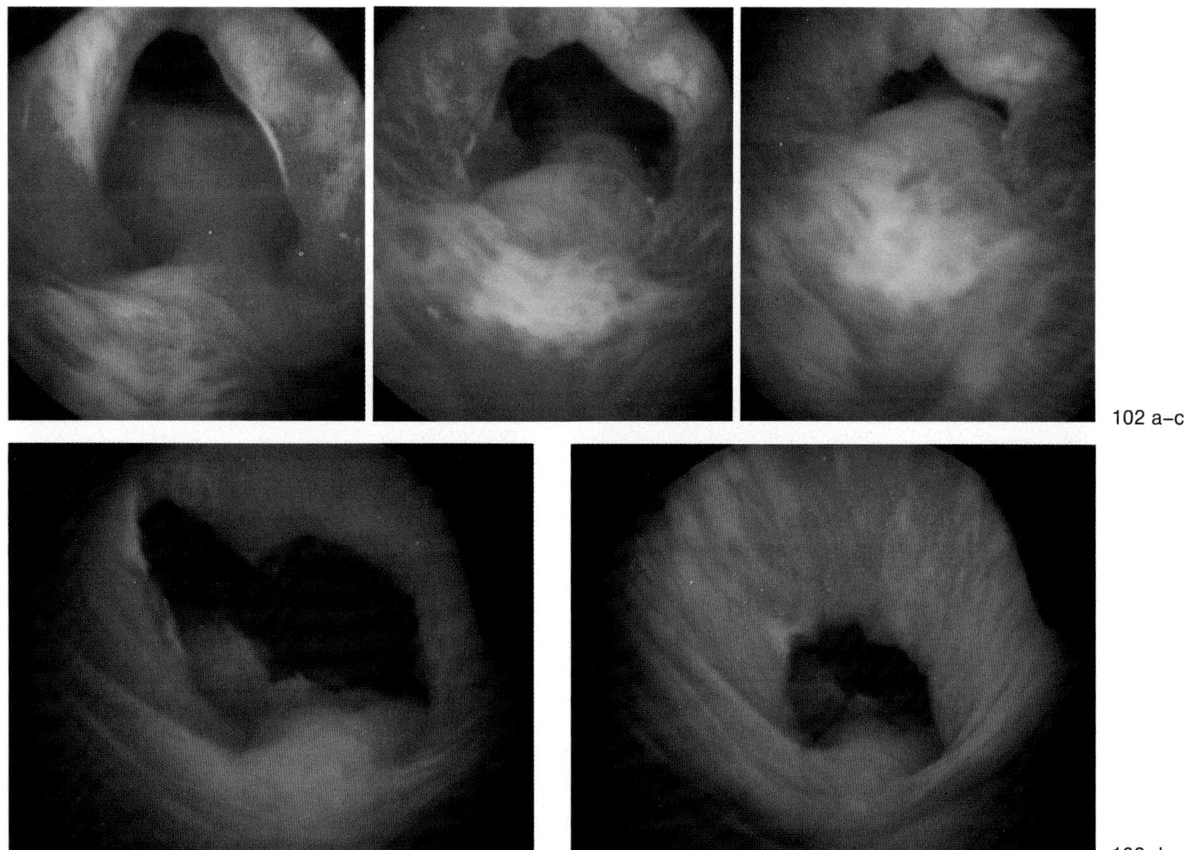

102 a–c

102 d–e

External Sphincter Before and After TURP

Fig. 103, a Opened sphincter mechanism with concretions. Conservatively treated hypertrophy.
The middle urethra is seprated from the prostatic urethra by a circular bulge. The verumontanum rides on this bulge. The adenoma has no marked lateral lobes, and the utriculus is only slightly developed. At the side are the punctate openings of the ejaculatory duct. The concretions (black spots) are small phosphate stones in the excretory ducts. These illustrations compare the external sphincter before the operation (Figs. 103, a and b) with the ureteral stump after TURP (Figs. 103, c and d). After TURP the fossa also is limited by the circular bulge. Therefore, the shape of the urethral stump during (and after) TUR is the most reliable expression of the quality of the operation. Repeated inspections of the internal sphincter and testing of its function therefore are obligatory, together with rectal palpation. These factors are of definite significance for a successful TURP.

Fig. 103, b Closing of the sphincter mechanism.
The verumontanum is actively lifted and drawn into the prostatic urethra by the muscle fibers of the external sphincter, which radiate into the middle urethra. The passive upper circumference of the urethra is plied into longitudinal folds. The bladder is closed from below by the contraction of the urogenital diaphragm, which lifts the urethra together with the verumontanum. The urethra here is not quite closed. Its lumen has the shape of a sickle (compare Fig. 103, d). Comparison with Fig. 103, a explains the mechanism of closure.

Fig. 103, c External sphincter after TURP.
A circular bulge between the middle urethra and prostatic fossa still persists, as it did before TURP (Figs. 103, a and b). The verumontanum projects into the fossa. The prostatic urethra, previously surrounded by the adenoma, has now disappeared completely (TURP, 40 gm net). It has been replaced by the hollow sphere of the fossa, which is well seen by trocar cystoscopy (compare Fig. 107, b) and in the cystogram (see Fig. 55).
The floor of the fossa is faintly illuminated and ends in a horizontal line at the bladder neck (trigone). Above it, the black lumen of the bladder is seen. At 12 o'clock the fold that was formed by the two lateral lobes meeting here still persists. The same result can be achieved with cryosurgery (compare Fig. 182, d).

Fig. 103, d Contracted external sphincter after TURP.
The lumen of the ureteral stump is almost closed. The verumontanum is pushed into the opening from below; the upper, passive part of the urethra is plied into longitudinal folds.

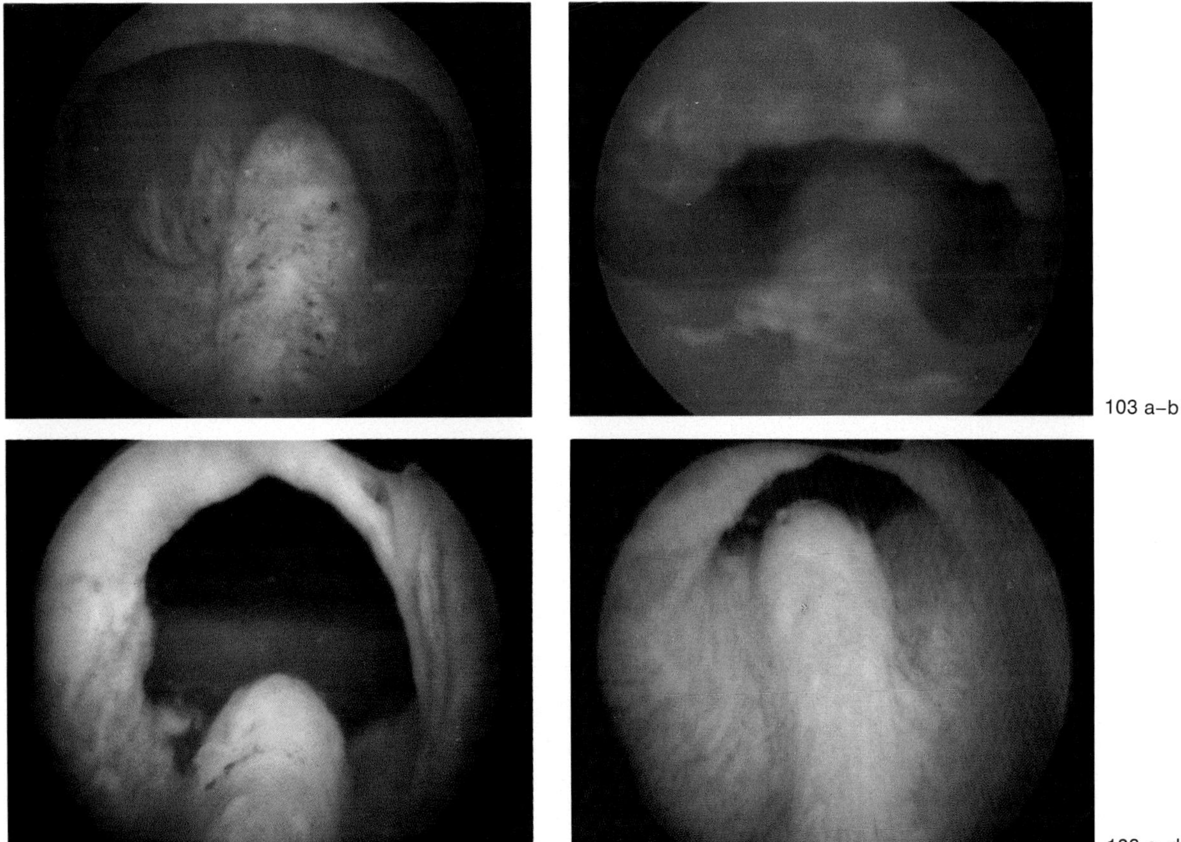

103 a–b

103 c–d

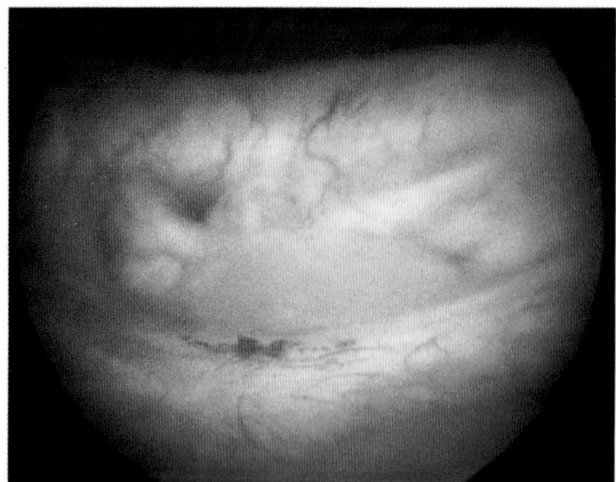
104 a

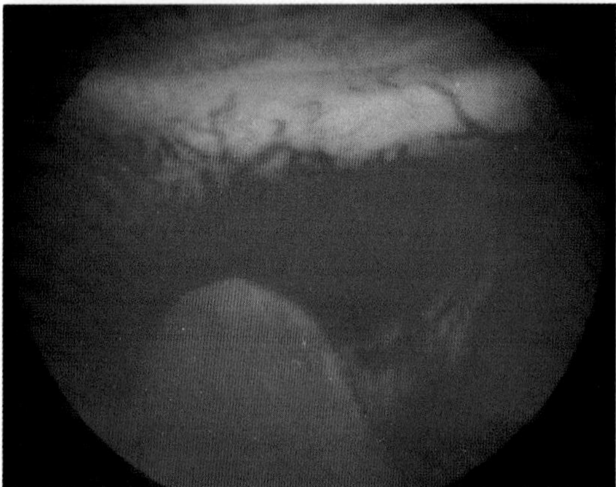
104 b

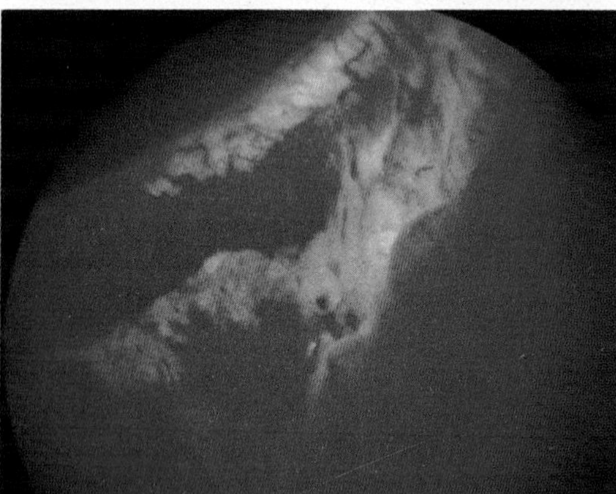
104 c

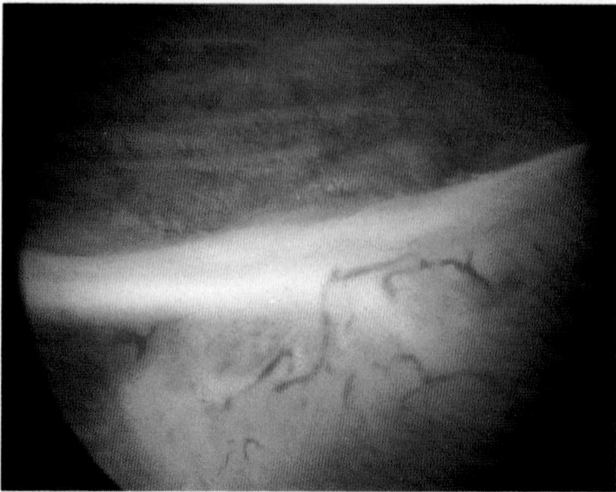
104 d

Bladder Neck and Prostatic Urethra After Transurethral Prostatectomy (TURP 30 gm net in 50 min; performed 19 years previously)

74-year-old patient with TURP and resection of a bladder tumor (T_A). Twelve years later chemical cystitis was diagnosed as due to the cytostatic instillation therapy used to treat the bladder tumors. Following cryosurgery of the mucosal infiltrations, the urologic status remains normal 19 years later; the patient is now 93.

Fig. 104, a Epithelialized fossa after TURP. The cystoscope is drawn back to the point where the prostatic urethra ends; it is then bent downward. The fossa, with its whitish, scarred epithelium, is demonstrated. Regenerated blood vessels run up to the bladder rim. At the center of the picture, the wall of an exposed seminal vesicle bulges up (compare Figs. 94, e and f). At the left, a yellow stone is seen in a sacculation. The trigone was largely resected because the median lobe of the adenoma had grown below the bladder floor (compare Figs. 92, b; 106, a–e).

Fig. 104, b. The prostatic urethra between the verumontanum and the bladder floor is shortened by the view. The untouched verumontanum projects toward the center of the picture; it is isolated completely by TUR. The prostatic fossa itself lies in the shadow of the flashlight, which is situated at the tip of the endoscope. It therefore has an unnatural dark red color. The prostatic fossa is confined by a transverse bar from the bladder (rim of the resected trigone).

Fig. 104, c. A seminal vesicle bulges into the fossa (center of the picture). The fossa here is resected somewhat too deeply. Distally, toward the endoscope, the velvet-like reddish mucosa of the fossa is lighted by a reflected flash. Above, in the re-epithelialized capsule, there are scar blood vessels.

Fig. 104, d. The brightly illuminated bladder neck is confined by a scarred bar, reflecting white light. Above, at the right, the interureteral crest and the orifice are scarcely recognizable. Below, the scarred epithelialized mucosa of the prostatic fossa is seen, together with regenerating vessels.

Comparison of TURP with Cryoprostatectomy

Fig. 105, a Bladder neck with epithelialized prostatic fossa after transurethral prostatectomy.
This view onto the bladder neck and the taut, full bladder (about 400 cc) is made up of five cystoscopic pictures. The epithelialized fossa is inflated to create a hollow sphere. The partially resected trigone is pictured below, as are the slit-shaped ureteral ostia and the posterior bladder wall with its mucosal blood vessels. An air bubble hangs above at the bladder roof. At the right, the wall of the completely resected prostatic urethra is seen (this sector is set more toward the center of the picture). The scar structure of the prostatic fossa is evident. The wide-open internal sphincter has lost its function. A forebladder with a wide connection to the main urinary bladder has formed (compare Fig. 106, b). TURP (40 gm net) and TUR of a bladder papilloma. Sixteen years later, this 63-year-old patient had no abnormal urologic findings.

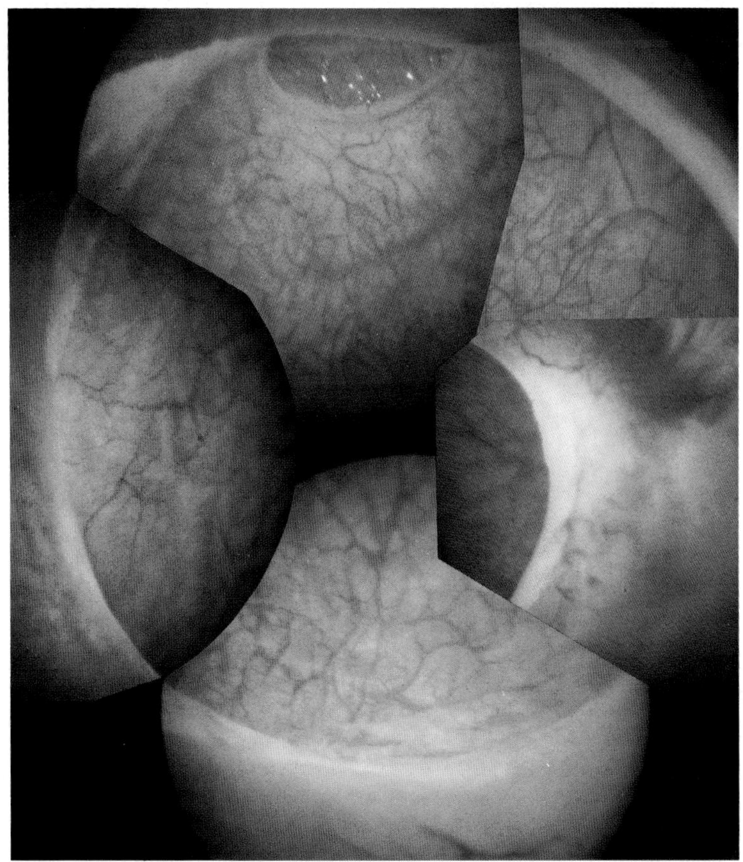

105 a

105 b–c 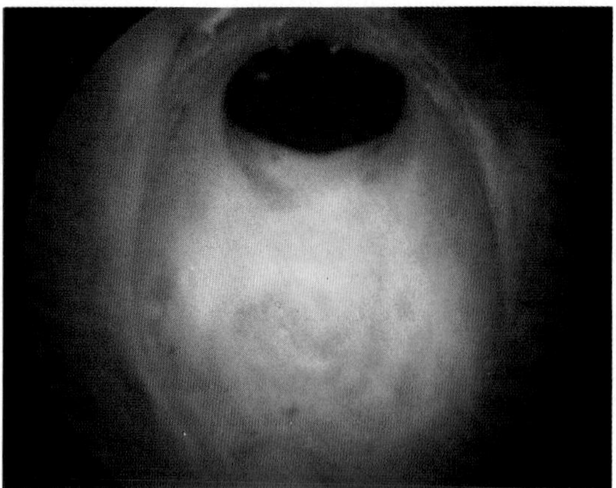 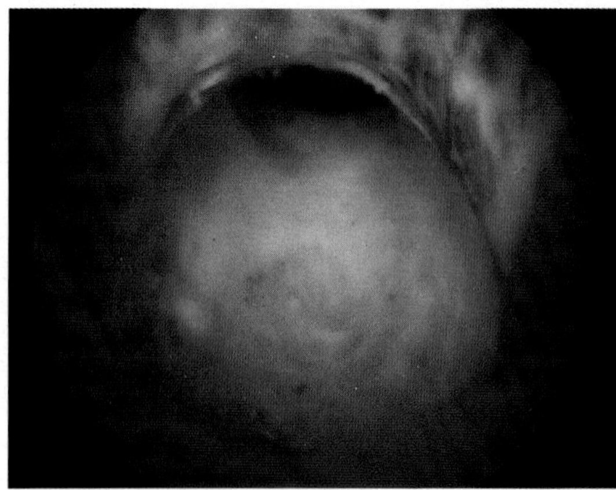

Fig. 105, b Wide-angle urethroscopy of the entire prostatic urethra and the spheric fossa after cryprostatectomy.

At the lower margin of the picture, the knob-shaped colliculus seminalis is seen at 6 o'clock, where the bulge of the external sphincter rises at both sides to form an oval opening to the fossa. Above, the black, round entrance to the bladder formed by the internal sphincter is pictured. Cryoprostatectomy had been performed five years previously (compare Figs. 103, c and d).

Fig. 105, c View from the middle urethra toward the bladder neck.

Below, the rim of the external sphincter covers the view onto the verumontanum. The transition from the middle to the prostatic urethra is recognized by this bulge of the external sphincter. It surrounds the scarred epithelialized fossa. It is covered distally by the mucosa of the middle urethra. Above, the partially disguised opening into the bladder is visible (bladder neck).

Bladder Neck and Seminal Vesicles

Fig. 106, a Spherical seminal vesicle.

The smooth untouched surface of a seminal vesicle is seen at the lower left. It was uncovered during TURP (15 gm net). At the right and above, it is surrounded by muscle fibers of the bladder wall. The trigone above the seminal vesicle was widely resected. It can be resected down to the interureteral crest when a subvesical adenoma or an infiltrating process must be removed. When it is cut too deeply, the connection between the prostatic capsule and the bladder floor is separated. A cleft is formed (compare Figs. 93, a–e). This is also caused by overdistention of the bladder due to high pressure irrigation. This increases the incidence of scarred strictures (over-resection; Figs. 119, h; 120 c–f).

Fig. 106, b Epithelialized seminal vesicle in the prostatic fossa after TURP of a giant adenoma (145 gm net in two sessions).

The epithelium has regenerated over the seminal vesicles. It is remarkable that blood vessels are missing in the region of its pale surface. Behind it, the transition from the prostatic fossa to the bladder neck is indicated by a bulge. Here, the vessels are well regenerated.

In this 61-year-old patient, adenoma remained at the apex after TUR of 110 gm. TUR was repeated (35 gm net) because of formation of residual urine (300 cc). Micturition was then possible with no residual urine. Eleven years later there were no abnormal urologic findings (Fig. 106, c).

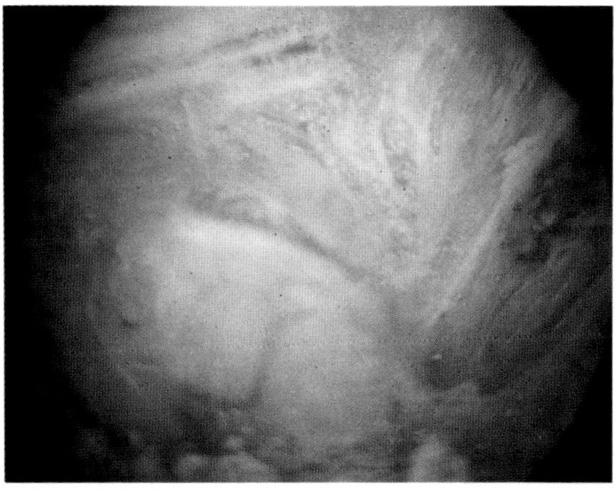

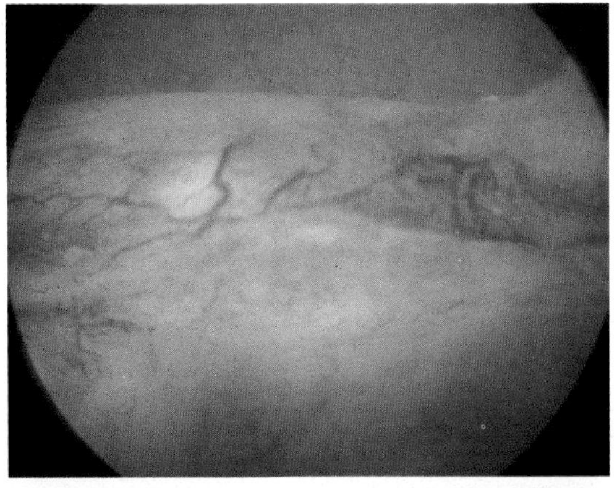

106 a–b

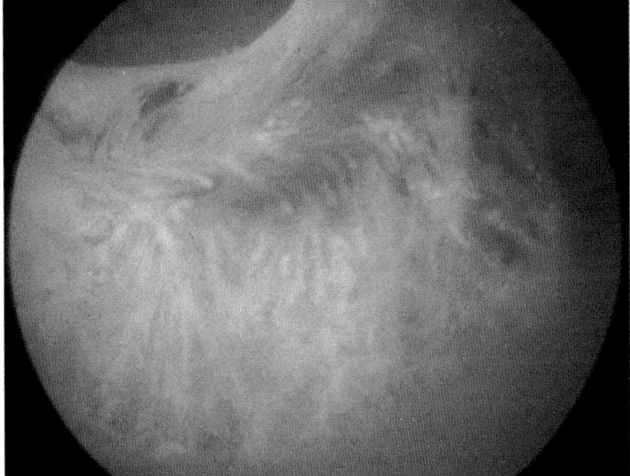

106 c

Fig. 106, c Epithelialized prostatic capsule and bladder neck after TURP.

The structure of the tissue below the regenerated epithelium is well realized in this illustration. Above, the internal sphincter delimits the fossa. The vertically running fibers of the capsule (true prostatic tissue) are well demonstrated. They form the hollow sphere of the totally resected fossa (forebladder). The middle layer of the capsule was resected too deeply at 5 o'clock, exposing the seminal vesicles (Fig. 106, b).

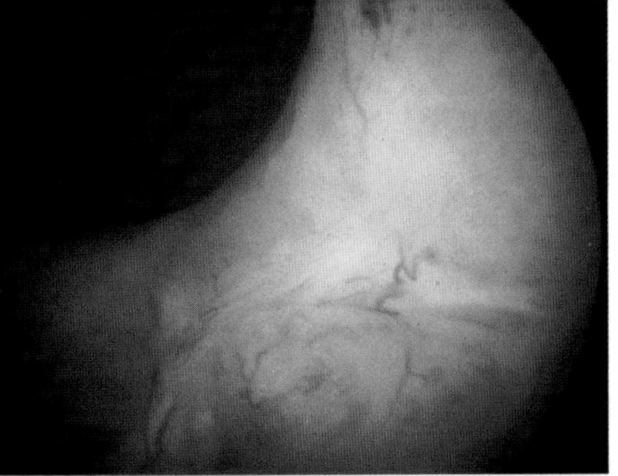

106 d

Fig. 106, d Epithelialized seminal vesicle in the fossa after TURP.

In the prostatic fossa at 5 o'clock (same as Fig. 106, a) a button-like structure is seen that is covered with scarred epithelium and fine vessels. It represents a hypertrophic seminal vesicle. The wide-open, circular bladder neck distinguishes the fossa from the bladder.

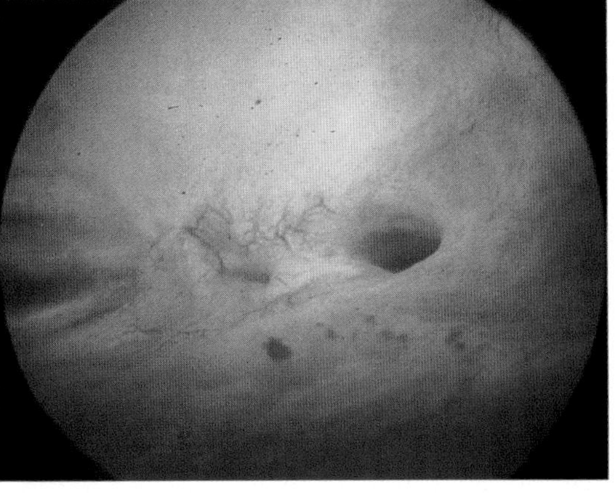

106 e

Fig. 106, e Open seminal vesicle after TURP (50 gm net in 35 min).

The prostatic fossa is covered with regenerated mucosa (below). At the right is the opening of a deep artificial connection between a seminal vesicle and the prostatic urethra. At the left are several folds with scar vessels. The different shades of red of the mucosa result from varying distances from the endovesical flash. The upper part is nearer to the flash and therefore is overexposed; the lower part is more distant and therefore underexposed.

Trocar Cystoscopy in Transurethral Prostatectomy (TUR 50 gm net in 40 min)

Fig. 107, a Prostatic adenoma.
The tumor widens the bladder neck. The spherical lateral lobes are separated from the pluglike median lobe by the Y-shaped urethra. Above, the narrow trigone is shown to be displaced by the median lobe. The left leg of the Y is covered by bleeding caused by catheterization. At the right there is a mucus flake. The cystogram demonstrates clearly the alteration of the bladder floor caused by the adenoma. We emphasize x-ray cystography of the fossa before *and* after TUR, because the quality of the operation may be judged and diagnosis of such later complications, recurrence, stricture, prostatitis, incontinence etc. is facilitated (see Figs. 61; 83, b).

Fig. 107, b Large prostatic fossa.
Three days after TURP, the spherical surface of the wound between the bladder neck and verumontanum is covered with fibrin and some necroses. The elastic bladder neck (internal sphincter) had been stretched to a diameter of 5 cm by the adenoma. The 20 Fr Mercier catheter appears from the urethral stump at the apex.

Fig. 107, c Prostatic fossa two weeks later.
The prostatic fossa has shrunk to about half its previous size. Necroses already are shedding, and the apex has begun to epithelialize. The colliculus seminalis can be identified below as a small knob. The interureteral crest was cut during TUR. The ureteral orifices are situated on both sides of the defect. The right one (at the left) carries an inflammatory nodule.

Fig. 107, d Prostatic fossa one month later.
The diameter of the fossa is reduced to 2 cm; its epithelium was largely regenerated. The catheter was introduced for demonstration. The defect of the interureteral crest is still recognized. The mucosa is somewhat inflamed at the rim of the fossa; the distribution of vessels in the bladder is normal.

Fig. 107, e Healed bladder neck.
Two months later, healing is finished. The bladder neck is not entirely closed, so that the verumontanum can be verified in the depth of the prostatic urethra. The vascularization of the mucosa at the bladder floor is still somewhat increased. The right ureteral orifice expelled a bluish colored urine jet. The left orifice is closed. Anatomy of the bladder neck is almost restored.

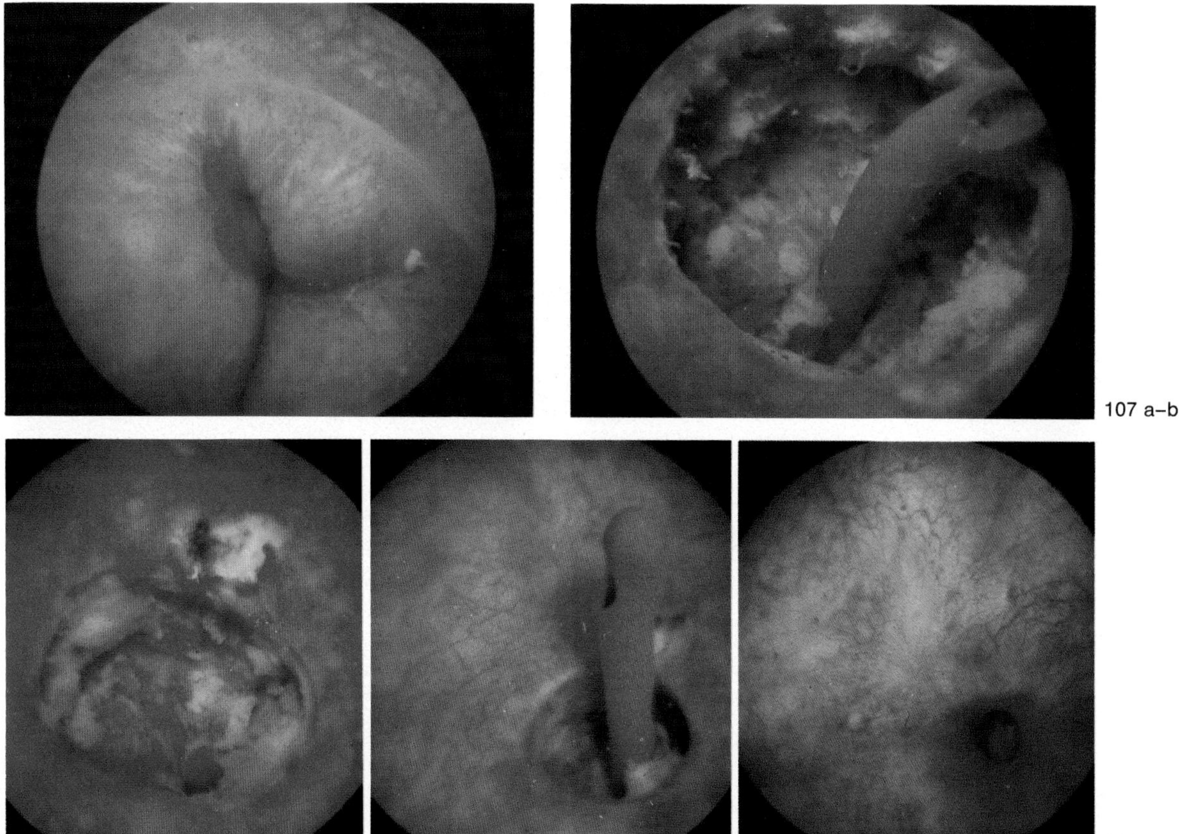

107 a–b

107 c–e

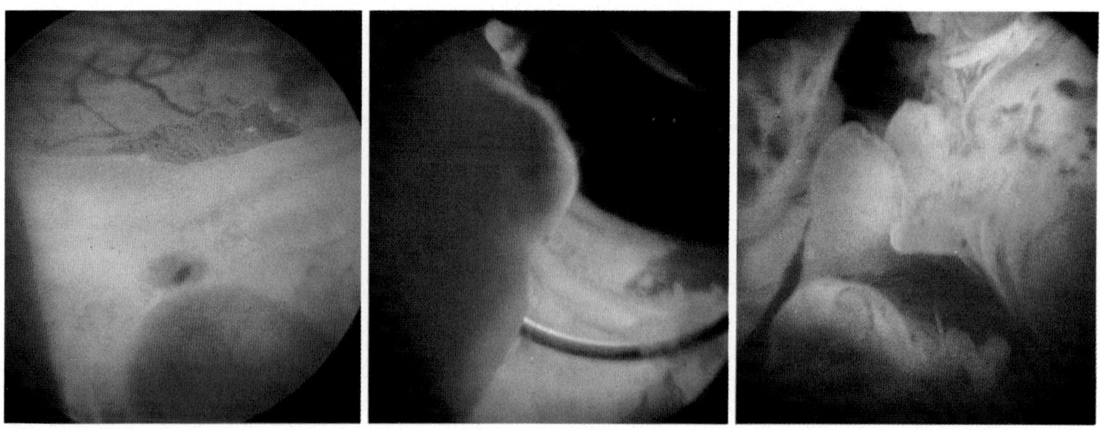
108 a–c

Partial TUR of Prostatic Hypertrophy (Urethroscopy)

Fig. 108, a Resected ejaculatory duct after subtotal TUR (30 gm net).
Above the verumontanum (below), the prostatic fossa spreads. It is covered with whitish scarred epithelium and is delimited by an oblique bar. Directly above the verumontanum, a cut ejaculatory duct is seen as a round defect. The pillar of the right lateral lobe has been left here. Inflammatory pseudopapillomas are situated at the transition from the fossa to the bladder mucosa (chronic urinary infection).

Fig. 108, b Adenomatous remnants after partial TUR.
At the left, a large nodule, a remnant of the right lateral lobe, projects into the fossa. The floor of the fossa is completely resected and is covered with pale epithelium. Near the trigone there is a small mucosal bleeder. The cutting loop of the resectoscope is hooked onto the node (TURP 60 gm net in 50 min). Parts of the adenoma remain (partial TUR) when the bladder neck is resected too deeply at 7 o'clock and the lateral lobes are undermined (Fig. 101, c). Secondary TUR is relatively easy, because the topography of the fossa does not change during TUR: the adenomatous nodes are indurated and therefore easy to cut. In secondary resection, mistakes are recognized and easily corrected.

Fig. 108, c Adenomatous remnants after partial TUR.
Remnants of the left lateral lobe are covered with an edematous, inflamed mucosa. We call such mucosal growths due to chronic inflammation "pseudopapillomas." They cause erythruria and sometimes hematuria and chronic urinary infection. Most do not require treatment. When they cause complaints they are easily resected transurethrally or treated by cryosurgery. The bluish polyp over the verumontanum is composed of edematous mucosa (compare Fig. 137). At its side there is a small bleeder caused by mechanical irritation.

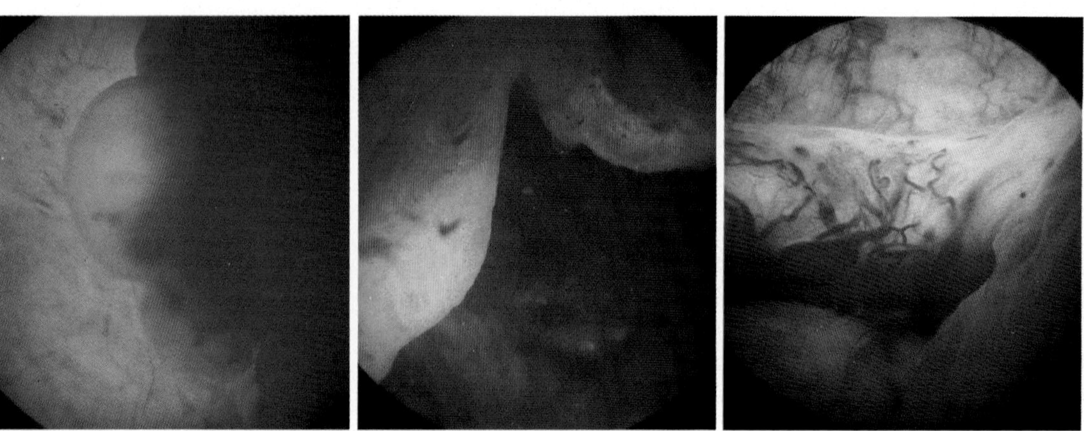
108 d–f

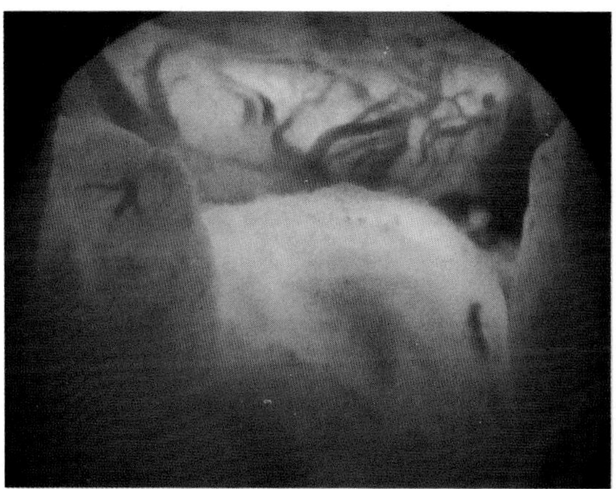

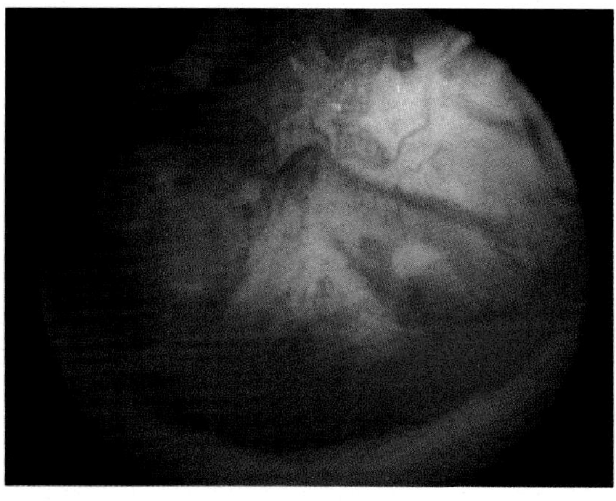

108 g–h

Fig. 108, d Adenomatous remnant after partial TUR.
The right side of the picture is filled by a large spherical adenomatous remnant of the left lateral lobe. It projects far into the lumen of the prostatic urethra. Its mucosa is edematous and diffusely reddened by inflammation (TURP 60 gm net).

Fig. 108, e Adenomatous remnants.
Bladder neck and anterior prostatic fossa. Large, spherical adenomatous remnants hang down from above. Below, the dark red posterior bladder wall is pictured (underexposed). At 12 o'clock the remnants meet and form the typical fold (compare Figs. 83, b; 85, b and c; 102, b and c) that connects the internal and external sphincters. Its end determines the margin of the adenoma at 12 o'clock near the external sphincter at the apex as reliably as does the verumontanum at 6 o'clock; i.e., the remnants of the lateral lobes should be resected until this fold is completely replaced by the round shape of the external sphincter (compare Fig. 103, c). In the upper prostatic fossa, all tissue hanging into the lumen is resected. The capsule itself (true prostatic tissue) is always concave like a hollow sphere. Result after four partial TURs in ten years in a 79-year-old patient; final TURP (90 gm net in 60 min).

Fig. 108, f Bar-like adenomatous remnant.
A part of the middle lobe is left, forming a bar (typical mistake of a beginner). It is connected with larger remnants of the lateral lobes. The bar is covered with scarred epithelium and regenerating blood vessels. The trigone is pictured above (compare Fig. 108, g).

Fig. 108, g Adenomatous remnants.
In the center of the picture, a large adenomatous node is seen on the floor of the fossa, below the bar described above. Nodes of the lateral lobes remained at both sides. TUR was performed mainly in the fossa near the bladder. The distal adenoma at the apex remained almost untouched (Fig. 108, f). The control knob at the resectoscope, rectal palpation (rectal sheath) and low pressure irrigation are of great assistance in safely resecting adenoma at the apex.

Fig. 108, h Undermined lateral lobes.
The external sphincter below is completely resected so that it is free of adenoma. The round lumen of the prostatic fossa is filled with two large spherical adenomatous remnants of different sizes whose mucosa is changed by inflammation. Their base is in the upper third of the fossa; their lower portions more or less float in the fossa. They meet in the middle urethra like two cushions. Fifteen years previously a TUR was done; now TURP of 60 gm net in 55 min was performed.

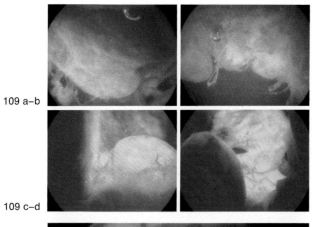

Palliative TUR of Prostatic Carcinomas
(Stage $T_4N_2M_1G_3$)

109 a–b

109 c–d

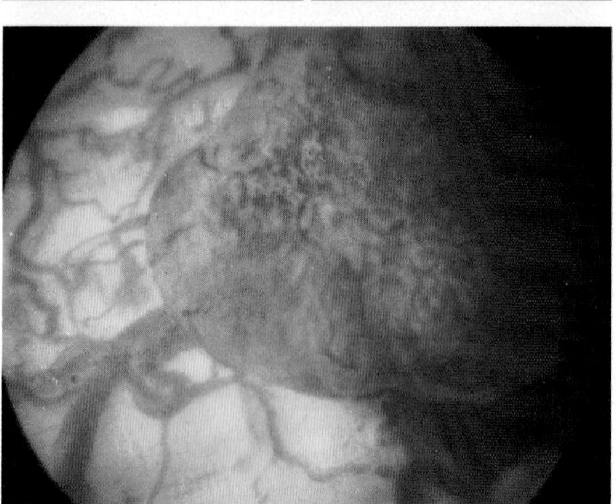

109 e

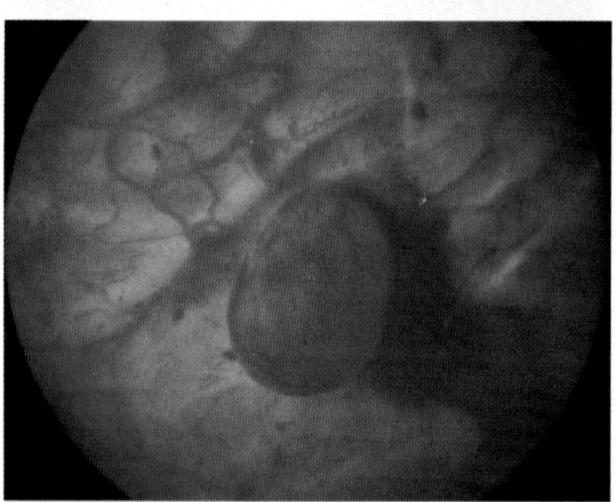

109 f

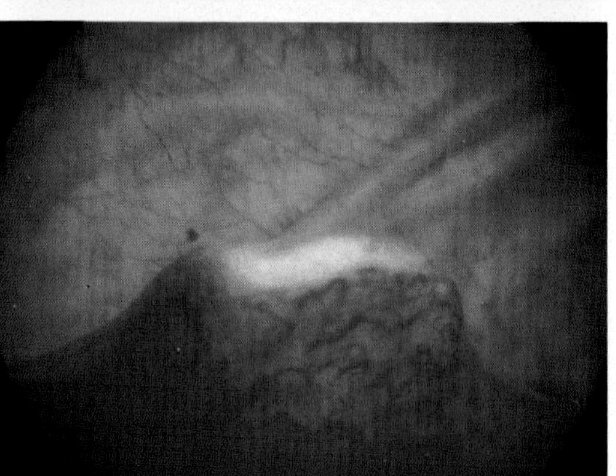

109 g

Fig. 109, a–d. Infiltration of the bladder neck.
This series, which demonstrates the rim of the bladder neck, is composed of four single pictures as seen through the urethrocystoscope. Two large prominent carcinomatous nodes project into the trigone (c, d). The node at the right lies in the shadow of the flash, whereas the left node is directly illuminated. Its carcinomatous tissue shines through the thin, stretched mucosa. In the background, behind the right node, the opening of a diverticulum is seen (d). At the bladder neck (left in c), further infiltration is recognized. Above, the fossa is irregularly infiltrated by cancer; a larger node has invaded the bladder wall (a, b).

Fig. 109, e Metastatic node with broad base on the lateral bladder wall.
The distended mucosa over the tumorous node is injected with atypical blood vessels. The bladder mucosa has a normal color, but its vessels are dilated owing to shrinkage of the bladder wall.

Fig. 109, f Polypoid metastasis.
The bean-shaped tumor hangs on its pedicle from the posterior bladder wall. Its shadow falls to the right onto the slightly trabeculated bladder mucosa with dilated vessels (still photograph taken from a movie; same as Fig. 95, a).

Fig. 109, g Infiltration over the left ureteral orifice.
A tumorous node rises from below. Its broad side lies in the shadow of the flash and carries atypical blood vessels. Its peak is covered with white mucosa that is poor in blood vessels. In the background the bladder wall is seen with oblique trabeculation. The bladder floor is well developed; therefore, it can be resected deep into the perivesical space without risk. The intramural part of the ureter is identified by its mucosal tunnel (compare Fig. 97, a). Attempts at radical TUR of such infiltrations are recommended when staging is more favorable than in this case.

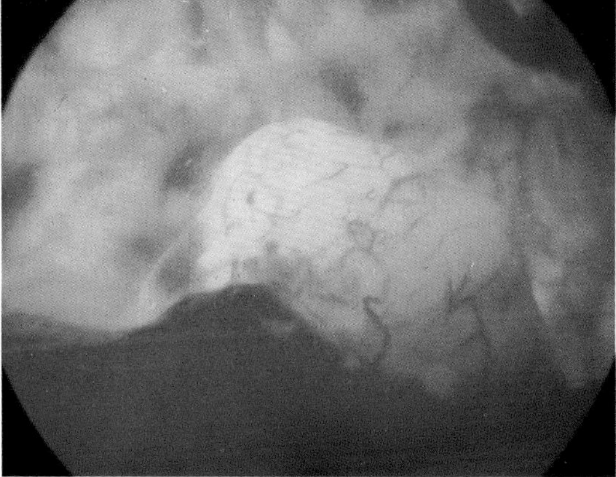
109 h

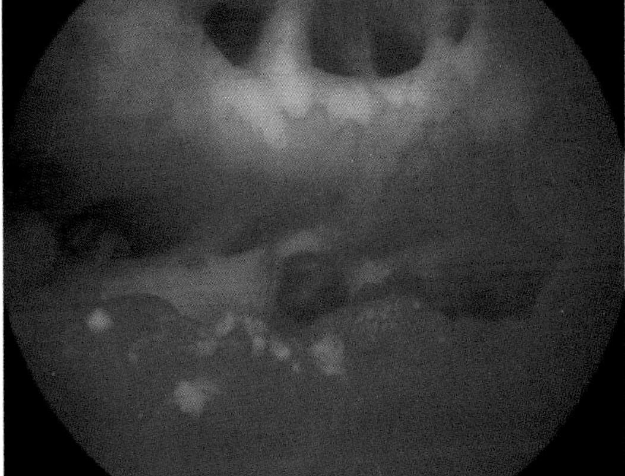
109 i

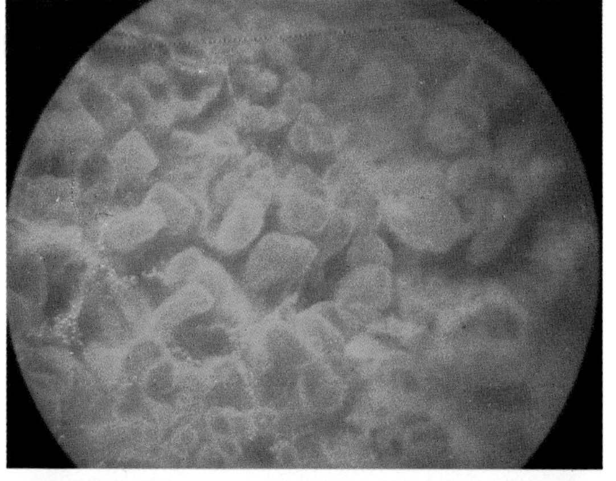
109 j

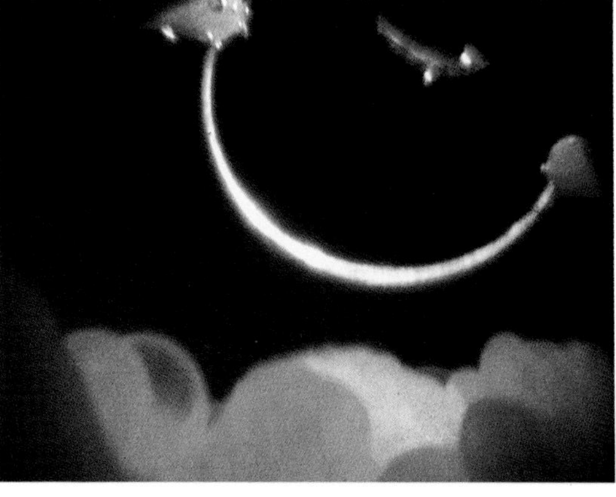
109 k

Fig. 109, h Metastasis over the left orifice.
The white, smooth tumorous node (stage $T_3N_xM_0$) has compressed the left ureteral orifice. This 72-year-old patient had been resected 11 years previously and been treated with 100 mg estradiol per month. Now, subradical TUR (35 gm net) was performed to relieve high residual urine. Three years later the patient died of generalized metastatic disease. Findings by rectal palpation were negative until then; micturition caused no complaints.

Fig. 109, i "Infiltrative cystitis" of the trigone (stage $T_4N_2M_1G_2$).
The mucosa is deformed (below) and infiltrated with white nodules that shine through the mucosa like tubercula. At the right, the bladder neck is infiltrated. On the bladder floor are some small oxalate stones. Above, the bladder is seen with trabecula and pseudodiverticula. Palliative TUR (60 gm net) was performed without success. Death occurred six months later.

Fig. 109, j "Infiltrative cystitis." (Erroneous diagnosis: "Prostatic cancer with shrinking bladder.")
The mucosa is swollen with edema; it has lost its vascular network. Correct diagnosis: Pseudopapillomas due to bladder stones.
This 77-year-old patient had been treated elsewhere for eight years with estrogens following the diagnosis of prostatic cancer. There is massive urinary infection without residual urine. Rectally, a medium-large but not hard prostate is palpated. The excretory urogram reveals prevesically dilated ureters, bladder stones and a small spherical bladder. At first, optic litholapaxy of five urate stones was performed, followed by TUR (45 gm net prostatic tissue in 50 min). Histologic study revealed an adenoma with chronic inflammation. At 82 years the patient died after a stroke. He had no urologic complaints; the urine was normal, there was no residual urine and rectal palpation also was normal.

Fig. 109, k Palliative TUR (60 gm net; stage T_0).
The mucosa of the trigone is edematously infiltrated. The cutting loop is fully extended and is set behind the bar for the first cut.

Subradical and Radical TUR of the Prostatic Carcinoma

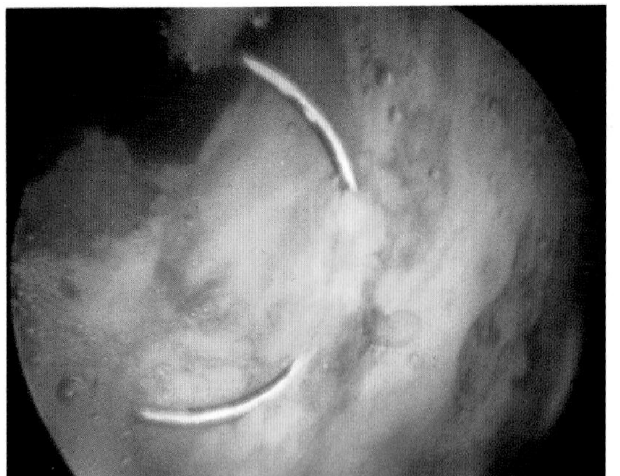

110 a

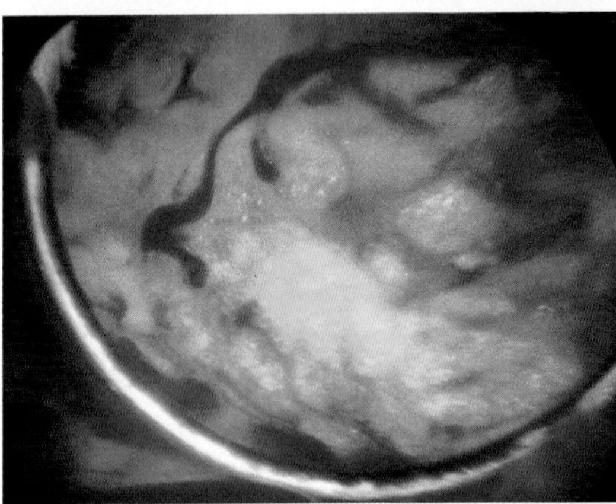

110 b

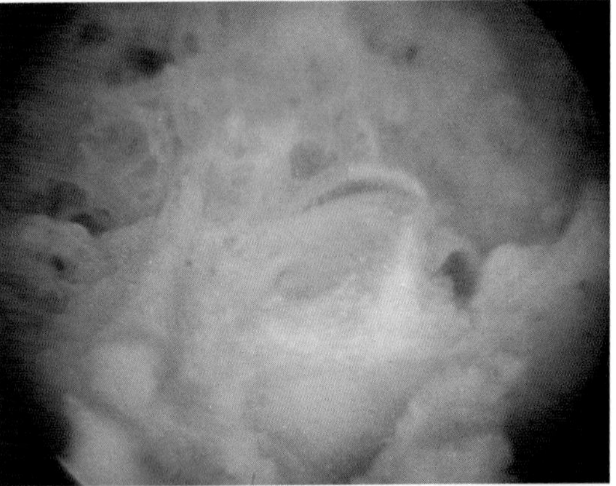

110 c

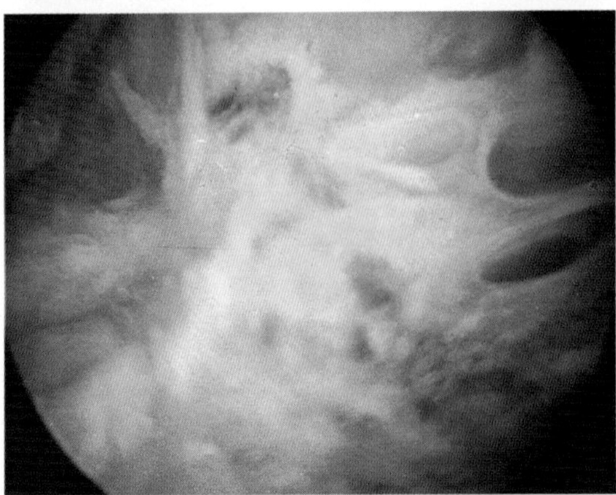

110 d

In this 71-year-old patient with hematuria, TUR of 50 gm in 20 min was performed. Two years later, a hard infiltration was frozen twice for 30 sec (repeated freezing). Cytologic examination following biopsy revealed Group V (Papanicolaou). Treatment was continued with cobalt irradiation (5000 R). Six years after the first operation, neither a prostate nor an infiltration was felt rectally. Excretory urogram: normal findings; large prostatic fossa. Urine and serum phosphatases are normal. No nycturia; patient voiding three times per day.

Fig. 110, a Subradial TUR in prostatic cancer (65 gm net in 55 min; stage $T_3N_0M_0G_2$).

The left side of the prostatic fossa is extensively resected. The cutting loop is inserted into the superficial capsule for cutting at three o'clock. The internal sphincter is seen at the left. Distally, at the right of the loop, there is amorphous tumorous tissue. TUR is continued until no more tumor is found.

Fig. 110, b Prostatic capsule infiltrated by cancer.

Cutting at the floor of the fossa has exposed nodular tumorous tissue with a structure similar to fatty tissue. In between, small veins are bleeding. At the upper left, true prostatic tissue, colored blue by indigo carmine, is recognized. With low pressure irrigation resection can be continued without risk until the entire tumor has been removed.

Fig. 110, c Radical TUR of prostatic cancer.

The right side of the infiltrated prostatic capsule is completely resected. The fossa is now delimited by the true fibrous capsule and the soft connective tissue of the periprostatic space (center). Bleeding of this tissue is negligible. It is colored blue by indigo carmine for better identification (see p. 20).

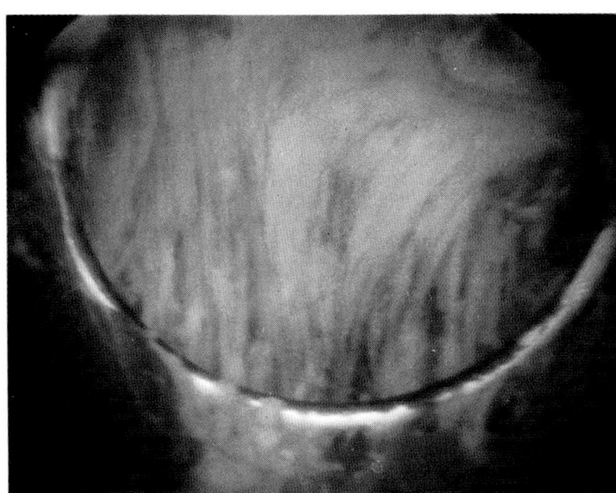

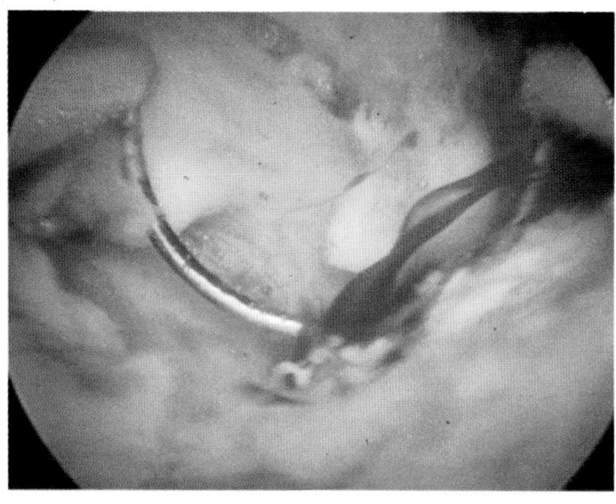

110 e–f

Fig. 110, d Periprostatic tissue exposed by radical TUR.
The periprostatic tissue has a yellow color. Between 1 and 4 o'clock, the fibers of the true prostatic capsule are recognized; they enclose hollow spaces, reminding one of vessels. Physiologic low pressure irrigation (see p. 25) prevents dangerous irrigant absorption (water intoxication syndrome).

Fig. 110, e Rectal muscle below the prostatic fossa after radical TUR.
At the floor of the fossa, longitudinal fibers of the outer muscle layer of the rectum are exposed. For better differentiation they are colored blue (indigo carmine). Complete resection of the capsule is possible, because the elastic wall of the rectum evades the cut. However, the rectal wall should not be pressed against the cutting loop by the finger, because then it is easily perforated (compare Figs. 94, g and 95, a). Even more extensive areas of the rectum can be exposed. The cutting loop is inserted into the distal stump of the capsule, which resembles the prostatic bar (Fig. 110, a).

Fig. 110, f Infiltrated suspicious prostatic capsule with bleeder.
The structure of the deep capsule is irregular. The cutting loop coagulates an arterial bleeder. In tumorous tissue, especially in the adenoma, the stump of the vessel retracts, thus rendering coagulation more difficult. Only in the sound capsule it is easily coagulated. When the capsule is either resected totally or perforated, the vessel must be sought in the stump of the capsule, not in the poorly vascularized periprostatic tissue. TURP of 50 gm net in 50 min. Histology revealed adenoma with chronic inflammation; cytologic examination of a biopsy of the periphery of the capsule revealed grade I (Papanicolaou).

Periprostatic Tissue Around an Atrophic Capsule (TURP of 70 gm net in 60 min)

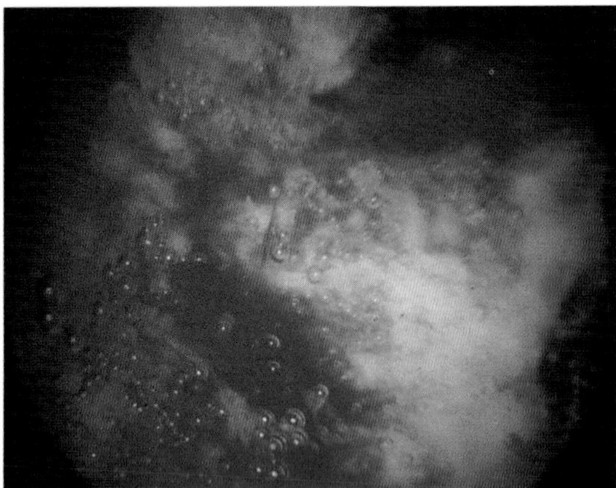

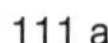

111 a

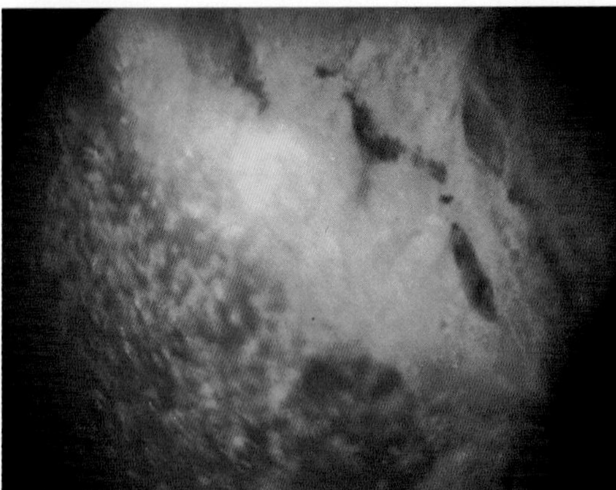

111 b

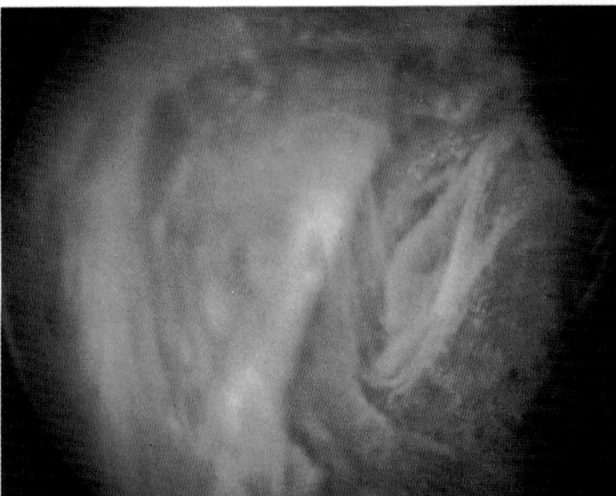

111 c

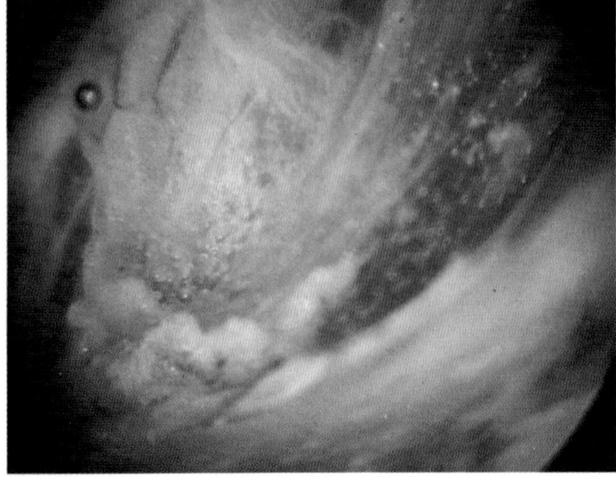

111 d

Fig. 111, a

The overdistended capsule (true prostatic tissue) has become atrophic following unintentional resection. The tissue is indurated by leukocytic infiltration and has a whitish color (typical aspect at the right). The tissue structures are lost. It bleeds diffusely. Small air bubbles tend to cling to this tissue. At the margin of the picture at 3 o'clock, the tissue has been coagulated. At 12 o'clock above there is an arterial bleeder. Its spray drifts off to the right; the blood is flushed toward the bladder by the irrigation (suprapubic trocar). The risks of total resection of the capsule are easily controlled by low pressure irrigation.

Fig. 111, b

At the upper right the resected stump of the prostatic capsule (true prostatic tissue) can be recognized. The line between 5 and 11 o'clock marks the transition into jellied periprostatic tissue. In this case, the capsule was mistaken for adenomatous tissue owing to loss of structure by inflammatory infiltration. Only the "perforation" into periprostatic tissue made the error apparent. This can be avoided when specific properties of the capsule (e.g., floating of the wall, difficulty in cutting the capsular tissue, thickness felt between the finger in the rectum and the cutting loop) are observed.

Fig. 111, c

At the right of the fossa the capsule is altered by inflammation. Here, a carcinomatous infiltration is suspected and the prostatic capsule therefore is cut in layers until periprostatic tissue appears between 3 and 5 o'clock. At the left, the fibers of the capsule are arranged in vertical layers; in the superficial layer they are close together (superficial and middle capsule). Toward the right, they become more and more loose (deep and fibrous capsule); between 3 and 5 o'clock, jellied periprostatic tissue appears.

Fig. 111, d

Extended resection of the left lateral wall of the capsule. The white stump of the fibrous capsule appears below. It runs into reddish periprostatic tissue above, which is covered with small air bubbles. In the upper center, part of the fibrous capsule still remains like a veil over the periprostatic tissue. In the background, the longitudinal fibers of the levator ani muscle can be seen shining through. Low pressure irrigation has prevented infiltration of the tissue with irrigant (compare Fig. 94, a).

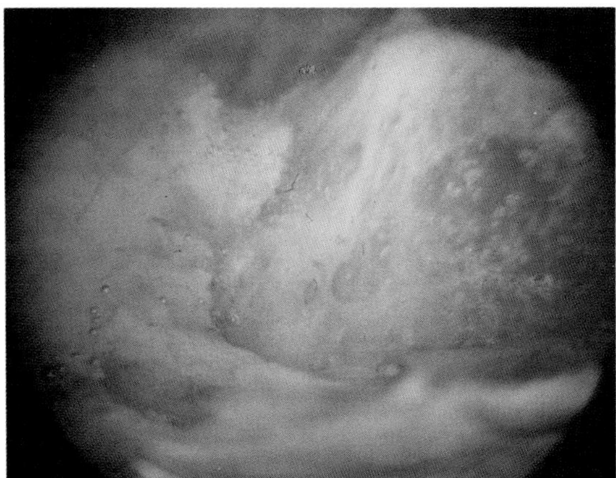

112

Prostatic Fossa After Combined Cryosurgery and TURP with High Pressure Irrigation

Fig. 112

This large prostatic adenoma was frozen in order to test the now obsolete blind technique of cryosurgery. Four weeks later, transurethral prostatectomy was performed. At the end of TUR it was realized (as illustrated here) that, mainly at the left, the prostate had been resected down into periprostatic tissue. Below, some oblique fibers of the fibrous capsule remain. Above, periprostatic tissue projects into the fossa; it has been jellied by infiltration of irrigant that resulted from the use of unphysiologic high pressure irrigation during TUR.

The combination of cryosurgery followed by TUR about eight weeks later is restricted to high-risk patients. In about 90 per cent of cases, however, cryosurgery alone has such a good result that supplementary TUR is superfluous. On the other hand, secondary TUR is an easy procedure because the remaining adenoma has been indurated by freezing. This reduces the time of TUR considerably (80 gm in 55 min).

Radical TUR of a Prostatic Carcinoma (50 gm net in 40 min); stage $T_3N_xM_0G_3$ (compare Fig. 94, c)

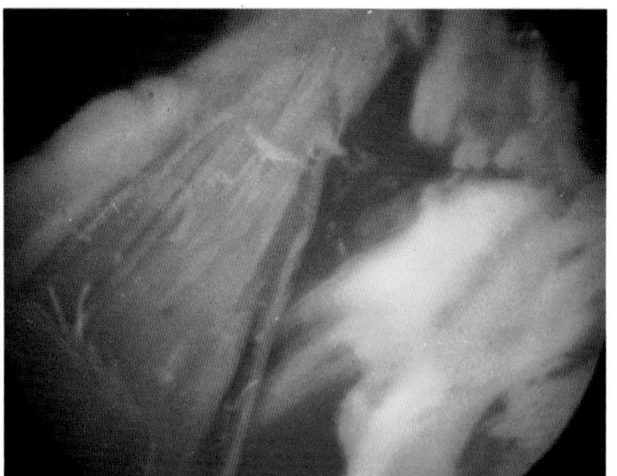

113 a

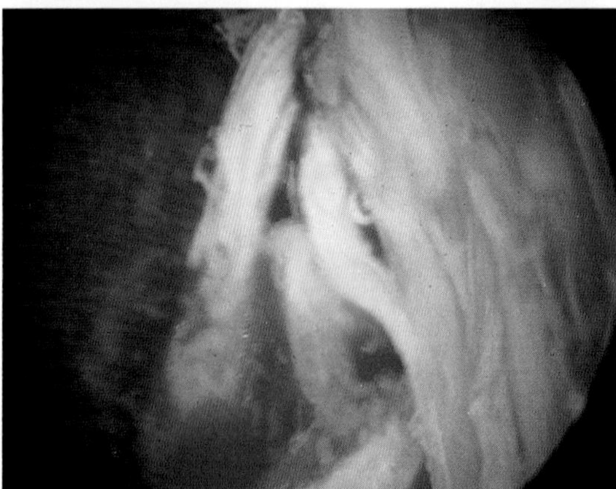

113 b

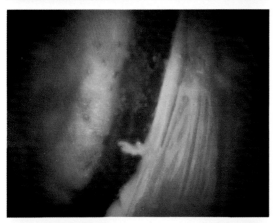

113 c

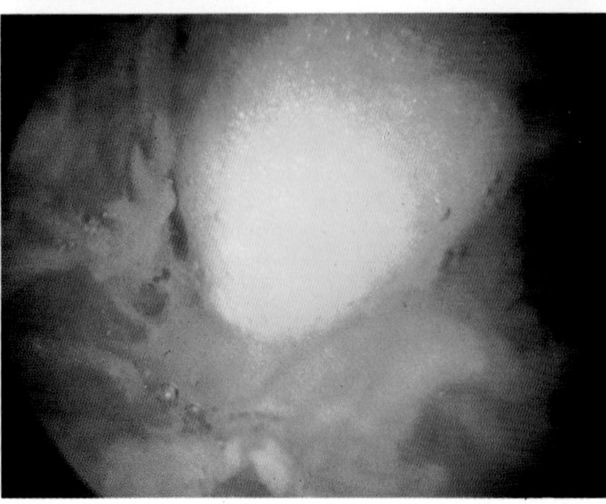

113 d

Fig. 113, a Prostatic fossa.
Here, a defect of the prostatic capsule is demonstrated that reaches far into the periprostatic space. A flesh-colored strip of the levator ani muscle with longitudinal fibers runs from 8 to 11 o'clock at the left. At the right, some prostatic tissue remains.

For subsequent radical resection of a carcinomatous infiltration, both low pressure irrigation and the three-dimensional orientation given by the finger in the rectum are necessary. Rectal palpation often is more reliable than direct vision. Thus, infiltrations over the rectum, especially when they are close to the external sphincter, are best resected over the rectal finger.

Fig. 113, b Periprostatic space.
The lateral wall of the fossa is seen after TUR of the prostatic capsule. At the right, long coarse fibers of the levator ani muscle run upward; at the left, watery infiltrated periprostatic tissue is seen. The muscle contracts upon electric irritation and lifts the fossa with a jerk. This is avoided by using the so-called "stutter-cutting" with reduced current.

Fig. 113, c Muscles of the pelvic floor.
Here, the prostatic capsule is resected totally in the region of the distal fossa (at the apex). Besides the tight muscle of the pelvic floor and the dark cleft, only periprostatic fatty tissue is seen (at the left).

Fig. 113, d Periprostatic fatty tissue.
The prostatic capsule is completely resected above. A large yellow fatty globe projects from the periprostatic space. Fatty tissue has different structures and colors, depending on the kind of infiltration (inflammation, cancer, water) and its content of connective tissue. A glimmering surface and a golden-yellow color are typical (compare Fig. 94, c), although both are not obligatory. When there is doubt, a small chip is cut and examined macroscopically with eye and finger.

Fig. 113, e Deep capsule.
Only a thin layer of the deep capsule remains. Its fine yellowish fibers run vertically over the illustration. Between them, periprostatic tissue shines through. The cancer is resected macroscopically down into sound tissue. This procedure is supported by the postoperative recovery. The structure of the tissue is not destroyed with low pressure irrigation. Thus, it may be readily differentiated (compare Fig. 91, a)

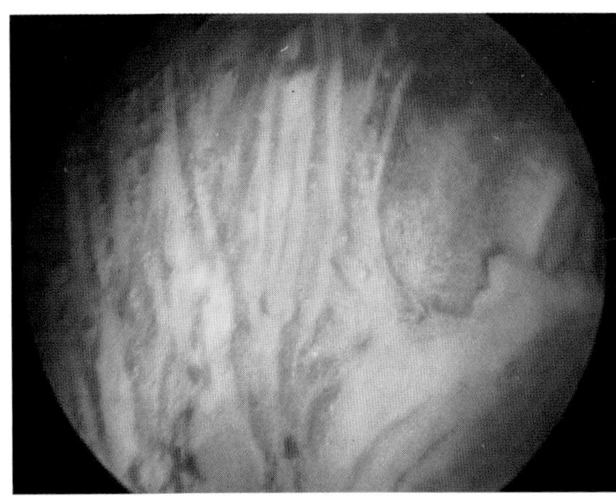
113 e

Fig. 114 Apex during TURP.
The stump of the resected prostatic capsule arises at the lower left. It is covered with black pigment. Toward the upper right it passes into periprostatic fatty tissue.
TURP of 60 gm net in 50 min. The capsule was resected too deep at the apex. Postoperative bladder atony developed: 800 cc of residual urine was present on the third postoperative day, 600 cc on the fifth and 50 cc on the sixth. Cystography showed a large, round subvesical excavation following TUR. Seven years later the patient was well. He urinated twice at night and three to four times during the day with a strong stream.

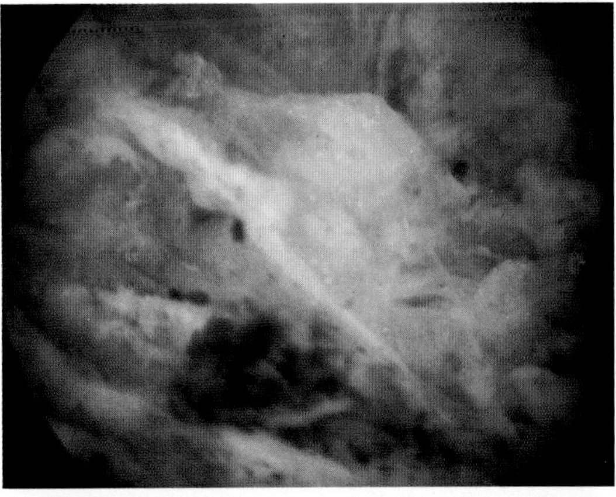
114

Fig. 115 Pigmented prostatic capsule due to siderosis.
At the left, tissue pigmented with colors ranging from brown to black is exposed (old hemorrhage into the capsule). Periprostatic tissue is at the right. Capsule still remained at the apex (compare Fig. 114).

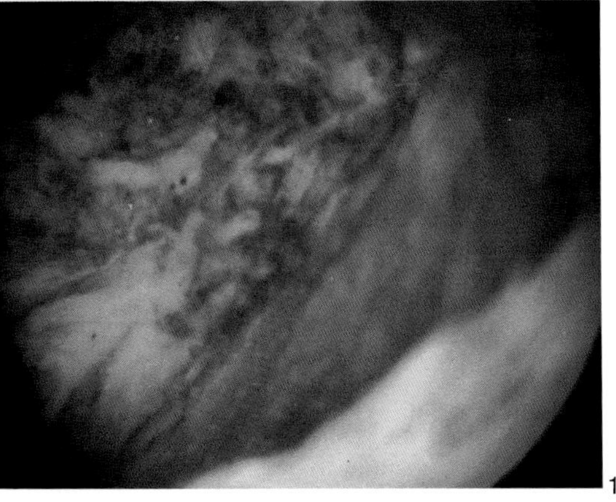
115

Perforation of the Prostatic Fossa into the Rectum

116 a

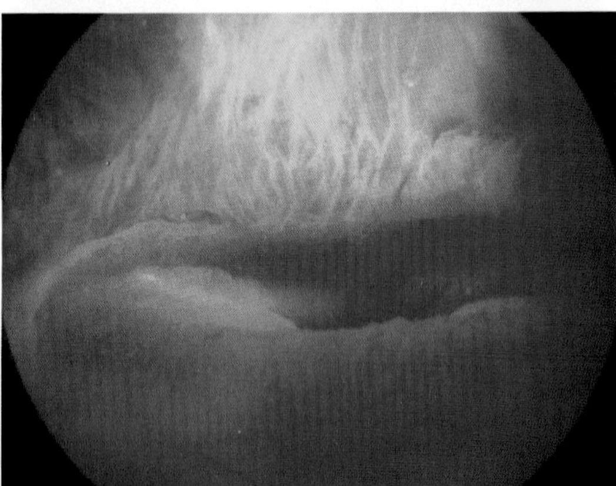

116 b

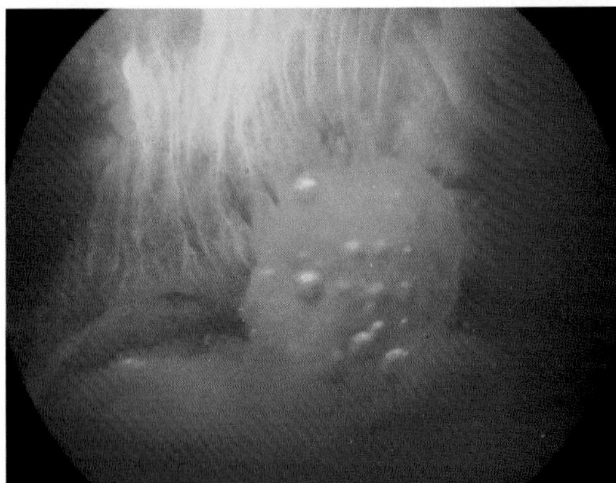

116 c

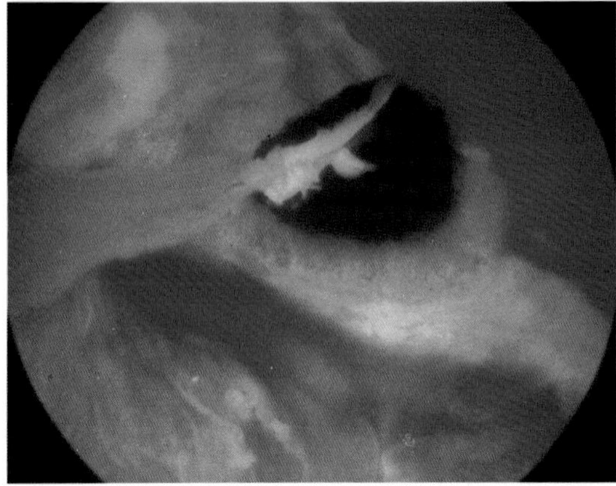

116 d

Attempt at radical TUR of a prostatic carcinoma stage $T_3N_2M_xG_2$ (130 gm in two sessions; Figs. 116, a–c). Postoperative recovery was without complications. However, a small rectal fistula was verified. No residual urine. The cystogram showed a large, completely resected fossa. Discomfort caused by the fistula necessitated an indwelling catheter. Three months later an artificial anus was made, and extended abdominal metastases were verified. Death due to embolism occurred on the eighth postoperative day. TUR of prostatic cancer in its final stage has not proved useful. We now prefer to use palliative cryotherapy, eventually in combination with irradiation.

Fig. 116, a Opening of the perforation.
The floor of the prostatic urethra is seen two months after TUR. In the upper half of the picture the longitudinal fibers of the rectum shine through the new epithelium of the urethra. The round hole in the middle of the fossa below represents the connection between the urethra and rectum (compare Figs. 95, a; 110, e)

Fig. 116, b
The perforation hole has contracted and forms a funnel between the urethra and rectum.

Fig. 116, c
Mucus is pushed from the rectum through the funnel-like opening into the prostatic urethra.

Fig. 116, d Perforation by transurethral catheterization between prostatic urethra and rectum after cobalt therapy and subradical TUR.
The prostatic capsule was resected completely at the bladder neck. Directly below the rim of the trigone (*above*), the thin rectal wall is exposed. Through the black opening a thread of mucus swims from the rectum into the urethra.

Cobalt therapy of a metastasis of seminoma in the prostate had been given one year previously. Now subradical TUR of a cancer stage $T_3N_2M_xG_3$ (65 gm in 70 min) was performed. Six days after TUR the thin rectal wall was perforated with a rubber catheter that had been introduced to determine the quantity of residual urine. This produced a permanent rectal fistula near the seminal vesicles. Three weeks later, an artificial anus was installed, and extended metastases were found in the small pelvis. One year later, the patient died of uremia.

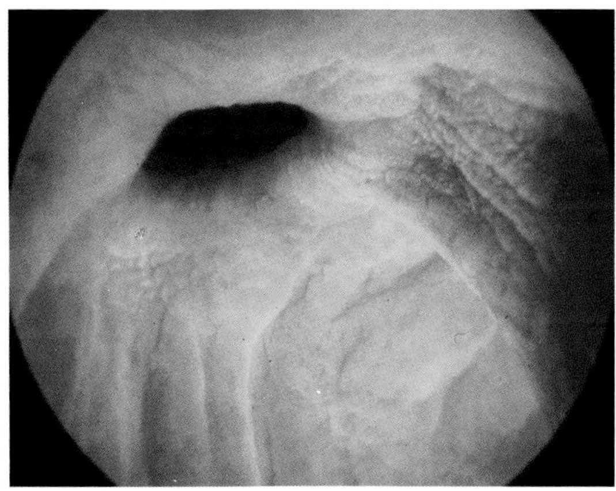

116 e

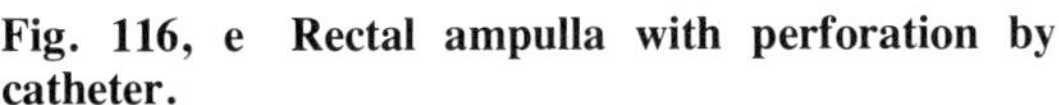

Fig. 116, e Rectal ampulla with perforation by catheter.

Rectoscopy in water (with the photocystoscope) shows the rectal ampulla slightly above the anus. It is connected through a round opening with the prostatic fossa. The foldings of the intestinal tube are clearly recognized; the rectal mucosa has a normal appearance (compare Fig. 116, d).

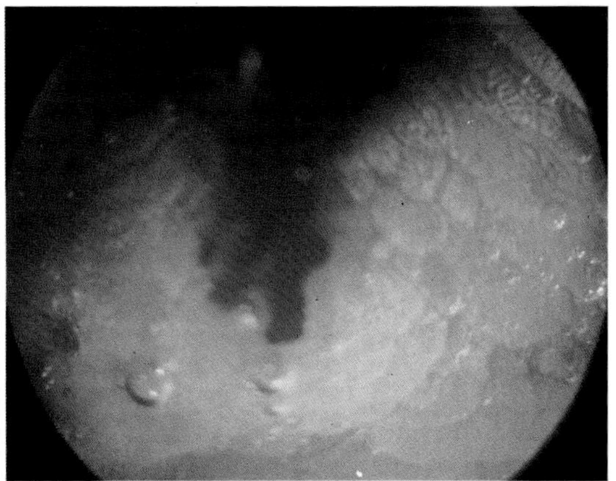

117

Fig. 117 Infiltrated, ulcerating intestinal mucosa due to prostatic carcinoma (stage $T_4N_2M_xG_2$).

Rectoscopy in water. The wall of the rectum protrudes into the lumen, where it is adjacent to the prostate. The rectal mucosa is edematously infiltrated. Above, near the anus, a large ulcerative defect is almost covered by the shadow of the rectal wall caused by the flashlight. The lower rim of the ulcer is bleeding after contact with the metal sheath of the endoscope.

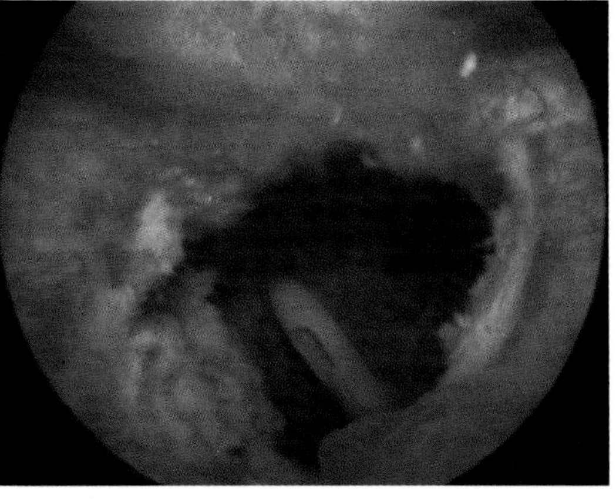

118

Fig. 118 Radical TUR of a prostatic carcinoma (stage $T_3N_xM_xG_2$) **after palliative cryotherapy.**

Trocar cystoscopy: a giant prostatic fossa four days after TUR. Above, the interureteral crest can be recognized; below lies the hemispheric fossa unfolded by the pressure of the irrigation. It is covered with superficially necrotic tissue. At the left, tumorous infiltrations of the bladder neck were resected (over-resection; compare Figs. 107, b, c). The diameter of the fossa (about 4 cm) may be estimated with the catheter (6.7 mm diameter). The mucosa at the rim of the fossa is inflamed.

In this 77-year-old patient a suprapubic bladder stab fistula and palliative cryosurgery were performed because of acute urinary retention. Four months later, 95 gm net were resected transurethrally in 60 min. The patient died at 82 years of age, but there was no further clinical evidence of prostatic cancer. Estrogen therapy with chlorotrianisene (Merbentul) was given.

Prostatic Fossa and Bladder Neck After Different Surgical Treatments of Prostatic Hypertrophy

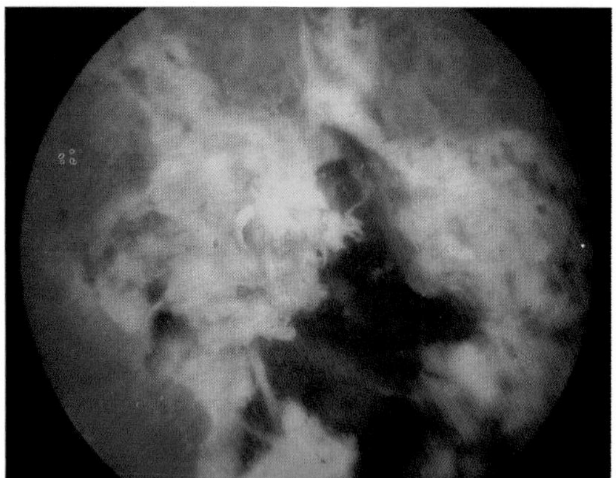

119 a

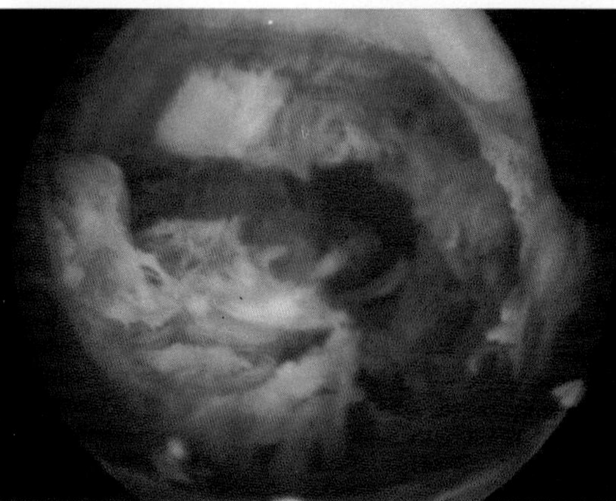

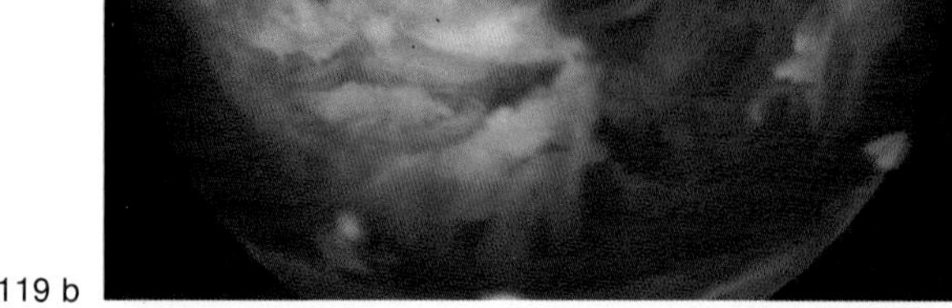

119 b

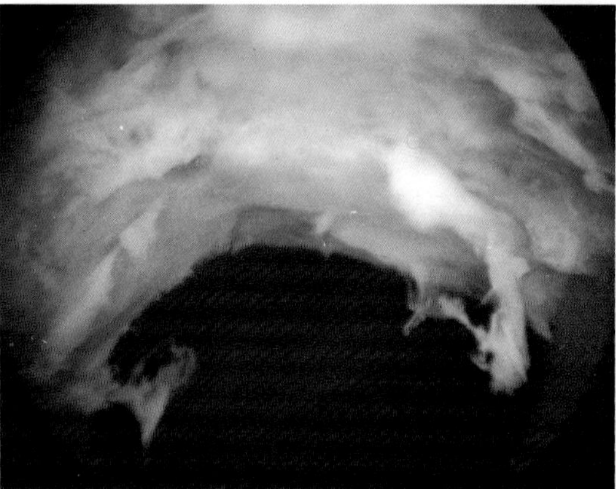

119 c

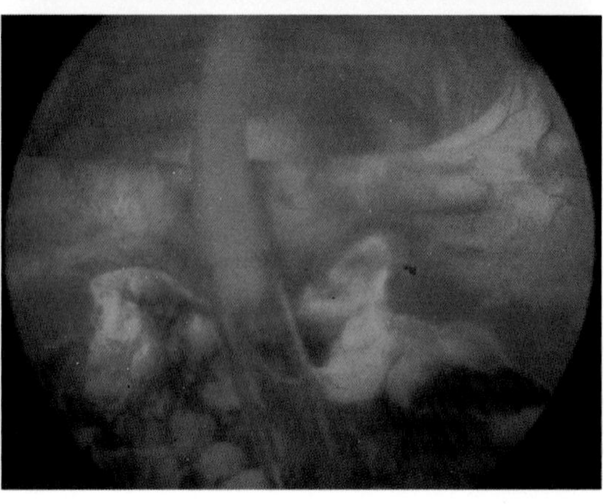

119 d

Fig. 119, a Prostatic fossa after transvesical prostatectomy (125 gm gross weight)

The bladder neck is seen one week following suprapubic cystoscopic surgery. It is deformed by the suture around the fossa and has the shape of a star. The fossa is extensively covered by necroses. The bladder mucosa is inflamed. Traumatization of the tissue during surgical manipulation should not be underestimated. Additional complications may result from the incision of the abdominal bladder walls — not necessary in TURP (for comparative mortality, see p. 235).

Fig. 119, b Bleeding prostatic fossa after TURP (25 gm net in 20 min).

The fossa is seen through the resectoscope when hemorrhage occurred one week after TURP. The concave fossa is opened wide by the irrigation pressure. It is covered with coagulated fibrin and old blood. This coating must be removed because it covers the source of bleeding.

Fig. 119, c Prostatic fossa after TURP (60 gm net)

The upper half of the fossa is covered with fibrin one week after TURP. Inflammatory reactions are recognized within the tissue. The fossa has the shape of a Roman arch. The adenoma is completely resected. For this reason the fold, which is formed by the intact lateral lobes at 12 o'clock (compare Fig. 85, c), has disappeared. The external sphincter also is perfectly round (compare Fig. 103, c).

Fig. 119, d Prostatic fossa after cryosurgery and radical TUR of a prostatic cancer (stage $T_2N_xM_0G_3$)

The bladder neck is seen by trocar cystoscopy one week after combined cryosurgery and TUR. The trigone has been resected subtotally, together with the infiltrated middle lobe. Unevacuated tissue chips remain in the fossa. On both sides of the translucent catheter (Tiemann tip), the interureteral crest is resected almost up to the ureteral ostia. The rim of the resected mucosa shows an inflammatory reaction. At 3 and 9 o'clock the ureteral orifices are recognized. Above, the bladder floor continues into a deep recess.

77-year-old patient. The prostate was frozen for 5.5 min and then immediately resected (70 gm net in 60 min). Death occurred at age 84; no further urologic treatment had been needed.

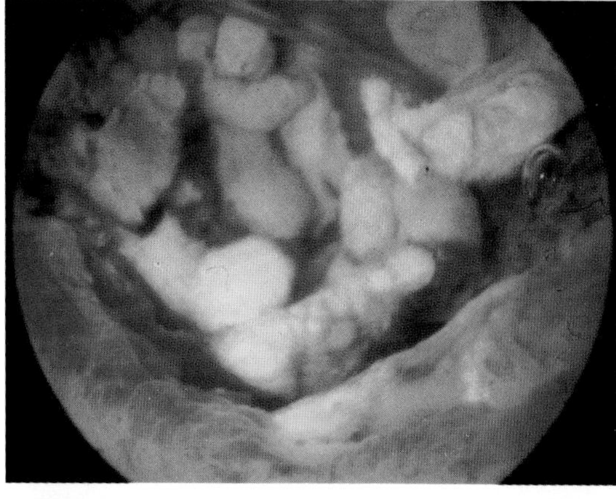

119 e

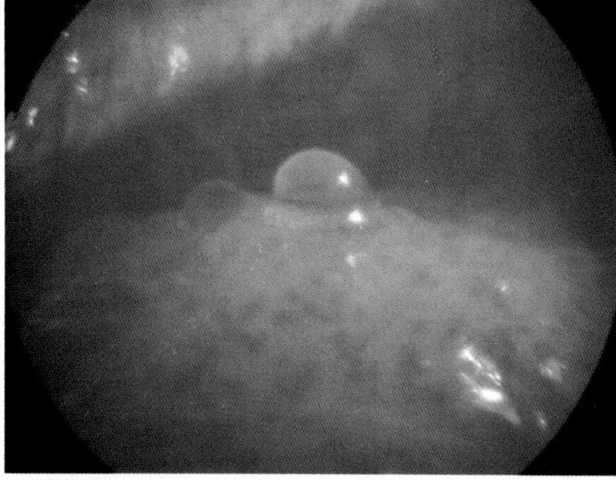

119 f

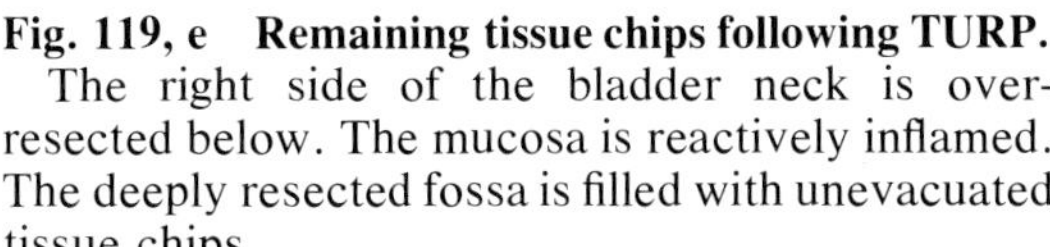

Fig. 119, e Remaining tissue chips following TURP. The right side of the bladder neck is over-resected below. The mucosa is reactively inflamed. The deeply resected fossa is filled with unevacuated tissue chips.

Fig. 119, f Bladder neck six years after partial TUR (80 gm net in 60 min)

Cystoscopy in air: at 7 o'clock there is an adenomatous remnant with inflammatory scarred mucosa. Two almost translucent granules reflect the flash. The bladder recess is filled with turbid fluid (red triangle). A flat adenomatous node of the middle lobe with chronic prostatitis remained. The result of partial TUR is often unsatisfactory. Subsequent TURP (70 gm net in 50 min) with low pressure irrigation was tolerated without complications (compare Fig. 119, g). Eight years later, a fatal cardiac infarction occurred.

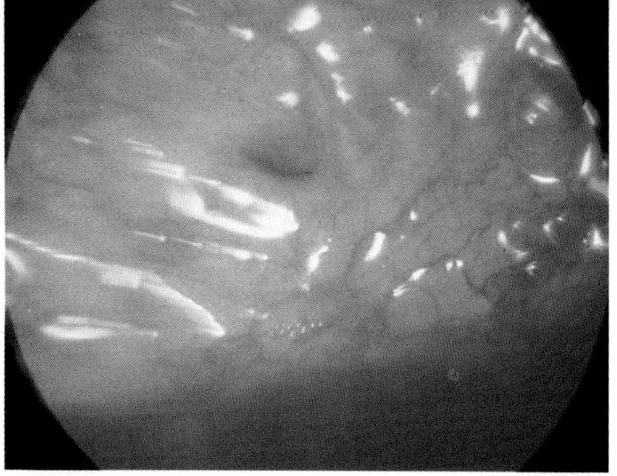

119 g

Fig. 119, g Bladder neck after TUR; second session (cystoscopy in air).

The prostatic urethra now is connected smoothly with the bladder floor. The flashlight is reflected from the mucosa. The dark red shadow of the light falls on the back wall of the urethra. The right ureteral ostium is closed. Some edematous granules are still found in the trigone (at 4 o'clock) at the end of a vascular tree (compare Fig. 119, f).

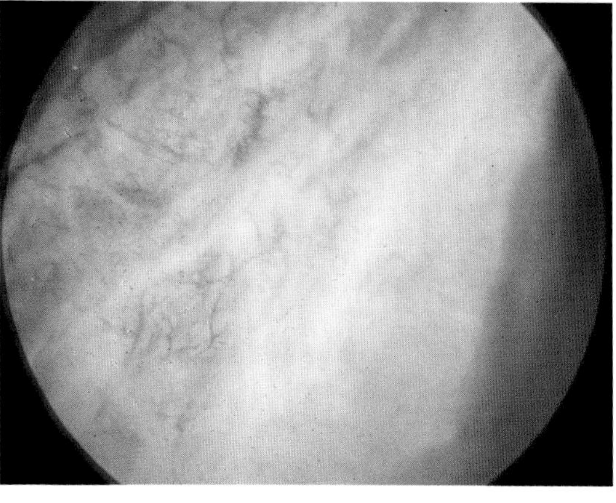

119 h

Fig. 119, h Scarred mucosa of the bladder due to over-resection seen in a second session after partial TUR.

The vessels of the mucosa are rarefied at the right. The fine muscle fibers of the bladder wall shine through. In the shadow of the flashlight the narrow bladder neck is continued by the prostatic urethra (compare Fig. 97, b).

TUR of Postoperative Bladder Neck Strictures (after TURP; trocar cystoscopy; compare Fig. 88)

Fig. 120, a Low pressure TUR with collapsed bladder.
Trocar cystoscopy shows the resectoscope in the depth of the bladder. The bladder walls hang into the lumen of the almost-emptied bladder, bulging in like cushions. The cutting loop is hooked onto the bladder neck. The small volume of the bladder (about 20 cc), the result of continuous trocar aspiration of irrigant, is sufficient for safe resection. The low volume of the bladder guarantees a physiologic pressure within the bladder. This prevents water intoxication.

Fig. 120, b Resected bladder neck.
The resected prostatic fossa now has the shape of a wide funnel. Some tissue adheres to the entirely extended cutting loop. At the right of the loop, an inflammatory nodule is on the mucosa of the ureteral crest. The rim of the concave fossa can be seen below the resected trigone.

Fig. 120, c Granulized prostatic fossa.
Here, the funnel-shaped fossa is seen within the bladder neck two weeks after TUR. Epithelialization has already started. The stump of the middle urethra is recognized, as is the verumontanum (directly above the lower rim of the fossa). Above, some necrotic tissue still remains around the apex of the already shrunken fossa. The tissue of the capsule is indurated and has a rough surface.

Fig. 120, d Epithelialized prostatic fossa.
The prostatic fossa has shrunk markedly four weeks after TURP. There is still some brown necrotic tissue at the apex. The interureteral crest is verified as an oblique, thick bar. In the filled bladder the tip of the 18 Fr rubber catheter points to the right orifice. The tissue around the fossa becomes more and more sclerotic, which is recognized by the increasing contraction of the bladder neck.

Fig. 120, e Recurrent bladder neck stricture.
Ten weeks after TUR, the fossa and bladder neck again have completely shrunk. The bladder outlet is located in the center of a star-shaped scar. Above is the interureteral crest with the two normal orifices.

Fig. 120, f Dilation of a postoperative bladder neck stricture with a semi-stiff 18-Fr catheter made of Rüsche-lit.
We no longer perform circular TUR of strictures (except in cancer; see Fig. 121). Today, we prefer endoscopic urethrotomy or cryosurgery (compare Figs. 122, c–e).

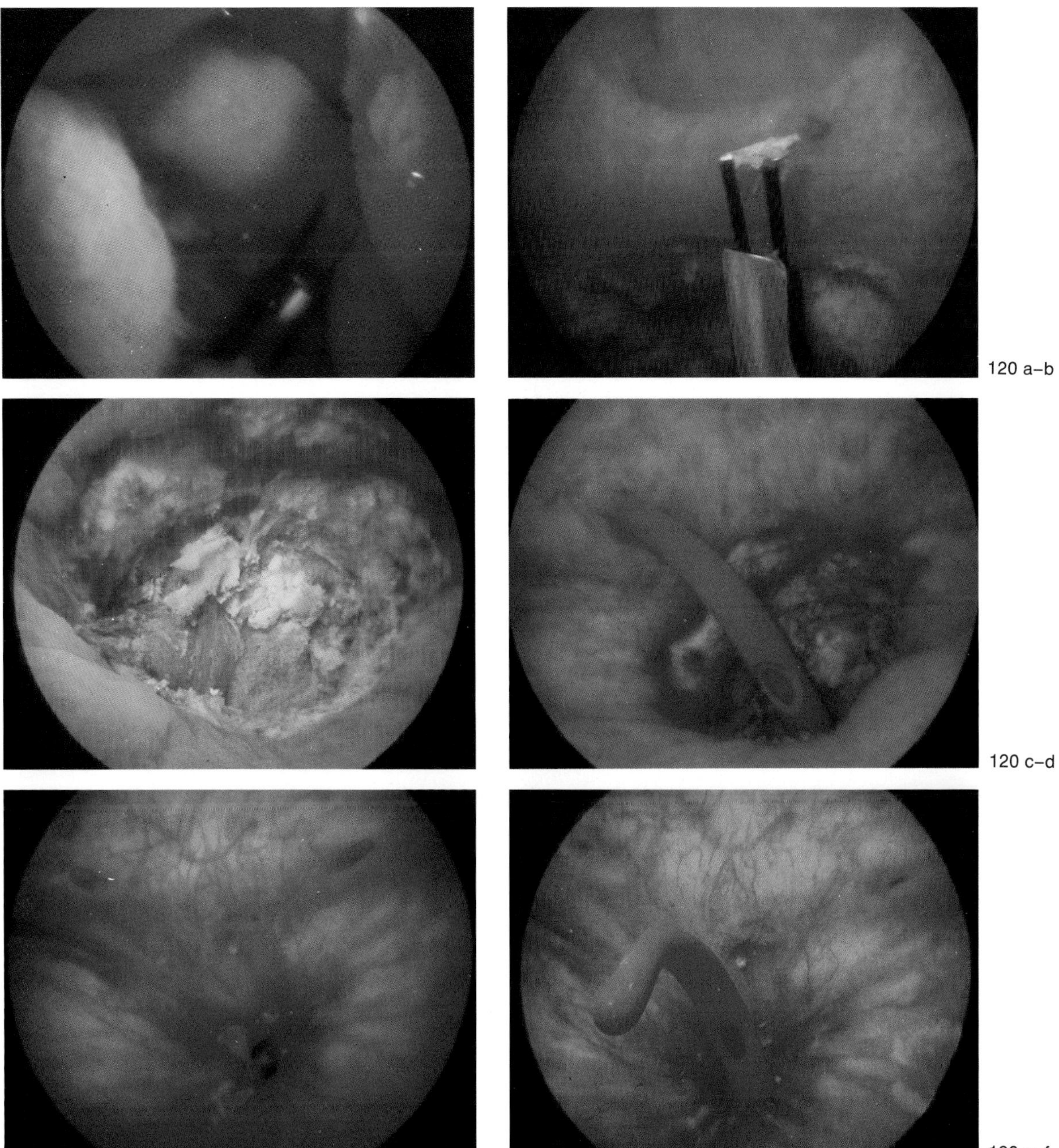

120 a–b

120 c–d

120 e–f

TUR of a Bladder Neck Stricture After Radical TUR of Prostatic Cancer (stage $T_2N_0M_0P_2$; 20 gm net in 25 min; four years previously. A second TUR (3 gm in 15 min) was performed, and nine years later the patient was clinically healthy and had insignificant incontinence).

Fig. 121, a Bladder neck stricture.
The resectoscope is introduced into the prostatic urethra — dilated first from 12 to 28 Fr — until the bladder entrance (internal sphincter) comes into sight. The cutting loop can just be introduced through the opening of the bladder neck. The first cut was made at 12 o'clock, because the scarred bar (at 6 o'clock) does not allow introduction of the loop. Above, the cut scar is verified, and the bladder floor can be seen through the opening.

Fig. 121, b TUR.
The upper circumference of the prostatic urethra is enlarged with a few cuts. The dimensions of the completely extended cutting loop are blurred by the wide-angle view. Its parallel bluish insulated wires are therefore shown at an angle. The cut surface of the scarred prostatic capsule is concave and smooth; the resectoscope (28 Fr) can now be introduced into the bladder.

Fig. 121, c Scar of the bladder mucosa.
The resectoscope is introduced into the bladder. The loop is set onto the scar infiltrated by inflammation. At the right of the loop, the interureteral crest with the left ostium is scarcely visible. Below, the mucosa is altered by scar formation (squamous cell metaplasia). The bladder neck is dissected between 4 and 8 o'clock.

Fig. 121, d Dissected trigone.
The infiltrated scar at the trigone is resected. The muscle fibers of the internal sphincter are exposed. The fossa is opened wide and is smoothly connected with the bladder floor (compare Fig. 91, h).

Fig. 121, e Hemorrhage due to chronic inflammation.
The right wall of the fossa is resected. White scarred tissue was cut; blood sprays from three arteries. The cutting loop (*below*) is partially covered by the rim of the mucosa. Hemorrhage in the depth of the capsule is stronger owing to chronic inflammation. TUR was performed with low pressure irrigation as radical sample excision.

The return-flow resectoscope is not advantageous here, because the narrow urethra obstructs the openings of the outlet channel. The suprapubic trocar is not absolutely necessary for this operation; however, without the trocar the bladder volume must be limited to a maximum of 200 cc with the aid of the irrigant dosimeter (p. 27).

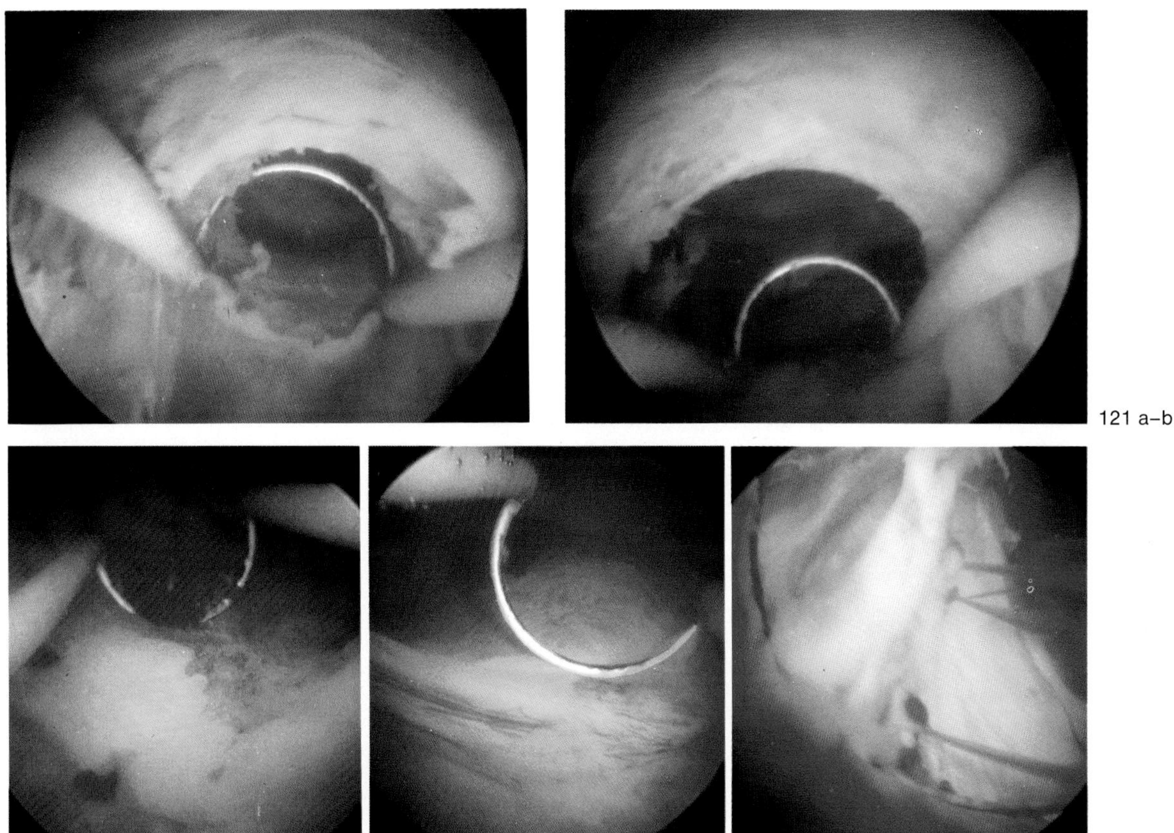

121 a–b

121 c–e

Endoscopic and Open Surgical Therapy of Bladder Neck Stricture

Fig. 122, a Postoperative bladder neck stricture with small adenomatous recurrence.
Trocar cystoscopy. A granuloma is growing on the bladder neck, which is contracted by scars that have drawn both ureteral orifices near the node. Between the orifices there is a blood coagulum caused by catheterization. It rises from the internal urethral meatus (compare Fig. 120, f).

Fig. 122, b Open surgical correction.
The scarred bladder neck is demonstrated by trocar cystoscopy after open surgical excision of an adenomatous prostatic remnant and ventral fixation of the longitudinally cut bladder onto the middle urethra. The 20-Fr rubber catheter was introduced without resistance. At the left a small scar granuloma shows slight inflammatory alterations. The orifices of the ureters are not verifiable.

Fig. 122, c Bladder neck stricture (TURP; Fig. 92, d).
The prostatic urethra as seen through the urethroscope has only a punctate connection with the bladder. The unlighted structure below represents the verumontanum and, to the right, the column of the left lateral lobe (between 1 and 5 o'clock). The brightly illuminated prostatic urethra is changed by scars and inflammation.

Fig. 122, d Endoscopic urethrotomy.
The beak of the urethrotome with return-flow irrigation is in the prostatic urethra. At the left, the concave fossa is smooth. At the lower right, scarred and inflamed mucosa covers a small adenomatous remnant. The irrigating chamber in front of the beak is not obscured because return-flow irrigation keeps it clear (see Fig. 53). The knife is extended and is about to cut the scar at 3 o'clock. At 12 o'clock the bladder neck is already incised. Further cuts are made at 6 o'clock (down into the perivesical tissue over the rectum) and at 9 o'clock. This method achieves results superior to TUR of the stricture, because the cut is cold and further damage of the tissue by electric current is avoided. A permanent indwelling catheter is obligatory for postoperative care.

Fig. 122, e Situation following dilation with metal bougie.
The internal urethral orifice has been forced open with the elbowed metal bougie (from 12 to 24 Fr) guided by the finger in the rectum. The verumontanum is at the 6 o'clock position; the urethral mucosa is inflamed (compare Fig. 122, i).

Fig. 122, f Scarred bladder neck after dilation.
A scarred bar (lower half of the picture) distinguishes the trigone from the prostatic urethra. Its mucosa is changed by inflammation. The bladder neck is opened wide to allow smooth passage of the endoscope (compare Fig. 122, g).

Fig. 122, g Scarred bladder neck after dilation.
The urethroscope has been drawn back into the distal prostatic urethra. Its upper wall is rigid and its lumen somewhat deformed. In the background, the right half of the trigone with the interureteral crest is seen (at the left in the picture). At the lower right, a red flake of mucus is floating in the irrigant. Below, the middle urethra obscures the view of the verumontanum (contraction of the external sphincter).

Fig. 122, h Prostatic urethra after dilation.
The urethroscope has been drawn far back into the middle urethra. The mucosa below is lifted by the external sphincter; the rigid arch of the scarred prostatic urethra is bent over it. The mucosa over the pillar of the right lateral lobe (at the left) is inflamed and covered by a fibrin flake.

Fig. 122, i Control by trocar cystoscopy.
The path of the elbowed metal bougie to the adenomatous urethra is surveyed. When the bougie is moved in the wrong direction, the bladder neck bulges asymmetrically. The instrument is guided under direct vision from the urethra into the bladder to be certain of avoiding a false path. The same technique is followed for the transurethral introduction of the lithotriptor in trocar lithotripsy (compare Fig. 126).

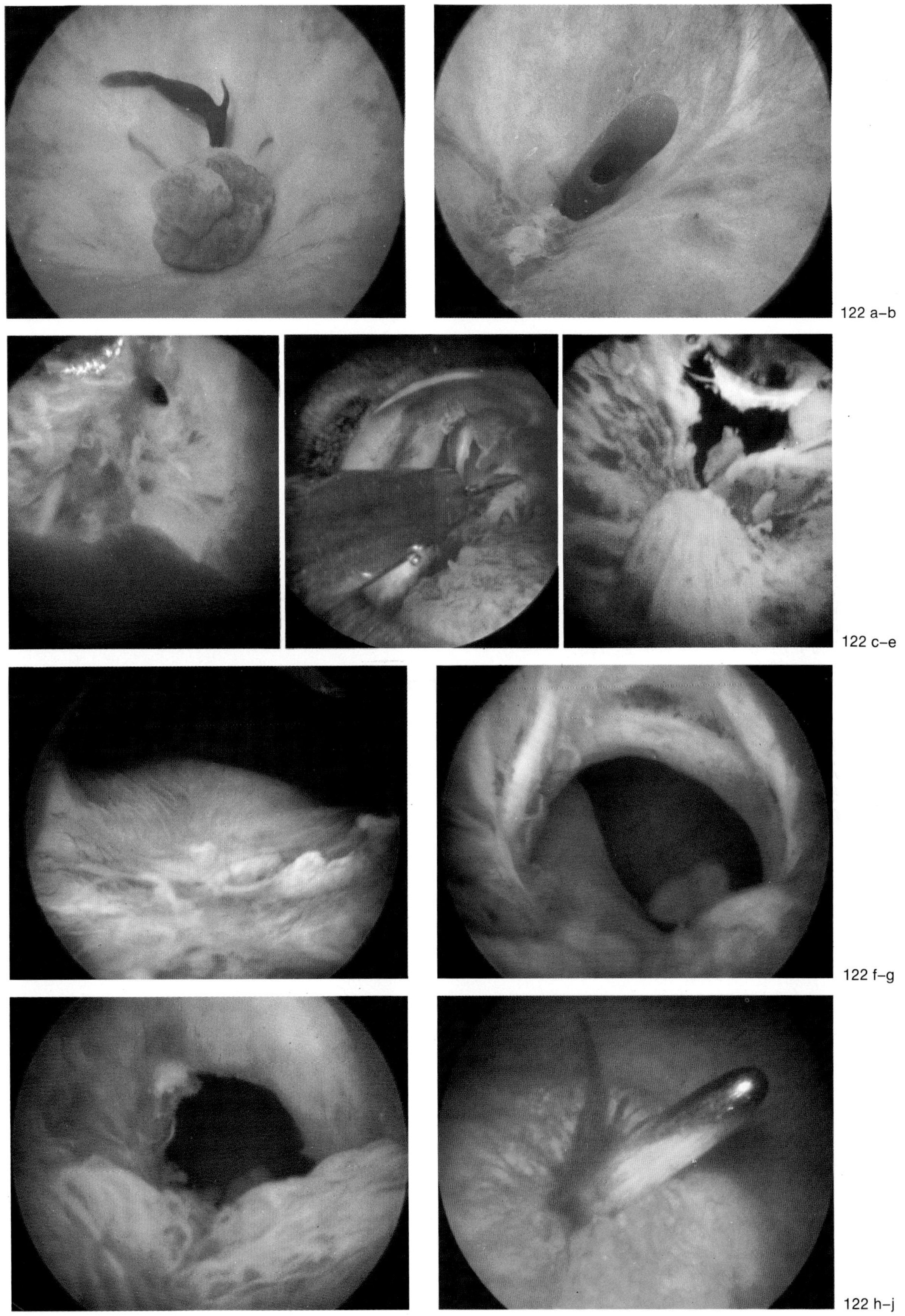

122 a–b

122 c–e

122 f–g

122 h–j

Perforations of the Urethra

Fig. 123, a Perforation of the strictured prostatic urethra by the resectoscope (TURP).
The false route has led into the tissue below the prostatic adenoma. Ruptured fibers of the prostatic capsule are seen within the perforation cavity. The disrupted rim of the mucosa is seen below; at the left, a part of the injured verumontanum is visible.

Preoperative stricture. Under control of the finger in the rectum, correct introduction of the resectoscope is managed and TURP (120 gm net in 90 min) performed.

Fig. 123, b Perforation of the middle urethra due to post-traumatic stricture.
The tip of the cystoscope has perforated the urethra from above and distal to the external sphincter. The large opening seen at the upper margin of the picture is the entrance into the incorrect path followed. A urethral catheter (6 Fr) was introduced into the retracted urethra. It serves to guide the introduction of a catheter or a hollow metal bougie.

Fracture of the bony pelvis occurred ten years earlier; small prostatic adenoma and chronic prostatitis. Conservative therapy was followed for ten years more.

Fig. 123, c Perforation of the middle urethra due to stricture.
The urethra is perforated above, where the resectoscope, introduced for TUR of a bladder tumor, has torn a hole. Below the transversally disrupted urethral mucosa (center) the narrow opening of the urethra is seen as a dark cleft. The verumontanum is visible through the opening in the background. Under urethroscopic control, the resectoscope is inserted transurethrally into the bladder.

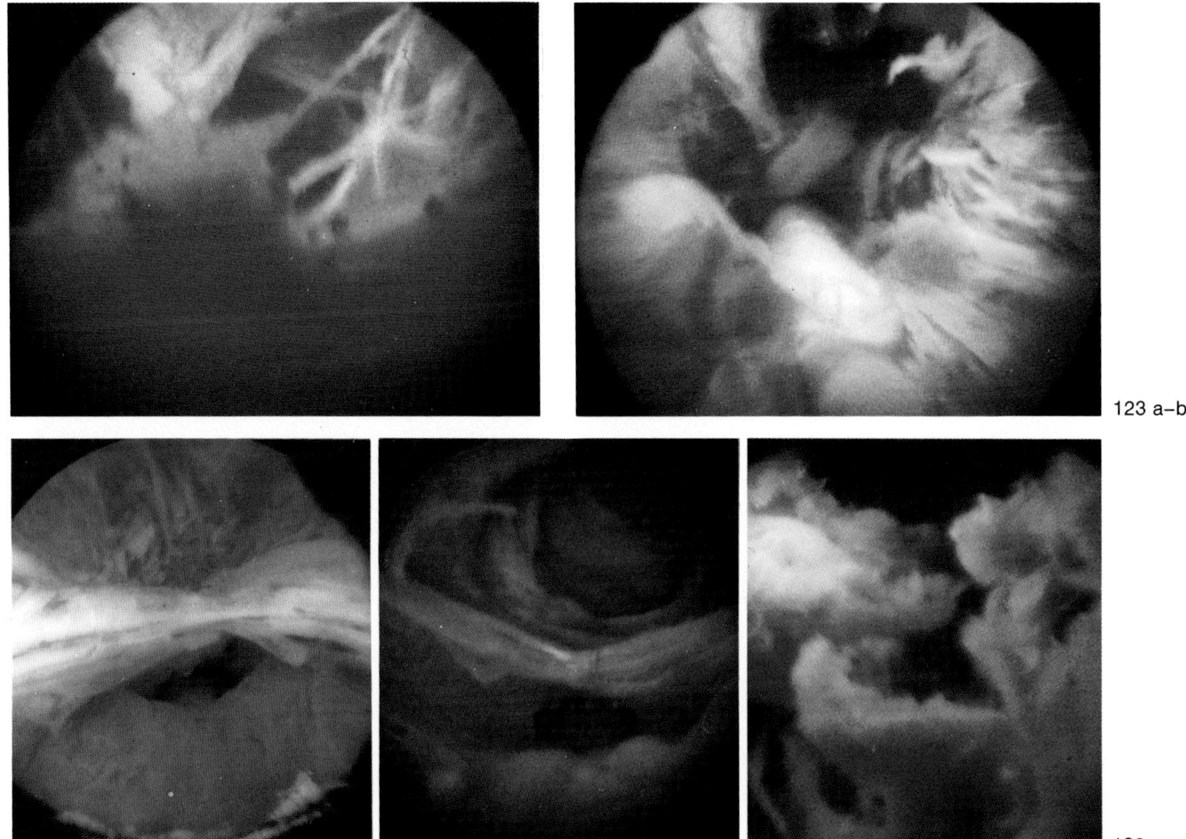
123 a–b

123 c–e

Fig. 123, d Perforation of the middle urethra due to preoperative stricture.
The resectoscope has been retracted from the false path seen above. Here, the opening of the compressed urethra is visible below the large entrance into the perforation. When the handle of the resectoscope is raised, the correct route into the bladder is found along the posterior wall of the urethra. Low pressure irrigation prevents excessive traumatization and infiltration of the tissue with irrigant. TURP is then performed without difficulty (15 gm net in 20 min).

Fig. 123, e Traumatic urethral disruption.
The middle urethra has been completely disrupted by fracture of the bony pelvis in an automobile accident. Urethroscopy shows shredded necrotic mucosa at the edge of the wound three weeks after the accident. The path through the stricture was found transvesically through an existing bladder fistula. Postoperatively, there was uncomplicated recovery of the urethra (compare Fig. 83, a).

124 a–c 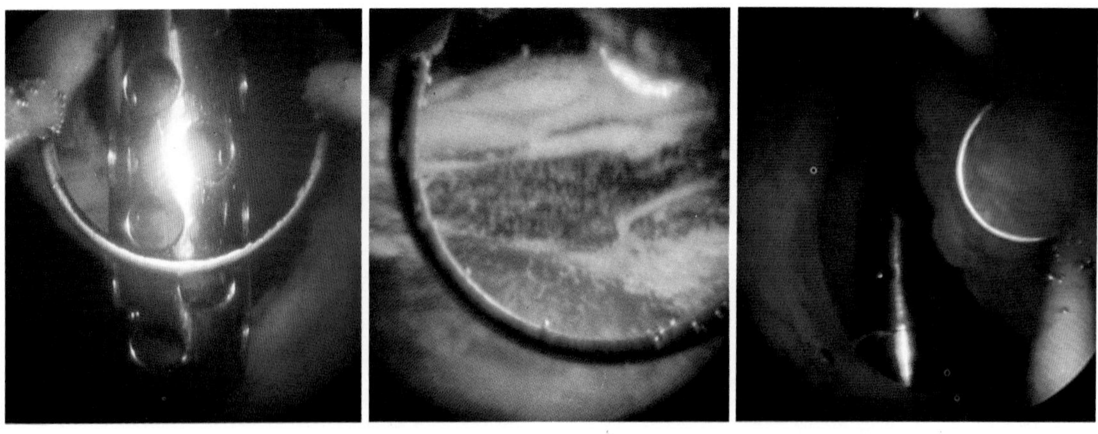

Comparison of Physiologic Low Pressure Irrigation with Unphysiologic High Pressure Irrigation (Low Pressure and High Pressure TUR)

Fig. 124, a Low pressure irrigation—TURP of a giant adenoma (about 300 gm gross weight).

The cutting loop is set on the bladder neck at 6 o'clock. Above, the rim of the resected prostatic fossa is visible. The trocar insert (16 Fr) is directly in front of the beak of the resectoscope. The irrigant is aspirated directly from the fossa.

The openings of the trocar insert are cleaned by moving the insert up and down within its sheath. Therefore, the trocar sheath should not be retracted from the bladder unintentionally. The bladder is almost empty, containing only about 20 cc of irritant. Thus, the fossa is not under the pressure that would occur with a tightly filled bladder. The relaxed prostatic fossa is easily moved, like a rubber cloth, as soon as the adenoma has been completely resected. Low pressure irrigation effectively prevents infiltration of the tissue by irrigant (compare Figs. 110–113; 124, b; 133, b).

In this 70-year-old patient, TURP (230 gm net in 110 min), trocar litholapaxy of about a dozen phosphate stones in the same session and blood transfusion were performed without complications. Over the next five years urologic follow-up showed no abnormalities.

Fig. 124, b Prostatic capsule infiltrated with water in high pressure irrigation (TURP of about 150 gm; Fig. 93, e).

The cutting loop is in front of the right wall of the capsule. The capsule is edematous and split by water infiltration. The irrigant is forced into the tissue with a high dynamic pressure because of the high pressure irrigation used. This can cause absorption of as much as 4 liters of fluid. Water intoxication and all its dangers (hyponatremia, urosepsis) result from this unphysiologic irrigation technique. (Compare Figs. 93, d; 94, b and d; 138, a).

Fig. 124, c Low pressure irrigation with suprapubic trocar; condition after blind cryosurgery with adenomatous remnant at the left.

The trocar insert is seen through the sickle-shaped opening of the prostatic urethra. The right wall of the prostatic capsule is free of adenoma (at the left). A spherical remnant of the left lateral lobe projects into the lumen at the right. The cutting loop pushes the adenoma toward the bladder for better visualization. This adenomatous node remained — probably because an insulating layer of air and water had formed between the cryoprobe and the surface of the adenoma. This insulation reduces the efficiency of freezing the adenoma. This complication of blind surface cryosurgery can be eliminated by repeated freezing and trocar cryosurgery (compare Fig. 89).

Cystoscopic Control of the Insertion of the Suprapubic Trocar for Low Pressure TUR and Trocar Litholapaxy

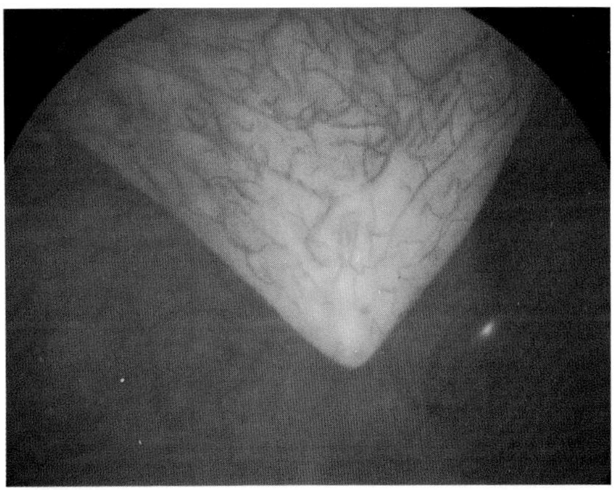
125 a

Fig. 125, a Projecting bladder roof.
The roof of the bladder projects over the tip of the instrument. The bladder can now be safely perforated by the trocar. Often the elastic bladder wall is pushed deep into the lumen until the trocar tip finally perforates (compare Fig. 128).

Directly above the symphysis the skin and the fascia of the rectus muscle are incised. Then the trocar is pushed into the filled bladder at an angle of 30° to the vertical (for technique, see Fig. 32). The perforation of the bladder by the trocar tip can be observed and corrected cystoscopically. This is necessary, especially when the bladder is insufficiently filled (below 300 cc).

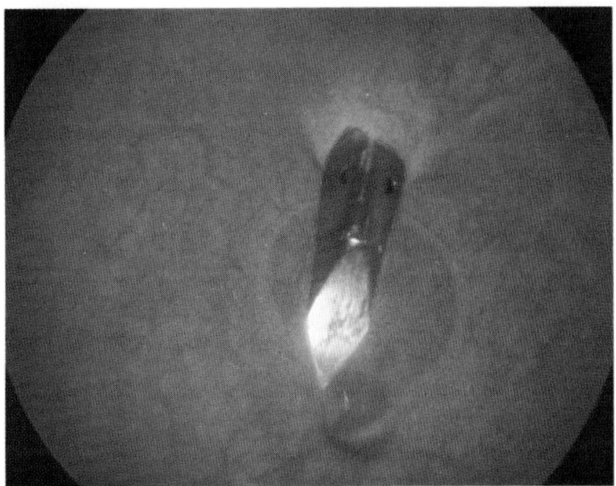
125 b

Fig. 125, b Trocar.
The trocar tip has perforated the bladder wall; the insert may now be exchanged by: (a) the optical system of a cystoscope for trocar cystoscopy or litholapaxy; or (b) the insert for aspiration during TUR (compare Figs. 124, 126).

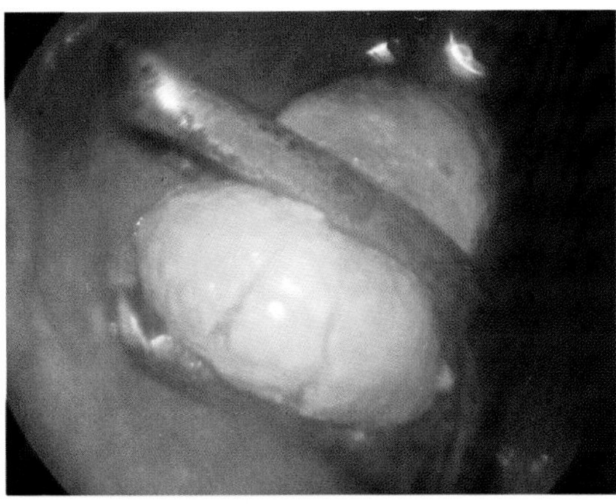
126

Fig. 126 Trocar litholapaxy with air insufflation; trocar cystoscopy.
This large urate stone was crushed in two minutes with a Bigelow lithotriptor, developed over 100 years ago, in the air-filled bladder. It was then evacuated with water.

Here, blind litholapaxy (Bigelow) and suprapubic trocar cystoscopy in the air-filled bladder were combined. This simple but effective method does not require great experience in endoscopy. It is safe because the surgeon always has excellent vision from above of both the stone and the lithotriptor. There is no risk of complications due to, for example, traumatization of the bladder wall. The wall may be traumatized mechanically by the lithotriptor when vision is impaired (obscured irrigant) or electrically by electrohydraulic litholapaxy. Trocar litholapaxy is the faster procedure, because the stone can always be clutched at its largest diameter under direct vision.

127 a–b 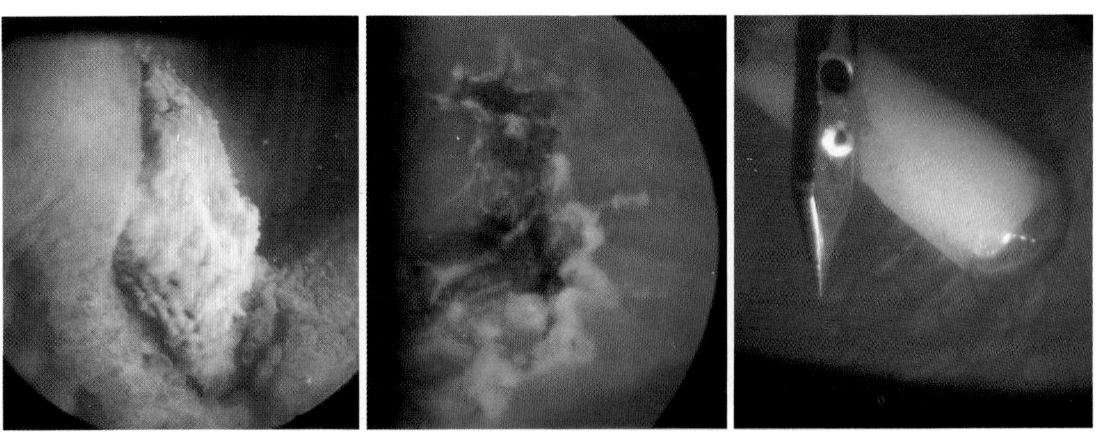 12

TUR of a Foreign Body Immigrated into the Bladder

Fig. 127, a Foreign body in the right bladder wall.
A suspension net made of nylon tissue has migrated into the bladder following incontinence suspension plasty.

Fig. 127, b TUR of the nylon net.
The part of the nylon net that has entered the bladder is resected. The mucosal defect is seen here. Three months later, an operation (after Marshall-Marchetti) for recurrent incontinence was performed with good results.

Fig. 128 Trocar extraction of a foreign body in the bladder (cytoscopy for control of the suprapubic introduction of a sheathless trocar cystoscope into the bladder).
The calcified body of a clinical thermometer lies obliquely within the bladder of a female patient. A suprapubically-introduced trocar cystoscope with optical system and cold light source is situated in front of it. The bladder is filled with 500 cc water. The tip of the thermometer is seized with a surgical clamp, introduced through the urethra, and extracted without difficulty.

The thermometer was introduced into the bladder three months previously by the patient herself. The condition was concealed until vaginal hemorrhage occurred due to traumatization of the bladder floor by the thermometer tip.

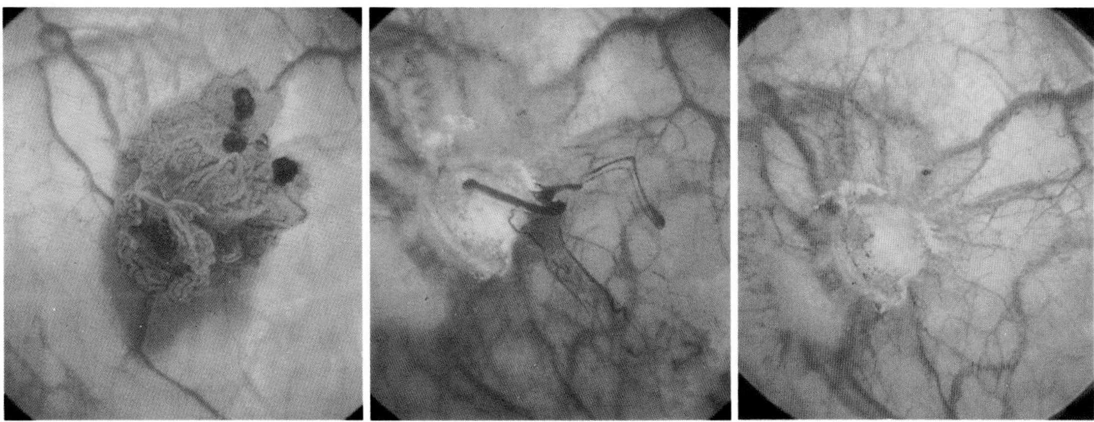

129 a–c

TUR of Bladder Papillomas

Fig. 129, a **Bladder papilloma, stage T_A.**
A pedunculated papillary tumors is noted on the right posterior wall of the bladder. Its villi are coarse; small vessels can be recognized in the mucosa of its surface. Several villi at the upper right carry dark red nodules (old hematomas). The tumor sits at the center of a star of obstructed veins. Like the old hematomas, these are an expression of increased activity of the tumor.

It is wrong to coagulate such a papilloma or to perform open surgery on it. By such management, tumor cells are implanted in the mucosa of the entire bladder (or into the abdominal incision).

Fig. 129, b Bleeding vessel of the pedicle.
The spouting pedicle artery can be recognized within the almost circular defect of the mucosa. The surrounding mucosa is hyperemic; its color becomes darker, and several veins appear.

Fig. 129, c Lesion of the bladder mucosa.
The pedicle artery and the margin of the mucosal defect are coagulated. Thus, the difference in color between the mucosa and the veins is made evident.

When the histology report shows a stage T_2, the circumference of the lesion may be frozen. Then the infiltrate within the vesical wall can be ablated (see Figs. 174–176). Recently, laser techniques have been used for this purpose.

Retrograde Cut for TUR of a Small Papilloma (Stage T_A) **Employing Return-Flow Resectoscope with Channel for Control of Bladder Pressure** (After M. A. Reuter)

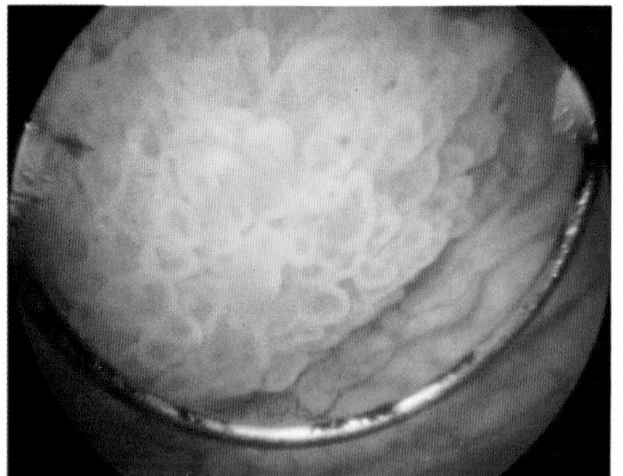

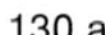
130 a

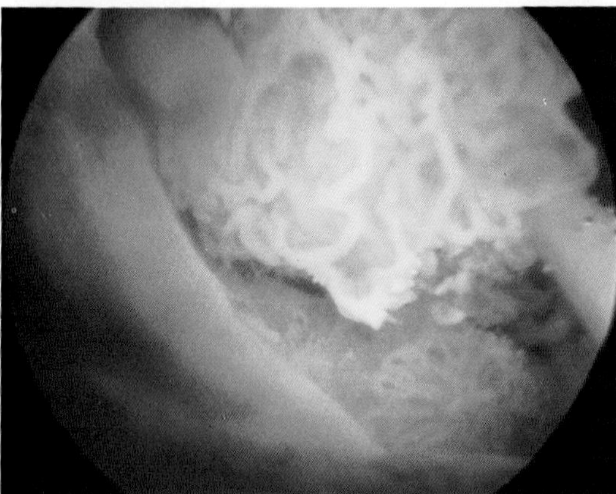

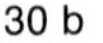
130 b

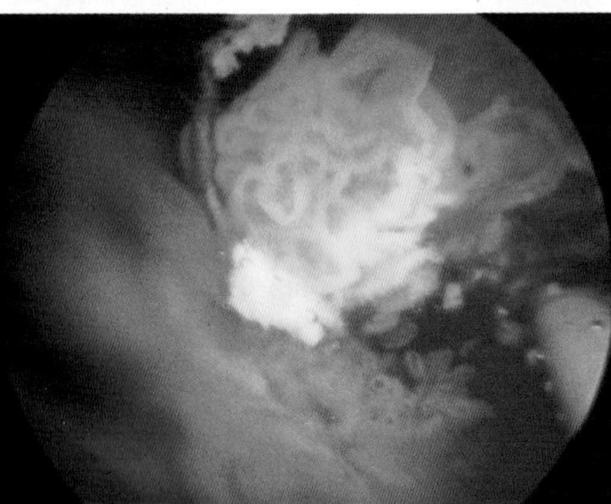

130 c

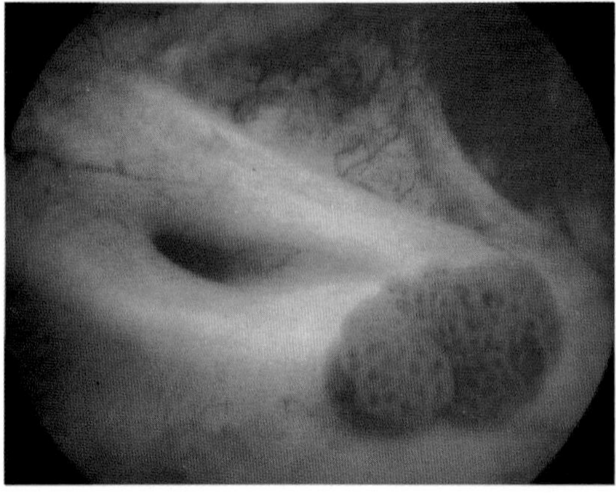

131

Fig. 130, a
The cutting loop is placed on the pedicle of the bladder papilloma at the level of the mucosa. The loop itself is almost retracted into the sheath.

Fig. 130, b
The base of the papilloma is cut from the mucosa with the entire resectoscope. The papilloma covers the wire, making direct vision impossible. The irrigation inflow is reduced (return-flow resectoscope; see Fig. 76).

Fig. 130, c
The loop has now passed below the papilloma. Irrigation is increased, and the cut papilloma is washed on the bladder floor. Below, the superficial wound of the mucosa can be recognized. TUR of the bladder requires some filling (50 to 100 cc), although the static pressure in the bladder should not exceed 15 cm water.

Fig. 131 Bladder after TUR of a giant papillary tumor (455 gm net; stage T_A).

The bladder is seen one year after TUR. The scarred ureteral crest runs obliquely through the center of the picture. The right orifice was superficially resected and is half-opened. A small recurrent papilloma is seen at the right on the trigone. Part of the posterior bladder wall is seen above.

In this 48-year-old patient, bladder papillomatosis, recognized for 10 years, has developed into a giant tumor (base on the bladder neck and the lateral walls). This mimicked bladder cancer with hydronephrosis of both kidneys. Because of initial uremia the patient was given up as hopeless by his physician. The tumor was resected in four sessions at intervals of a few days, and the patient quickly recovered. One year later the small recurrent papilloma shown here was resected. Over the following 15 years there was no recurrence. The excretory urogram was normal.

Today we first freeze such giant tumors (see Figs. 175, 176). One week later the base is resected (histology, residual tumor).

Radical Low Pressure TUR of a Solid Bladder Cancer, Stage $T_2N_0M_0G_3$ (cytoscopy)

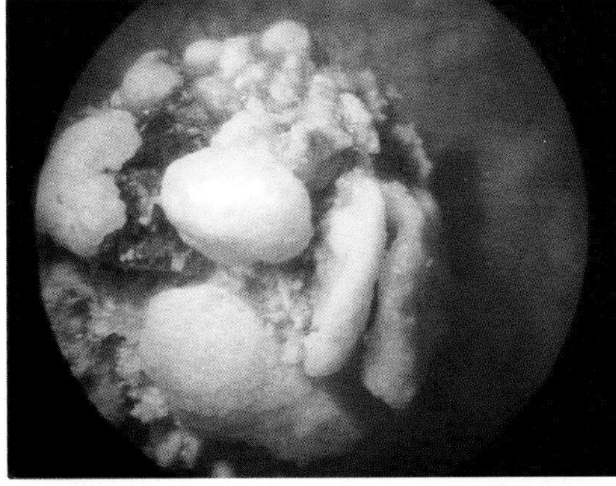

132 a

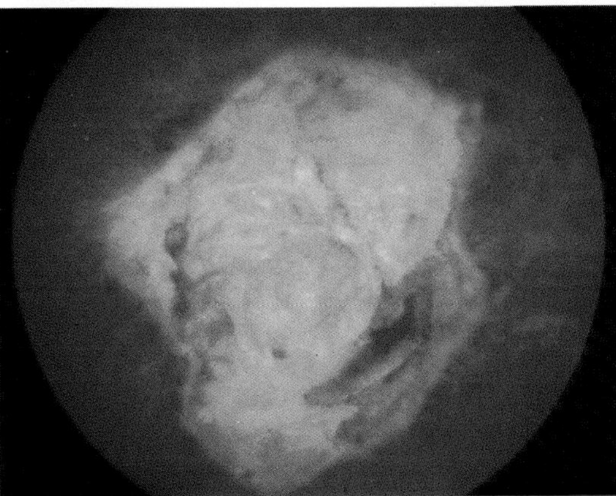

132 b

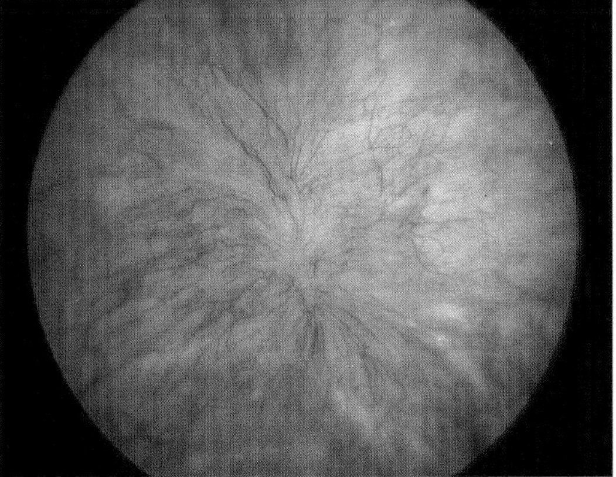

132 c

Two grams (net) of tissue were resected and several stones crushed. The patient was dismissed on the fourth postoperative day. Cobalt irradiation (5200 R). Two months later, open surgery was performed and part of the bladder wall resected; a scarred ulceration with central necrosis was found. Histology revealed inflamed tissue with foreign body granulomas. Control studies in the following years revealed no pathologic findings (cystoscopy, x-ray). Four years later the patient died of cardiac infarction.

The return-flow resectoscope with continuous, active aspiration of irrigant and measurement of bladder pressure (measuring channel) proved to be the most useful instrument here.

Fig. 132, a Solid bladder tumor.
The fungiform solid tumor rests on a broad base on the left lateral wall of the bladder. Its necrotic surface is covered with several bean-shaped calcifications.

Fig. 132, b Wound after TUR.
The bladder wall is resected down to the middle layer. There, bladder muscle with narrow fibers without infiltration is exposed. TUR is now continued until the outer layer of the bladder wall is reached, which is resected totally.

The muscle fibers of the bladder are thicker and more distinct than the fibers of the prostatic capsule. The paravesical tissue is similar to the periprostatic (compare Fig. 111).

Fig. 132, c Scarred bladder wall after open surgical resection.
One year after open surgery a scar is found in the bladder wall, where the vessels of the mucosa form a star around its center. The bladder is not irritated and there is no recurrence of tumor.

133 a–b

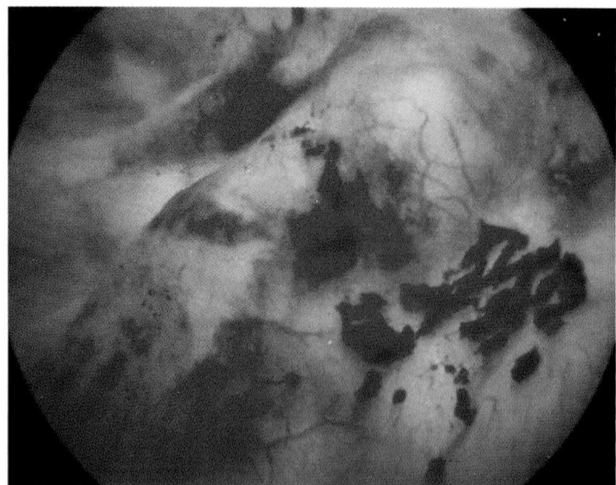

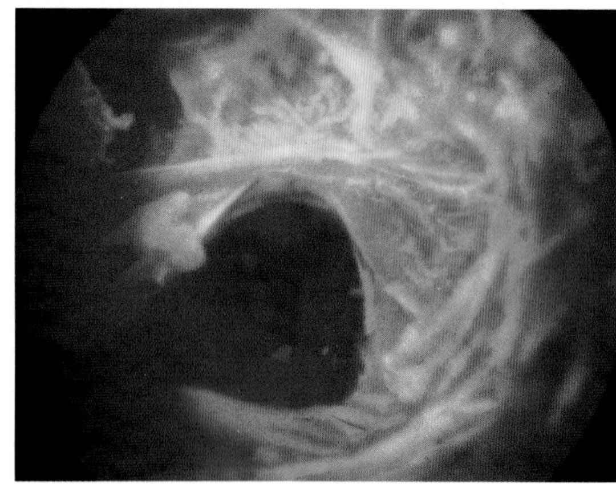

Radical TUR of an Intramural Solid Bladder Cancer, Stage $T_{3a}N_2M_xG_3$

This 81-year-old patient had had anuria for two days. Retrograde catheterization of the left ureter revealed an absolute block. Large volumes of urine came from the ureteral catheter at the right when an obstruction 2 cm above the orifice was eliminated. Two days later the retrograde pyelogram demonstrated tender renal calyces and a small defect in the lower ureter. A urate stone was suspected.

Radical TUR was performed down to the perivesical fatty tissue. The patient was dismissed ten days after the operation. Because of his poor general condition, further treatment was abandoned. The patient died 15 months later of metastases.

Radical TUR of the bladder tumor is mainly performed on the bladder floor. Here, the bladder wall can be resected completely down into perivesical tissue without danger, when the bladder pressure is kept within physiologic limits and the bladder is not overdistended. Today this is possible with low pressure irrigation and continuous aspiration of irrigant. We use the back-flow resectoscope with monitoring of the bladder pressure for the bladder tumor (whereas trocar TUR is performed for the large adenoma). The pictures that follow demonstrate well that the tissue is not infiltrated by water.

Fig. 133, a Hematuria from the left ureteral orifice.
The area surrounding the orifice is irregularly swollen. The mucosa does not show any defect; however, above and at the left of the slightly opened orifice a small node shines through from the depth. At the right of the orifice lies a threadlike coagulum.

Fig. 133, b **TUR of an intramural papillary tumor (15 gm net; stage T_A).**
The left orifice is resected into the shape of a funnel. The rough fibers of the bladder muscle wind around a central opening; this is coated with reddish mucosa. The opening represents the right ureter; a giant bladder papilloma has grown in its intramural part. The tumor was resected as far as the lumen was freed of papillomatous nodules.

This 74-year-old patient survived for six years without abnormal findings.

TUR of the ureteral orifice is not difficult when the finger in the rectum is used as in TUR of large prostatic adenomas. Bleeding vessels are coagulated at once, because several simultaneously bleeding arteries are difficult to find. The function of the resected ureteral orifice is usually unimpaired, even if it is deeply resected (see Figs. 97, a; 131; 135). We have investigated the results after TUR of the ureteral orifice in 56 patients. Here we found that in 25 per cent of the benign papillomas (24 patients) postoperative pyelonephritis occurs, which healed completely except in one patient. When resection was performed for cancer (22 cases), pyelonephritis occurred in 60 per cent; in 10 patients with clinical cure of the cancer the pyelonephritis was cured. Palliative TUR was performed in 12 patients, whose infection was not cured. In 10 patients the orifices were resected because of inflammatory disease, and only one pyelonephritic episode was observed. Today, we dilate the orifice with a metal bougie (like that in Fig. 122, i) and try to resect the papilloma within the ureter (resectoscope for children).

134 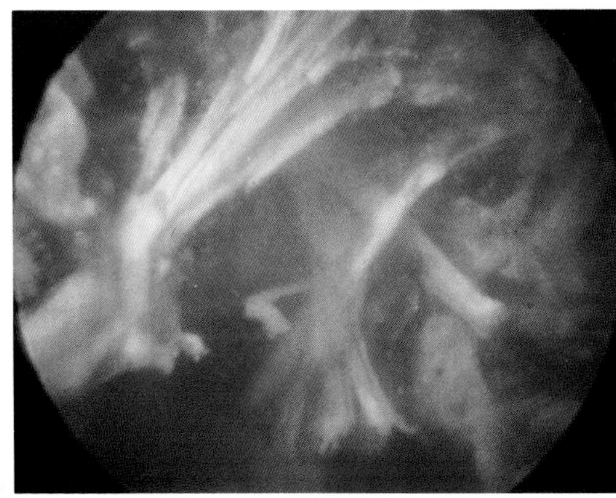

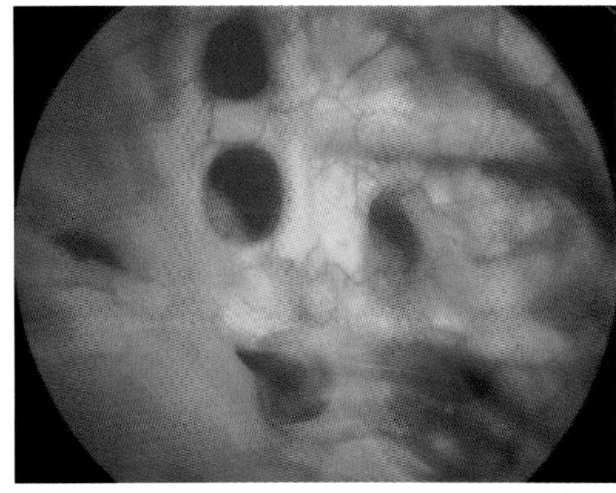 135

Fig. 134 Radical TUR of the bladder wall.
The tumor is resected down to the healthy tissue of the peripheral bladder wall. The picture demonstrates cut bundles of the peripheral muscle; in between, there is loose connective tissue of the perivesical space (compare peripheral capsule of the prostate, Figs. 91, 92, 111).

Fig. 135 Result after radical TUR of a bladder carcinoma (stage $T_2N_0M_0G_3$).
The scarred right ureteral orifice voids blue-colored urine. The trigone has a smooth, scarred surface. From the left bladder wall a scar comes down to the orifice. The scar reaches up into the three diverticula, which surround the orifice.

Three years previously an ulcerating tumor 4 cm in diameter situated on the right orifice was deeply and completely resected. On the first postoperative day an artery had to be coagulated. Nine years later the urine was normal; excretory urography and cystoscopy revealed no evidence of recurrence.

136 a–b
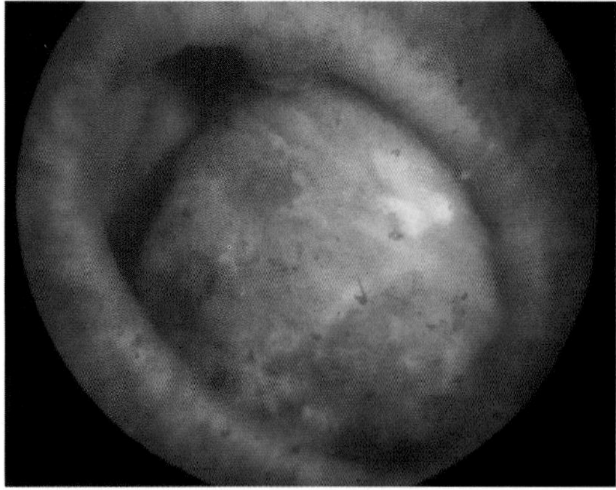
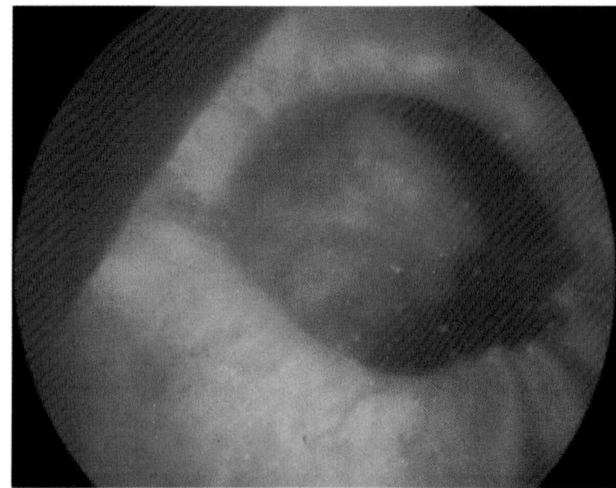

Radical TUR of a Spherical Bladder Carcinoma Within a Diverticulum
(Stage $T_{2m}N_0M_0G_1$)

Fig. 136, a
The tumor is the size of a walnut and nearly fills the wide-open diverticulum. A small papilloma rests at the rim of the diverticulum at 12 o'clock. At the left of the tumor, the depth of the diverticulum is realized.

Fig. 136, b
Three weeks after TUR the entire depth of the diverticulum is visible — here, however, from a greater distance than in *a*. The outlines are blurred by the slightly obscured irrigant. However, it is seen that the base of the tumor at the right in the diverticulum (at 3 o'clock) and the small papilloma were resected. The red shadow at the left represents part of the bladder neck. No recurrence after six years.

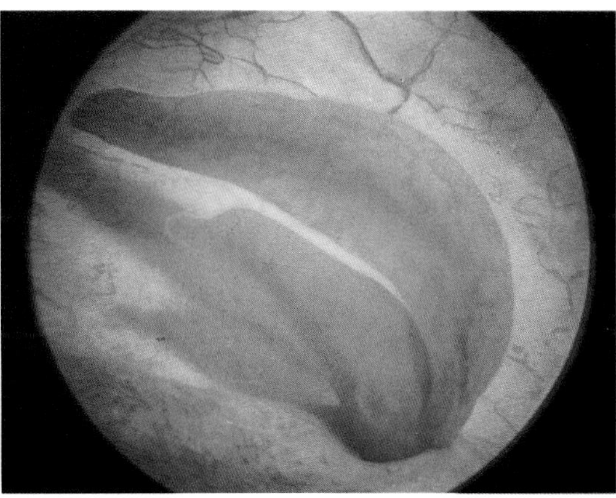

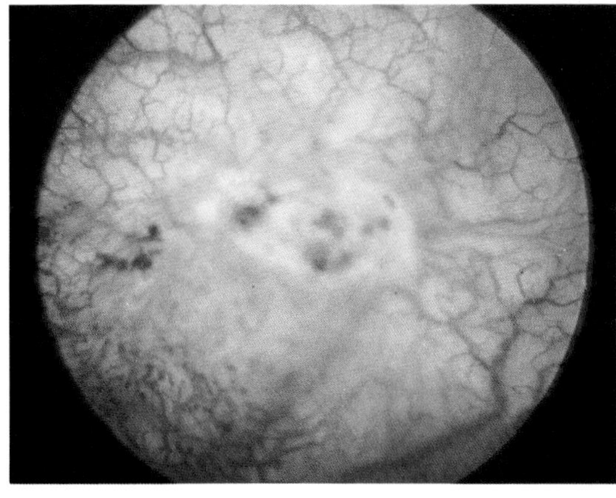

137 a–b

TUR of a Polyp in the Ureteral Orifice (Stage $T_0P_0G_0$)

Fig. 137, a

The interureteral crest is seen at the lower margin of the picture. A polyp arises from the left orifice; its two branches are almost translucent and are interspersed with fine blood vessels. The flashlight threw the shadow seen on the bladder floor.

Fig. 137, b

Illustrated here is the wound of the surprisingly small base of the tumor seen after TUR. The ureteral orifice is below the wound. The bladder shows a typical hyperergic vascular reaction (compare Fig. 129).

This cut was performed retrograde to create the smallest possible wound surface. Simple polyps of the urinary bladder are rare; unlike papillomas they consist only of edematous mucosa.

138 a–b 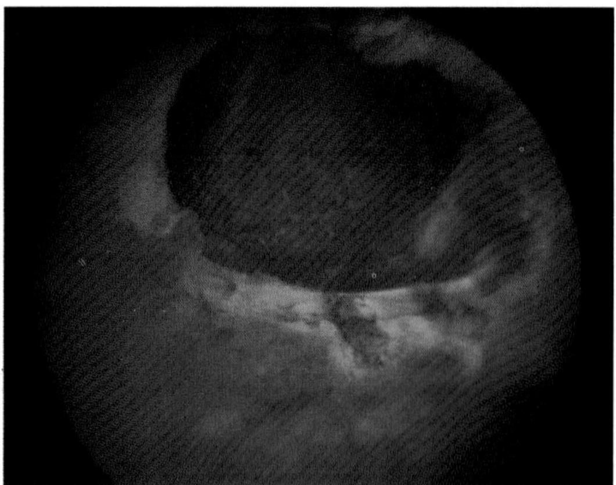

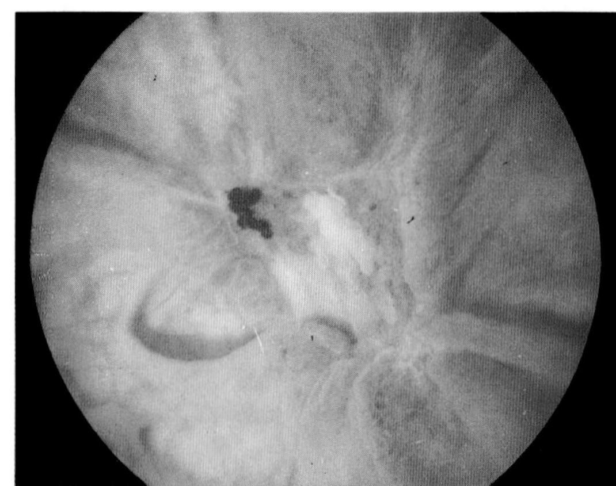

Perforation of the Bladder Wall During High Pressure TUR of a Large Papilloma (5 gm; Stage T_A)

Fig. 138, a Fresh perforation.
A wide, round opening can be seen at the right in the lateral bladder wall about the bladder neck. In the depth of the wound, dark red paravesical connective tissue is pictured. This is the result of an unintentional total bladder wall resection below the base of the tumor.

Perforation of the bladder was favored by two factors: 1. High pressure irrigation was applied, throwing a sharp jet of irrigant onto the defect; this tore it wide open, quickly forming a wide cavity in the perivesical space filled with irrigant. 2. The tumor was resected in the tightly-filled bladder. Thus, the bladder wall is under great tension and becomes even thinner. The cut then ruptures the stretched wall and perforates it. This can be completely avoided by using physiologic low pressure irrigation and continuous aspiration through the return-flow resectoscope. Even when the bladder is perforated, no irrigant is deposited in the paravesical space. This allows TUR of the entire bladder wall in the region of the tumor.

The bladder often is much thinner in the female than in the male—especially in patients with bladder atony and atrophy due to incontinence. TUR of bladder tumors perforates such a bladder relatively easily. Therefore, the loop must remain exactly within the level of the bladder mucosa when cutting. Retrograde cuts are more dangerous and must always be carefully guided.

Fig. 138, b Ulcerated scar.
A star-shaped scar remains two months after perforation of the bladder wall. In the center of the scar a defect of the mucosa is still evident. Its upper left rim is bleeding (compare Fig. 132). The perforation healed spontaneously after exclusive treatment by an indwelling catheter kept in place for two weeks.

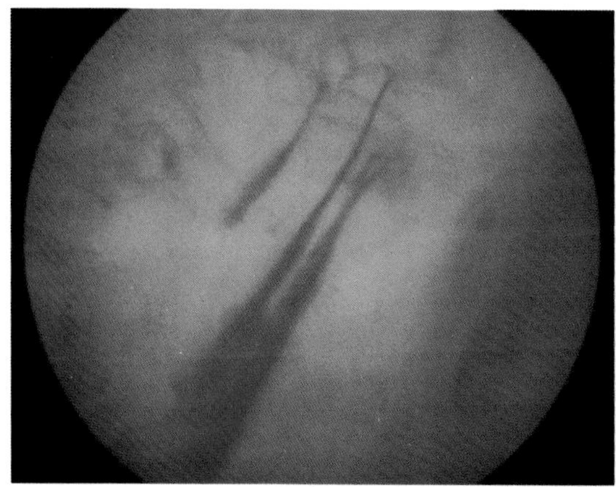

39

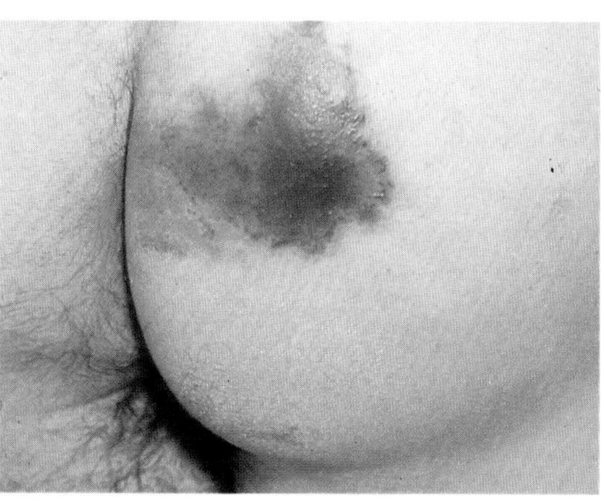

140

Fig. 139 Cytotoxic hemorrhage in a bladder with recurrent bladder tumors (stage T_A) after repeated TUR (chemical cystitis).

Three streaks of blood run down the posterior wall of the bladder that has been filled with slightly obscured irrigant. The bladder extravasates spontaneously from the mucosal veins. Unlike the irradiated bladder, the vessels are hyperemic, but without visible ulceration.

Electrical coagulation of these vessels usually is not successful. They have to be resected very superficially within the mucosa. As a result, larger sections of mucosa are removed; the regenerated epithelium is poor in vessels and does not bleed. Cryosurgery with moderate freezing temperatures (−20 to −40° C) is equal to TUR in result (compare the bleeding irradiated bladder, Fig. 183, a). Laser rays also can be applied for coagulation.

In this 38-year-old female, recurrent "benign" bladder tumors had been recognized for 11 years. Irrigation therapy of the bladder with cytostatic drugs was begun. Three years previously a pregnancy was carried to term without complications. Now chemical cystitis has occurred, causing persistent bladder hemorrhage and anemia. The bleeding vessels were coagulated and resected in five sessions at intervals of one to six months. This finally healed the disease; no papillomas recurred. At the age of 45 the patient died in a traffic accident, but shortly before her death urologic findings were normal (cystoscopy, isotope nephrogram, urine examination).

Fig. 140 Cytotoxic necrosis of the buttocks after permanent intra-arterial infusion of cytostatic drugs.

An irregular necrotic region is seen here in the skin of the right buttock.

The patient presented with a bleeding, shrunken bladder due to cancer, stage $T_4N_1M_xG_3$. The disease was so far advanced that operative therapy was not expected to be successful. Thus, the right internal iliac artery was tied and a transfusion tube introduced. Over the following two weeks the artery was permanently infused with cytostatic drugs until it became obliterated. The hemorrhage stopped spontaneously.

The patient recovered so well that he got married, but six months later he suddenly died.

The necrosis of the buttocks was caused by simultaneous irrigation of the external gluteal artery. In the following reported cases this artery was tied up (Z Urol *59*:125, 1966).

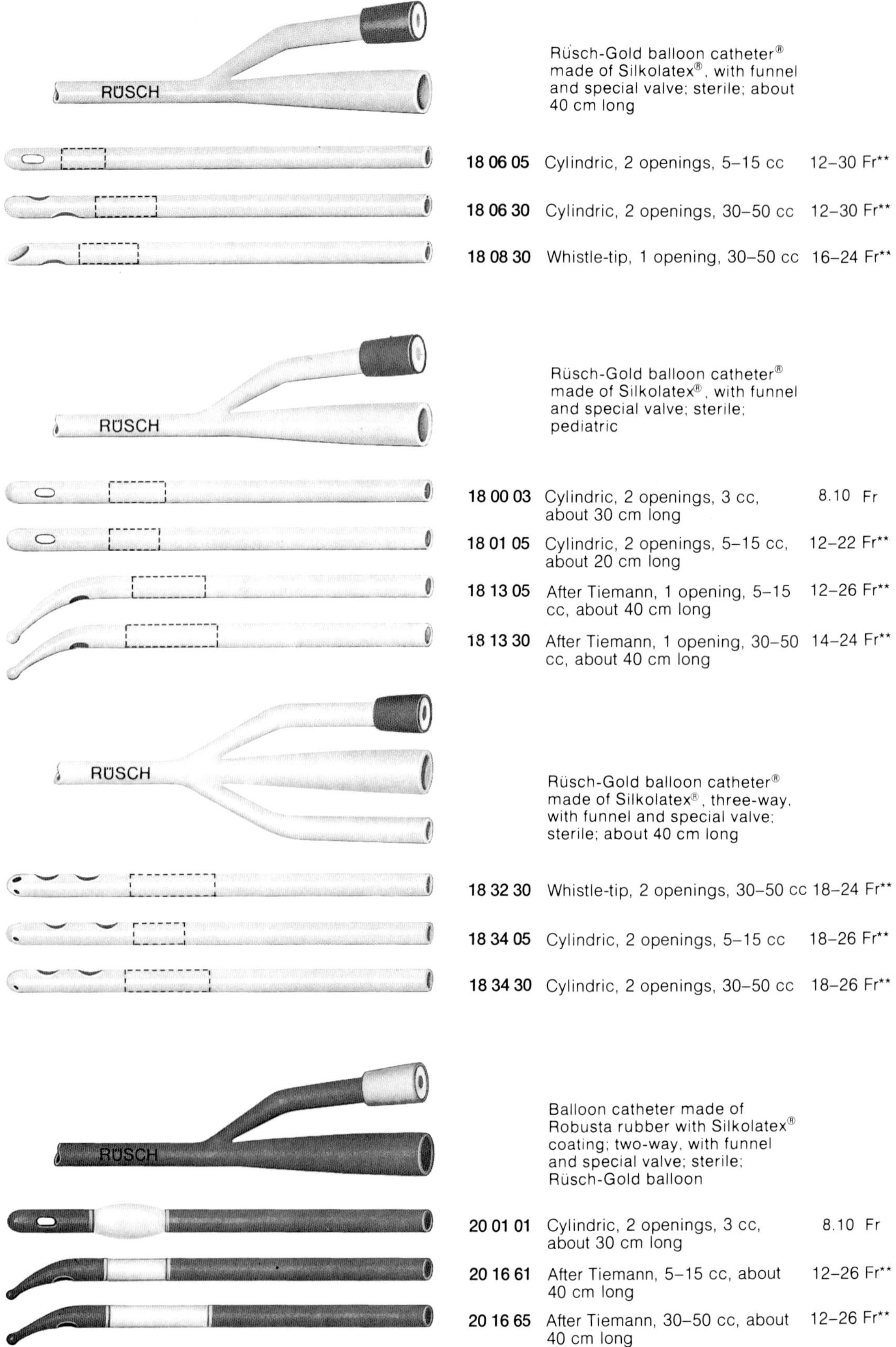

RÜSCH
Rüsch-Gold balloon catheter® made of Silkolatex®, with funnel and special valve; sterile; about 40 cm long
18 06 05 Cylindric, 2 openings, 5–15 cc 12–30 Fr**
18 06 30 Cylindric, 2 openings, 30–50 cc 12–30 Fr**
18 08 30 Whistle-tip, 1 opening, 30–50 cc 16–24 Fr**
RÜSCH
Rüsch-Gold balloon catheter® made of Silkolatex®, with funnel and special valve; sterile; pediatric
18 00 03 Cylindric, 2 openings, 3 cc, about 30 cm long 8.10 Fr
18 01 05 Cylindric, 2 openings, 5–15 cc, about 20 cm long 12–22 Fr**
18 13 05 After Tiemann, 1 opening, 5–15 cc, about 40 cm long 12–26 Fr**
18 13 30 After Tiemann, 1 opening, 30–50 cc, about 40 cm long 14–24 Fr**
RÜSCH
Rüsch-Gold balloon catheter® made of Silkolatex®, three-way, with funnel and special valve; sterile; about 40 cm long
18 32 30 Whistle-tip, 2 openings, 30–50 cc 18–24 Fr**
18 34 05 Cylindric, 2 openings, 5–15 cc 18–26 Fr**
18 34 30 Cylindric, 2 openings, 30–50 cc 18–26 Fr**
RÜSCH
Balloon catheter made of Robusta rubber with Silkolatex® coating; two-way, with funnel and special valve; sterile; Rüsch-Gold balloon
20 01 01 Cylindric, 2 openings, 3 cc, about 30 cm long 8.10 Fr
20 16 61 After Tiemann, 5–15 cc, about 40 cm long 12–26 Fr**
20 16 65 After Tiemann, 30–50 cc, about 40 cm long 12–26 Fr**

Fig. 141 Catheters often used after TUR, cryosurgery, urethrotomy and for bladder fistulas.

20 20 00	Cylindric, 2 openings, 50 cc, about 40 cm long	18–26 Fr**
20 21 01	2 openings, 5 cc, about 40 cm long	18 Fr
20 21 02	2 openings, 30 cc, about 40 cm long	20–24 Fr**
20 22 01	Elbowed (after Mercier); 2 openings, 50 cc, about 40 cm long	18–24 Fr**

Balloon catheter made of Robusta rubber with Silkolatex® coating; two-way, with funnel and Rüsch-Gold balloon; special valve; sterile; about 40 cm long

20 23 00	Elbowed after Mercier; whistle-tip, 2 openings, 50 cc	20.22 Fr
20 24 01	Elbowed after Mercier; 2 openings, 50 cc	24 Fr
20 24 02	Elbowed after Mercier; 3 openings, 50 cc	22–26 Fr**
20 25 00	Whistle-tip; 2 openings, 50 cc	20–24 Fr**
20 26 00	2 openings, 50 cc	20–26 Fr**

Balloon catheter made of Robusta rubber with Silkolatex® coating; three-way, with funnel and special valve; sterile; about 40 cm long

20 43 00	Cylindric, 2 openings, 50 cc	20–26 Fr**
20 44 01	Elbowed after Mercier; 3 openings, 50 cc	20–26 Fr**
20 44 02*	Elbowed after Mercier; 3 openings, 75 cc	24 Fr
20 45 00	2 openings, 50 cc	20–26 Fr**

*Not illustrated.
**Available only in even Fr sizes.

Endoscopic Cryosurgery

"Any new technique is at first thought to be inferior to perfected, conventional procedures." (W. P. SCHUCK)

"The utilization of endoscopy as an aid in localization during cryosurgery, as emphasized by Reuter, is extremely interesting and emphasizes that urologic cryosurgery can be done under direct vision with improved accuracy when combined with other modes of examination. Certainly these techniques need to be refined and made more sophisticated.

The utilization of cryosurgery as part of the armamentarium for the management of extensive prostatic carcinoma is in its infancy. There is no question that the perineal approach to the main mass of the prostatic carcinoma can produce extensive destruction and elimination of the main mass of the prostatic tumor more satisfactorily than any other technique available at the present time. This is far superior to transurethral cryosurgery for prostatic cancer in that it approaches the neoplasm in its area of growth and does not have to destroy the urethra and base of the bladder to reach the tumor itself." (R. H. FLOCKS)

INTRODUCTION

Endoscopic cryosurgery of prostatic and bladder tumors has become a routine procedure because of its obvious merits. It differs from conventional operations in essential features. It is relatively uncomplicated and there is little stress to the patient, making the procedure ideal for the large adenoma in a high-risk patient, for carcinoma in its early stages and as palliation for an inoperable carcinoma. It also can be indicated for the treatment of large bladder tumors that otherwise require highly sophisticated transurethral techniques. The complications of endoscopic cryosurgery occur mainly because of improper patient selection, choice of instruments and technique.

If cryosurgery still meets with skepticism and rejection today, it is the negative experiences with the blind technique that are cited. We readily concur. The blind technique with its overlong freezing time was part of the experimental stage of cryosurgery (see Figs. 161, 165, 169, 170). We reject blind cryosurgery because of our own unsatisfactory experiences and its inherent low efficiency (see Tables 12, 14). On principle we insist on controlling all the phases of the process of freezing tissue within the body. This is not possible without optical and other aids. Therefore, we have developed the following methods: 1. endoscopic cryosurgery (with trocar cystoscopy); 2. determination of the distance between the frozen area and the rectum; 3. repeated freezing with short freezing times (one to four minutes at the most) is obligatory; 4. trocar cryosurgery for central freezing of the tumors (e.g., in the peripheral prostatic capsule, Fig. 172); 5. partial burning of the tissue after freezing reduces the volume of the cryonecrosis (Cryocaustic).

After ten years of experience, endoscopic cryosurgery with repeated freezing has become a routine procedure in our hospital. With a frequency of 25 per cent, it now ranks second only to TUR. This represents a frequency about 10 per cent higher of indications for cryosurgery than one would expect to find in an average hospital. Open prostatic surgery has a frequency of about 2 per cent.

Each of these three methods has its own indications, distinct from each other. Application of each of the three, observing proper indications, has led to a decrease in postoperative morbidity and mortality. The choice of the correct operative procedure is made on an individual basis, considering the operative risk-degree (see p. 6).

To achieve satisfactory results with cryosurgery, the following postoperative measures are necessary (obligatory in patients with a large adenoma over 4 cm in diameter and in those with carcinoma and in poor-risk patients).

1. A suprapubic bladder fistula is maintained with an 18 Fr catheter over a two- to three-month period as a "safety valve" when voiding is obstructed (easily changed).
2. No transurethral catheter is used. Necrotic materials are voided transurethrally (the bladder fistula is closed during the day from the third week on).
3. Ambulatory suprapubic cystoscopy of the air-filled bladder is performed through the fistula without anesthesia to check on postoperative progress after four, six and (if necessary) eight weeks. The fistula is closed only when the bladder is free of necroses and residual urine.
4. When residual urine or poor voiding continues, a second session (cryosurgery or TURP) is performed after two or three months under the protection of the suprapubic bladder fistula (necessary in about 10 per cent of cases).

Historical Background

1961 Cooper JS, Lee A StJ: Hypothermic coagulation in neurology.

1963 Gonder MJ, Soanes WA: Cryoprostatectomy.

1968 Sesia G: Nitrogen oxide cryoprostatectomy, repeated freezing.

1968 Schrott KM: Carcinoma and freezing speed.

1968 Reuter HJ: Endoscopic cryosurgery of prostate and bladder, trocar cryosurgery, rectal distance measurement.

1970 Ablin RJ: Cryoimmunologic response.

1972 Flocks RH: Open perineal cryosurgery for prostate cancer.

1976 Keller AJ, Völter D: Cryocaustic.

Blind Cryosurgery

This technique is now obsolete. We have found postoperative complications to be eight times higher after blind cryosurgery than after endoscopic cryosurgery of prostatic hypertrophy. These failures are caused by a number of factors; a few are listed here:

1. An overlong freezing period of about 20 minutes without objective control of the freezing process. As a result, extended areas of sound tissue in the bladder neck, including the ostia, can be frozen and destroyed.
2. The rectal control knob of the probe does not permit precise placement of the freezing element on the tumor.
3. The overlong "Standard" cryoprobe is suitable for only about 10 per cent of the cases (i.e., the large adenoma over 5 cm long).
4. In most cases surface cryosurgery permits only partial destruction of the tumor.
5. Blind cryosurgery can be employed palliatively only in the prostatic urethra. Processes in the bladder and the peripheral capsule of the prostate cannot be treated.

Inadequate equipment is another reason for the failures of blind cryosurgery. Several new cryosurgery units and cryoprobes have promised more than they could provide (see Table 20, p. 242).

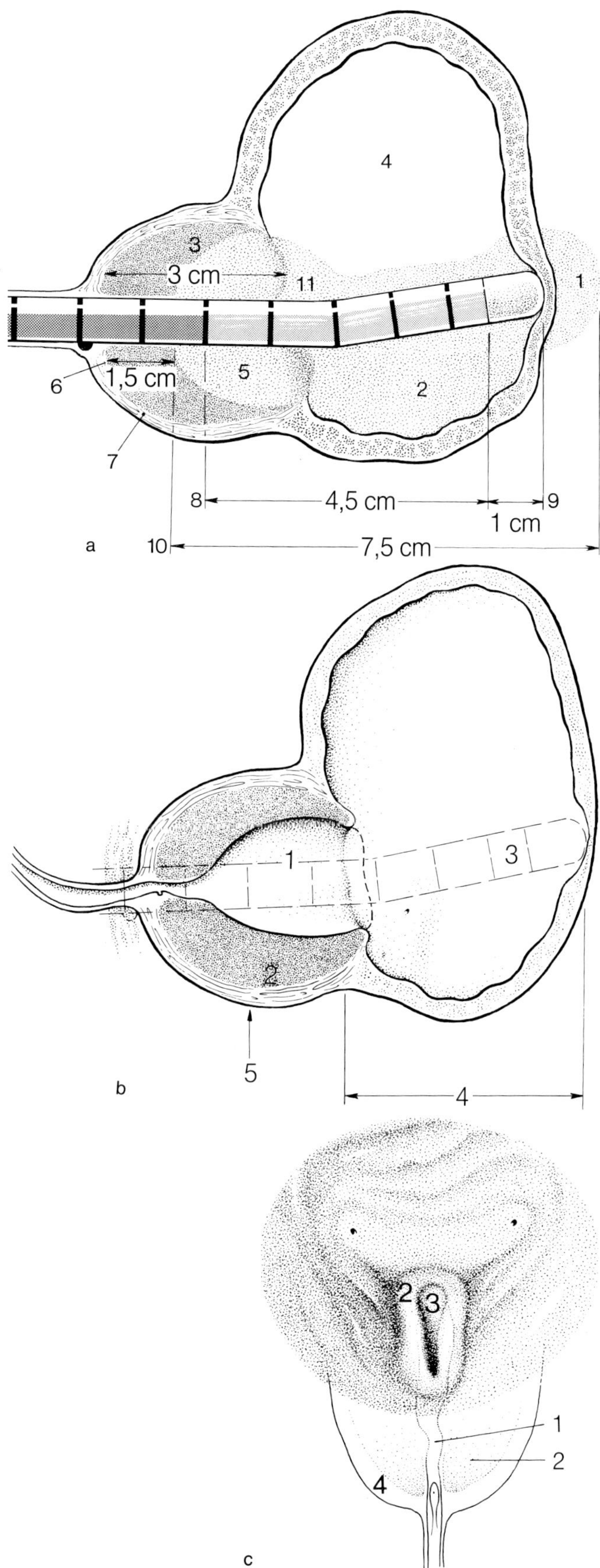

Fig. 142, a–c Complications and results of blind cryosurgery with the "Standard" cryoprobe (24 Fr; 4.5 cm length of freezing element; isolated tip; compare Fig. 165).

(a) Complications: 1 = Freezing element of the "Standard" cryoprobe is too long for most adenomas. Thus, the tip is pressed inadvertently against the posterior wall of the bladder. Its inadequate insulation fails to prevent freezing of the bladder wall at that point (as seen in the color film, "Cryosurgery," shown at the A.U.A. meeting, New York, 1973). 2 = The urine on the bladder floor freezes unnoticed, damaging the bladder wall and the ureteral orifices (compare Fig. 169). Diuresis is induced by cryosurgery, and in a few minutes 50 cc or more urine may collect on the bladder floor. 3 = Prostatic adenoma 3 cm long. The freezing element of the probe is about 2 cm away from the apex (control knob); therefore, it extends only about 1.5 cm into the prostatic urethra. The remaining 5.5 cm (including 1 cm of the insufficiently insulated tip) project over the bladder floor and can be harmful (so-called "harmful length"). The "Standard" cryoprobe is useful only for adenomas more than 5 cm long (compare Fig. 163). 4 = Gas (air). 5 = Frozen area within the adenoma (about 1.5 cm). 6 = Unfrozen adenoma (1.5 cm). 7 = Capsule. 8 = Freezing element (4.5 cm). 9 = Insulation (1 cm). 10 = Total length of the frozen area (7.5 cm). 11 = Length of the adenoma (3 cm). The results of blind cryosurgery with the wrong cryoprobe ("Standard"; partial cryoprostatectomy) are inadequate, leaving a saber-shaped urethra (compare Figs. 152, 165, 170).

(b) Longitudinal section through the prostatic fossa showing defect after cryosurgery (1). 2 = Remaining indurated adenoma surrounded by the capsule (5). 3 = Position of the "Standard" cryoprobe during freezing (compare Fig 165). 4 = Dangerous length of the projecting cryoprobe (4.5 cm).

(c) Trocar cystoscopy: Bladder neck with residual adenoma after incorrect freezing technique (blind cryosurgery). 1 = Prostatic urethra with frozen funnel (3). 2 = Remaining adenoma. 4 = Capsule.

FUNDAMENTALS OF CRYOSURGERY

Cell death is accomplished only if the tissue is frozen rapidly to −40°C and lower, down to −180°C. The effect is simultaneous formation of ice crystals in the extra- and intracellular spaces (homogeneous enucleation). Slow freezing prevents cell death by lyophilization (heterogeneous enucleation with temperatures up to −15 °C). A high freezing speeds is therefore essential (see Table 20, p. 242).

All our experiments have shown that the therapeutically effective depth of tissue freezing is reached after about three minutes (see Fig. 143). The drop of temperature slows as the area of freezing extends into the periphery, and the certainty of cell destruction is decreased.

We have further demonstrated that a frozen area is formed in the tissue around the cryoprobe. A well defined border exists between this area and the adjacent unfrozen tissue (see Distance Measurement, p. 179).

Further investigations have shown that cells surviving in this area die only after repeated freezing; slow thawing has a similar effect. In view of these studies, we freeze and thaw two or three times, limiting freezing time to three minutes as a rule. The distance between the well defined border of the frozen area and the rectum is measured with a needle transrectally.

If nitrous oxide (N_2O) is used for cryosurgery, freezing must be repeated up to eight times. The slow freezing speed (maximum cold, -90 °C) is about compensated by this means.

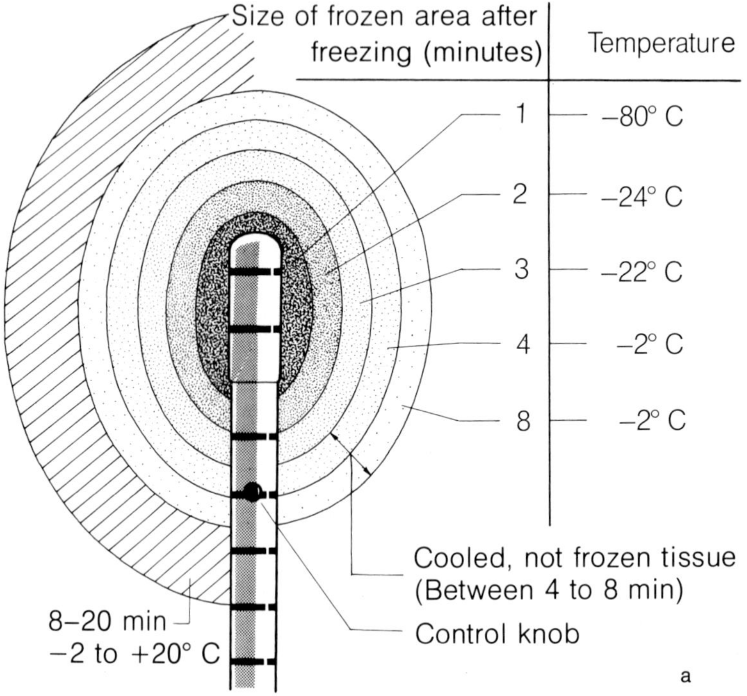

Fig. 143, a–d Freezing zones and partial cryoprostatectomy.

(a) Relation of freezing time and temperature in the frozen area during cryosurgery performed with the most commonly used cryoprobe, the "Special" (freezing element 28 Fr diameter and 2.5 cm lenght without useless insulation of the tip). The rate of expansion of the frozen area is markedly reduced three minutes after the start of freezing by the insulating effect of the frozen tissue (−22° C); it is completely stopped after four minutes (−2° C). When freezing is continued for more than four minutes, the tissue is only cooled, not frozen. In this peripheral zone (4–8 min; respectively, 8–20 min), tissue destruction leads to the formation of sloughs. Repeated freezing for three minutes at most is preferred over longer freezing times, because, in our experience, solid sloughs are not formed (see Table 20).

(b) Frozen area 5.7 × 3.9 cm around the "Special" cryoprobe (28 Fr; 2.5 cm freezing element). The tip of the probe was chilled for four minutes in water at 20° C.

(c) Frozen area (1) and cooled zone (2) within the prostatic adenoma (3). 4 = Capsule.

(d) Frozen funnel (5) within the prostate with indurated adenomatous coating (cooled zone) and the remainder of the middle lobe (6); partial cryoprostatectomy. 7 = verumontanum and middle urethra.

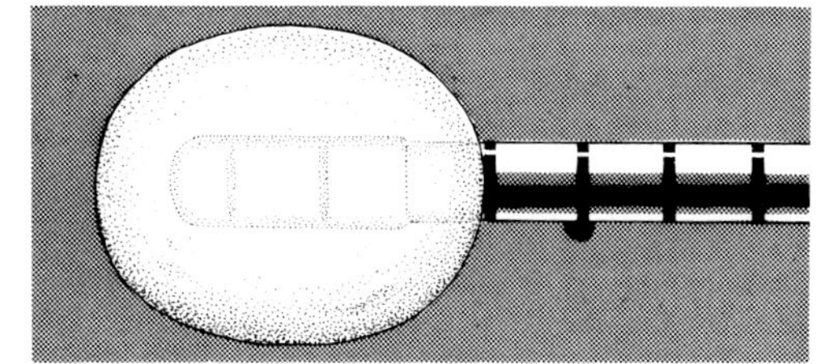

b

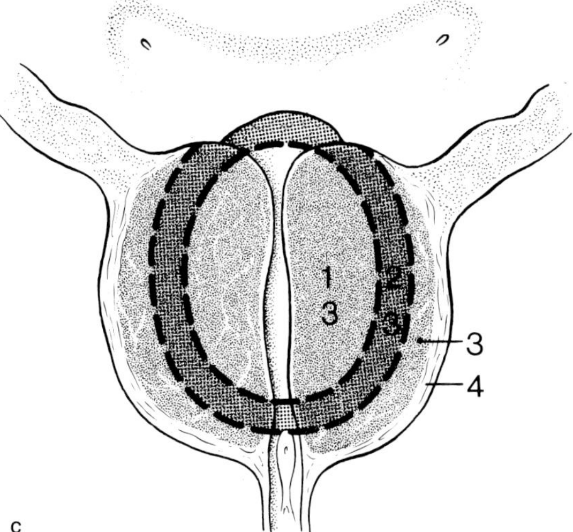

c

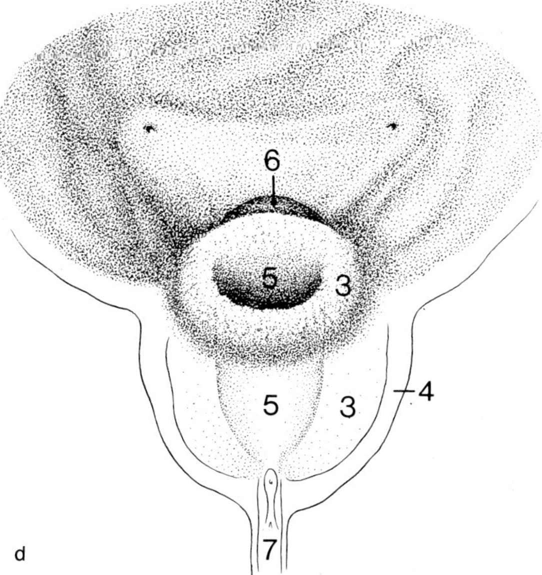

d

THE CRYOSURGERY UNIT

The cryosurgery unit freezes to a temperature of −196°C, with liquid nitrogen being evaporated in a chamber within the tip of the cryoprobe. The unit should be able to reduce the temperature at the tip in a short time to very low readings. All technical processes are controlled automatically. Liquid nitrogen is stored in an isolated Dewar container. We have had favorable results with the CE-4 unit (Frigitronics). The effectiveness of the unit can be checked easily by following these steps:

1. Freeze the cryoprobe tip to −180°C to cool the lining.
2. Thaw the tip to +20°C.
3. Now calculate the time needed to freeze the cryoprobe tip from +20°C to −180°C (an efficient unit freezes the cryoprobe in less than 30 seconds). The "Special" cryoprobe is frozen with the CE-4 unit to −180°C in 15.1 seconds in air and in 24 seconds in water at 20°C.

The different cryoprobes are also checked by determining the freezing time. Next, the size of the frozen area is measured: after a freezing time of three minutes in water at 20°C the most effective size is reached (see Table 20, Fig. 143). The temperatures of the individual layers of frozen tissue can be measured with thermoelements (see Table 20 and p. 180). The shape and diameter of the frozen areas depend on the circumference and length of the freezing surface of the cryoprobe (Figs. 142–151). Only probes of wide diameter (24 or, better, 28 Fr) are sufficiently effective in urology.

a

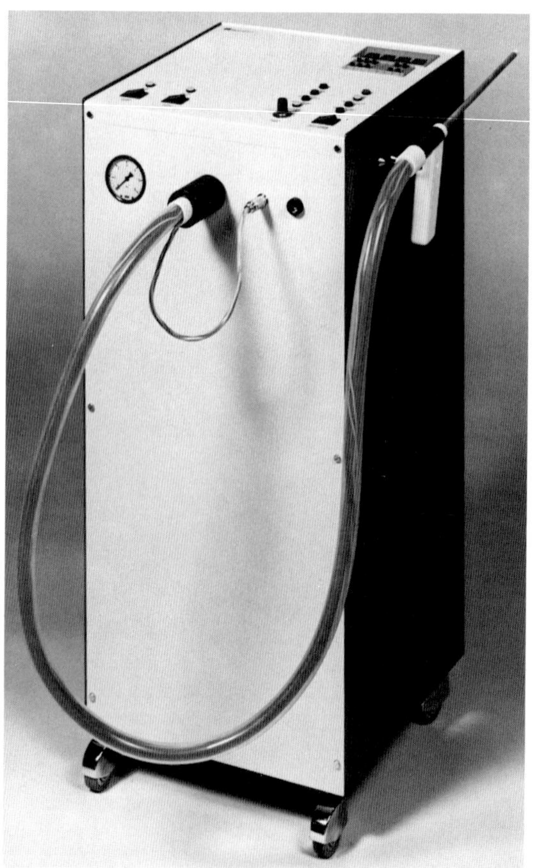

Fig. 144, a–c

(a) **Erbocryo OP.** Cryosurgery unit with special equipment for cryocauterization of the prostate. The reliable unit is fully transistorized and is equipped with a special attachment for refilling the 25-liter reservoir with liquid nitrogen; there is also a timer and an automatic thawing device. The temperature on the probe tip is displayed digitally from −196° to +200° C. (Erbe Elektromedizin, Tübingen, W. Germany.)

(bI) **Erbocryocaustic probe for prostatic and bladder tumors.** The temperature here also ranges between −196° and +200° C. The cryoprobes have diameters between 24 and 28 Fr and are coated with Teflon. This coating prevents tissue from sticking to the probe during cauterization. A lubricant is not needed for passage of the urethra. The control knob is 2 cm away from the freezing element. This element is 3 cm long in the short cryoprobe and 4.5 cm in the longer cryoprobe. Both do not have an insulated tip.

(bII) **Attachment for rectal distance measurement.** This measures the distance between the frozen area and the rectal mucosa from the apex (external sphincter). It is attached to the handle of the probe. Thus, the needles for measurement always touch the surface of the frozen area.

(c) **Erbo-Trocar Cryocaustic probe (after M.A. Reuter).** This probe is used for trocar cryocautery of prostate and bladder tumors; available diameters are 18, 21, 24 (and 28) Fr. The freezing element is 2 or 3 cm long. The available temperature range corresponds to the other probe.

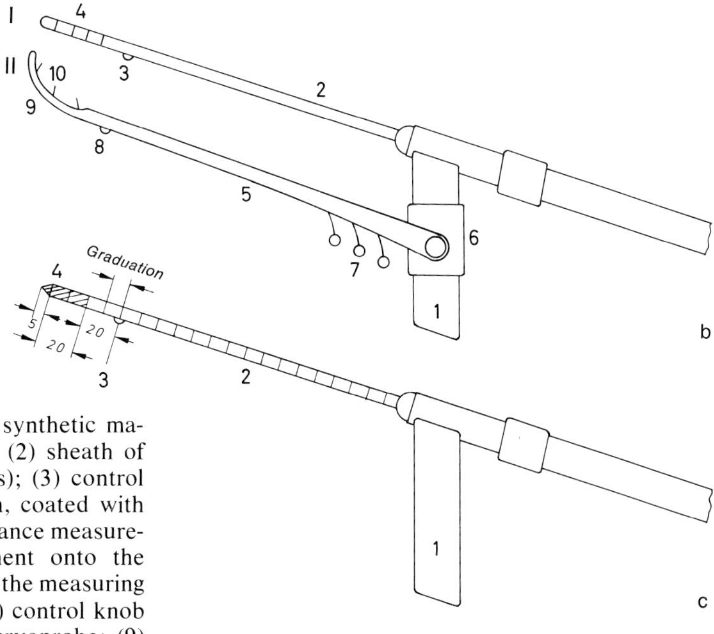

(1) Handle made of autoclavable synthetic material with hole for attachment (6); (2) sheath of the probe (graduated in centimeters); (3) control knob; (4) freezing element (3–4 cm, coated with Teflon); (5) attachment for rectal distance measurement; (6) fixation of the attachment onto the handle of the probe; (7) distal ends of the measuring needles graduated in millimeters; (8) control knob corresponding to the knob on the cryoprobe; (9) measuring end with five control needles; (10) tip of the control needles.

CRYOPROBES

Three different cryoprobes are required for cryosurgery. Shape, length and diameter of the freezing surface are important factors, because the freezing speed in tissue increases with the diameter of the probe. Two different probes are needed for surface cryosurgery; the trocar cryoprobe is used for the central freezing of tumors.

1. We prefer the "Special" cryoprobe. Its freezing section has a diameter of 28 Fr; its shaft is 1.6 mm thinner. This permits palpation of the distal rim of the freezing surface much like a control knob. This is important, for example, in freezing bladder neck strictures (see Fig. 182). The freezing surface of the probe is 25.4 mm long, and its unisolated tip is rounded. We use it for surface freezing of prostatic and bladder tumors less than 5 cm in diameter (see Fig. 174).

2. The "Standard" cryoprobe has a diameter of 24 Fr; the freezing surface is 4.5 cm long. It is used to freeze large prostatic tumors over 5 cm in length. Total cryosurgery in the sense of a prostatectomy usually is not possible in one session because the freezing effect is not sufficient to destroy adenomas with a total diameter of over 4 cm. Large adenomas, therefore, often are frozen by using both the "Standard" and the trocar cryoprobes. This allows central freezing of the lateral and median lobes and is more effective than surface freezing alone (see Figs. 149; 163).

3. The "Trocarcryoprobe," developed by us, has a diameter of 24 Fr; its freezing surface is 18 mm long. It is used to complete or to replace surface freezing (see p. 180) by central freezing (trocar cryosurgery, p. 182).

4. The silicone cryoprobe (Fig. 144) can be used without a lubricant. After cryosurgery frozen tissue is heated up to 160°C to avoid postoperative bleeding (cryocaustic; Keller and Völter).

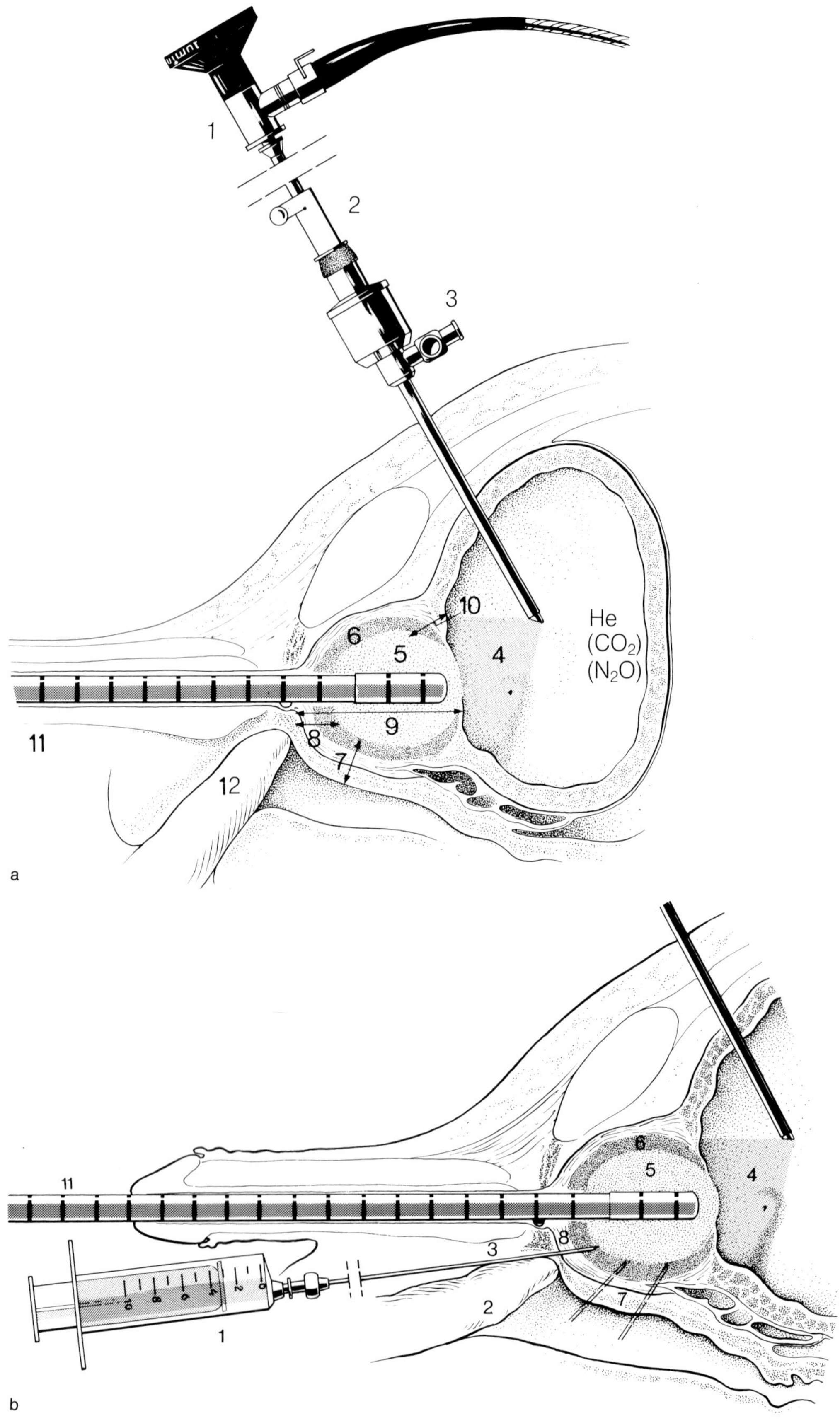
1
2
3
10
6
5
4
He
(CO_2)
(N_2O)
9
8
7
11
12
a
11
6
5
4
8
3
2
1
b

Fig. 145, a–e Endoscopic cryosurgery.

(a) Trocar cystoscopy for control of the endovesical freezing process. 1 = Optical system (of a regular cystoscope); 2 = screw for fixation of the optical system; 3 = trocar sheath with air-tight valve and stopcock (R. Wolf); 4 = field of vision of the 110° illuminated lens; 5 = frozen area within the adenoma around the freezing element of the cryoprobe; 6 = adenoma around the frozen area; 7 = distance between the frozen area and the rectal mucosa; 8 = distance between the frozen area and the external sphincter; 9 = distance from the apex to the bladder neck (length of the prostatic urethra or, as the case may be, the adenomatous prostate); 10 = distance between the bladder neck and the frozen area; 11 = "Special" cryoprobe with control knob and thickened freezing element on the tip (28 Fr) graduated in centimeters; 12 = palpation of the control knob at the apex, and endoscopic measurement of the length of the prostate in centimeters (see arrow); He = helium gas.

(b) Measurement of the distance between the rectum and the frozen area for exact control of the subvesical freezing process. 1 = Syringe with biopsy needle (3) for measuring the distance between the rectum and frozen area (7 and 8) and for aspiration biopsy; 2 = operator's index finger in place to indicate the rectal mucosa line on the needle when withdrawn. (4–8 and 11 are the same as in Fig. 145, a).

(c) Measurement of the distance between external rectal sphincter (apex) and the frozen area with the aid of the fingertip (compare Fig. 145, a and b; 2–11 as in Fig. 145, a).

(d) Trocar sheath with air-tight valve and obturator (R. Wolf). The sheath is used for suprapubic trocar crystoscopy with a regular optical system, which is introduced after removing the obturator. 1 = Valve with tip of the trocar obturator; 2 = total view.

(e) Trocar cystoscopy for endoscopic cryosurgery. 1 = Trocar cystoscope; 2 = aspiration of urine from the bladder floor under endoscopic control; 3 = ureter catheter in trocar cystoscope with side channel (1).

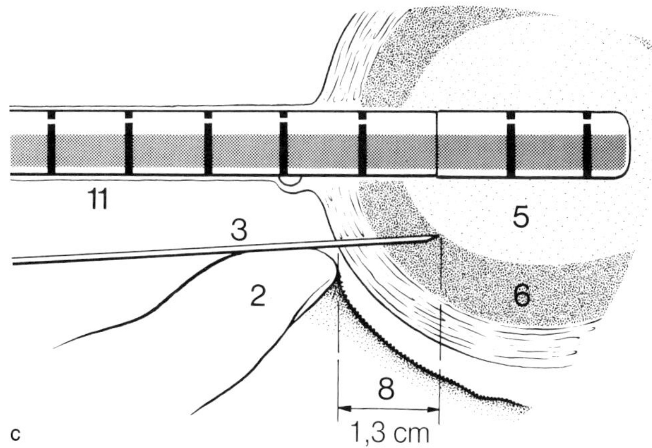

c

d

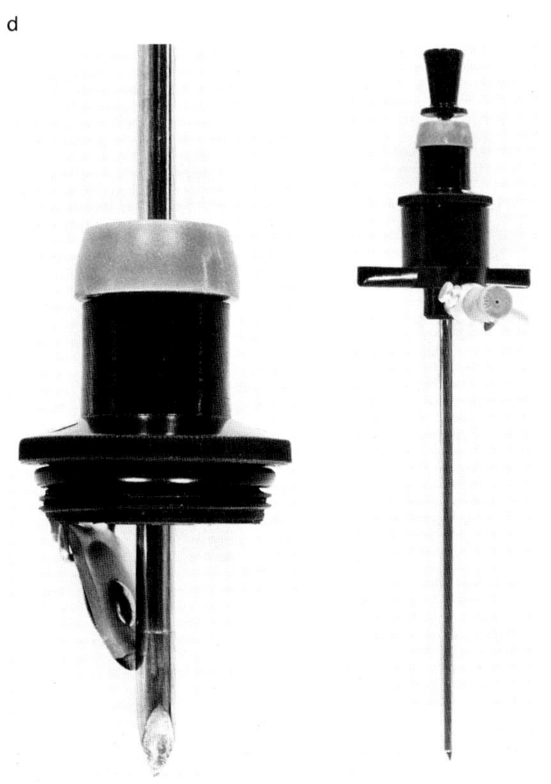

e

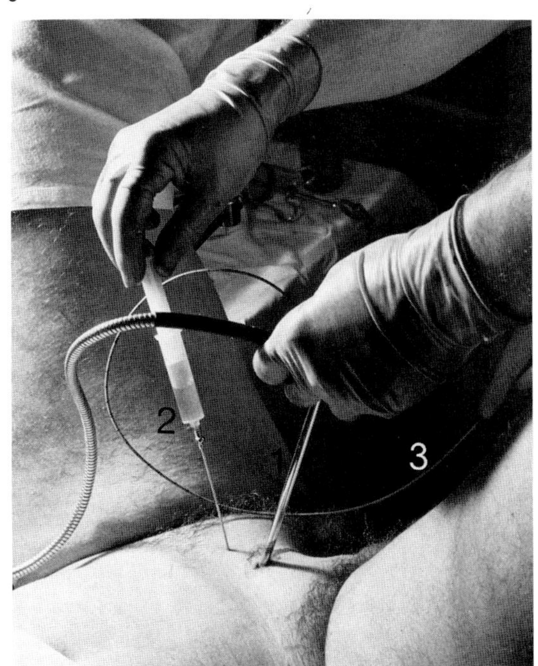

ENDOSCOPIC CRYOSURGERY

This method was developed by us to control freezing in all phases. Endoscopy (trocarcystoscopy) allows continuous visualization of the bladder neck during cryosurgery. The frozen tissue always forms a well defined border against the unfrozen mucosa. Every phase of the freezing process therefore can be controlled and can be stopped as needed. The freezing process hidden in the depths of the prostate is controlled by further measures: rectal distance measurement, probe twisting and thermostatic control.

Suprapubic Trocar Cystoscopy (Fig. 145)

For trocar cystoscopy we use air-tight trocar cystoscopes without operating channels. The procedure is easy to perform and is without risk if the following conditions are observed: The bladder must be filled to a volume of 300 to 400 cc (minimum 150 cc). The incision must be at the upper rim of the pubic bone; the trocar is introduced toward the bladder at an angle of 30 degrees, not vertically. (This is to avoid puncturing the enlarged prostate.) The abdominal musculature must be relaxed; the patient cannot strain or cough. Peridural or local anesthesia in combination with preoperative Valium is therefore preferred. If the patient strains, gas or water extravasates beside the trocar into the perivesical space, and the bladder loses volume. However, the bladder can be refilled, and the extravasated gas (or water) is resorbed without complication. Diuresis should not be induced before cryosurgery (furosemide infusion), because then the bladder floor must be dried repeatedly by a suprapubic cannula.

Exploratory puncture of the bladder and cystoscopic guidance of the suprapubic introduction of the trocar into the bladder are important controls for the inexperienced operator. Quick action during cryosurgery is favorable, because diuresis and hemorrhage obscure the view. Suprapubic cystoscopy also can be performed through a bladder fistula, which should be made at least one week before cryosurgery. The suprapubic stab incision also can be made on the tip of a transurethrally-introduced curved bougie (J. Alvarez).

Complications. We now have performed more than 3000 suprapubic punctures for cystoscopy, cryosurgery and low pressure irrigation (during TUR) and so far have experienced no serious complications with disagreeable consequences for the patient. However, it is of interest to know what kinds of complication may occur:

1. Puncture of the peritoneum (in the sense of a laparoscopy) because an emptied bladder was not noticed.
2. Puncture of the enlarged prostate because the angle of the stab incision was too vertical (Fig. 149).
3. Puncture of the paravesical space because the tip of the intruding trocar slid unnoticed sideways on the bladder wall.
4. Withdrawal of the bladder wall from the tip of the trocar because the trocar was introduced too slowly or because an atonic bladder was not adequately filled. Paravesical fat is then seen through the optical system (Fig. 171, d).

These complications (1–4) can be avoided by exploratory puncture and cystoscopic control during the incision.

5. Loss of gas by straining occurs only when patient preparation for the operation is inadequate.
6. Hemorrhage of a vein in the bladder mucosa due to the incision. Blood runs over the lens, obstructing vision. The bleeding can be stopped in a few minutes when the trocar cystoscope is held as flat as possible (rare complication).
7. Blurring of vision by the bladder contents (mucus, urine, blood, foam). In this case the lens can be wiped at the mucosa of the lateral bladder wall or can be drawn out of the air-tight sheath (Fig. 145) for cleaning.
8. Rapid covering of the bladder floor by urine or blood, so that it can no longer be seen. Urine or blood can then be aspirated through a needle introduced suprapubically, through the trocar or through a catheter.
9. Accidental withdrawal of the trocar from the bladder. A new incision is always possible when the bladder volume is sufficient (300–400 cc.), because the bladder musculature contracts and closes the small incision (about 12 to 18 Fr) at once.
10. Postoperative complications: Purulent infection of the site of incision is rare; it heals spontaneously (we have seen no instance of abscess formation).

Escape of gas can result in local crepitation under the skin, but without untoward consequences. We have never seen a large paravesical extravasation of water that required surgical intervention. Scrotal edema or hematoma is rare, and more often these complications are due to cryosurgery (the tissue was overfrozen) than to trocar cystoscopy. We have never seen dangerous complications following trocar cystoscopy or indeed any other suprapubic puncture of the bladder for TUR.

In the male child we prefer trocar cystoscopy over transurethral trocar cystoscopy (12 Fr trocar); pediatric cystoscope (after Reuter).

The technique of suprapubic cystoscopy is shown in Figures 10, 49, 145, 149 and 151.

Perineal Trocar Cystoscopy

Trocar cystoscopy can be performed through the perineum in bladder cirrhosis or urethral stricture. The technique is similar to perineal introduction of the trocar cryoprobe (Figs. 147, 148).

Rectal Distance Measurement (Fig. 146)

Rectal distance measurement ensures endoscopic control (see Figs. 145, 149). The principle is simple. The distance between the rectal mucosa and the surface of the frozen area within the prostate is measured with a fine cannula. Using the same technique employed for fine needle biopsy, the cannula is pushed deep into the prostate until it touches the frozen area. With his fingertip, the operator marks the point on the needle where it entered the mucosa. When the needle is removed from the rectum, the distance between the mucosa and the frozen area can be measured exactly (the distance between the fingertip and the needle tip). Before the puncture, we inject 20 ml of 10 per cent povidone-iodine in the rectum.

In addition, we routinely check the distance between the frozen area and the apex (the external sphincter) and the other limits of the prostate — e.g., the bladder neck. Although several incisions are necessary for continuous control, we have not seen any postoperative complications. Transvesical distance measurement (suprapubic) is also possible. The needle is introduced alongside the trocar cystoscope and pushed into the bladder neck under endoscopic control until it meets the frozen area.

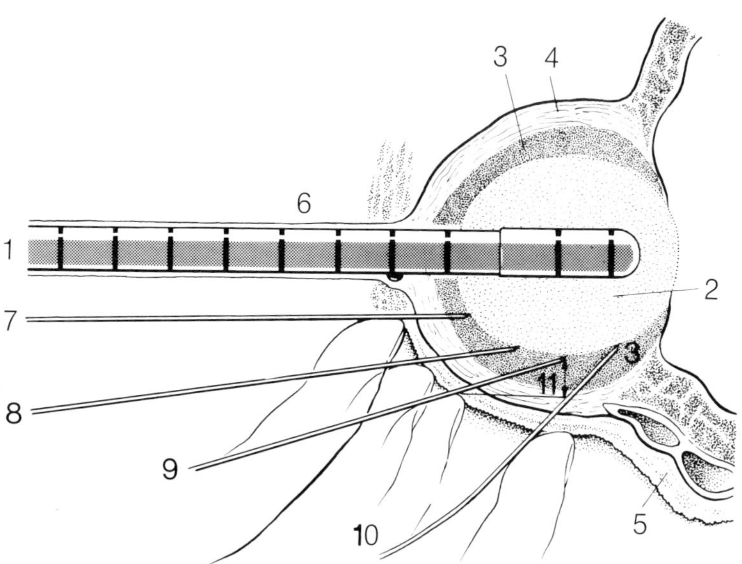

Fig. 146 Control of the subvesical iceball by rectal distance measurement.
The distance between the rectal mucosa (5) and the frozen area (2) is measured repeatedly (compare Fig. 149). When the expanding area of freezing approaches the rectum, the distance is reduced (11). 1 = Cryoprobe ("Special," 28 Fr); 2 = frozen adenoma; 3 = unfrozen adenoma; 4 = prostatic capsule; 5 = rectal mucosa; 6 = urethra; 7 = fine needle for measurement near the external sphincter; 8 = distance measurement at the apex; 9 = distance measurement in the middle prostate; 10 = distance measurement near the seminal vesicles (trigone); the needle is bent with the finger; 11 = the greater distance measured when the needle is introduced obliquely must be considered and corrected.

Temperature Controls

With the aid of needle-like thermocouples, the temperature of the tissue can be determined. This technique is useful only when the site of the needle tip is known exactly. Therefore, we recommend that the operator mark the needles with small spheres 5 to 10 mm from the tip to avoid uncontrolled introduction deep into the prostate. However, we prefer the simpler measurement of rectal distance.

The Probe Twisting Control

The frozen area in the prostate is fixed around the cryoprobe by the freezing process. However, when the probe is twisted slightly around its axis, the frozen area in the depth of the prostate can be palpated rectally. Caution is recommended, because twisting too forcefully ruptures the frozen blood vessels, causing considerable postoperative hemorrhage.

In conclusion, the advantages of endoscopic cryosurgery with distance measurement and repeated freezing are as follows:

1. The surgeon can see what he is doing.
2. The cryoprobe can be positioned exactly and can be readily adapted to the tumor.
3. Sound tissue (e.g., ureteral orifices, bladder wall, rectum) can be protected from freezing.
4. Bladder tumors are frozen without open surgery.
5. New procedures like trocar cryosurgery or cryocautery improve the quality of the cryosurgery.
6. Necrotic complications are seldom seen.

GENERAL TECHNIQUES OF CRYOSURGERY

Freezing is performed with four different techniques:

Surface Freezing

Surface freezing is most frequently applicable (Figs. 161–171). The freezing element of the probe is placed on the surface of the tumor. Therefore, the effect of the cold is strongest at the tumor surface. At a depth of 1 or 2 cm in the tumor, the freezing effect nearly vanishes (Fig. 143). All probes can be used for surface freezing.

We introduce the cryoprobe transurethrally, like a metal bougie, into the gas-filled bladder. Following rectal palpation, the control knob is set on the apex of the prostate; the optimal position is endoscopically controlled. Freezing is begun and is surveyed continuously both endoscopically and rectally (distance measurement). At the same time, fluid is aspirated suprapubically from the bladder floor to keep it from freezing (Fig. 149).

Freezing is stopped when the frozen area reaches a distance of 3 to 5 mm from the rectal mucosa at the apex (external sphincter; Fig. 145) and when a freezing time of 3 minutes has been reached. If the rectal distance still is more than 5 mm, the probe is thawed and placed more distally. The rectal control knob can then be as much as 10 mm distal to the apex. Freezing is repeated until the correct distance between the frozen area at the apex and the rectal mucosa has been reached. If the adenoma is too long, it is not completely frozen. After freezing of the apex, the tip of the cryoprobe is repositioned endoscopically on the bladder neck. The bladder neck is then frozen separately from the apex.

As a rule, the tissue is frozen at least twice to guarantee a sufficient cryosurgical effect. Finally, the tissue is thawed to allow the transurethral introduction of a catheter (20 Fr; 5 cc balloon) into the bladder. This takes about 5 to 10 minutes, and is controlled endoscopically. A suprapubic fistula can be made through the sheath of the trocar with a small disposable tube (see Fig. 48, a).

Central Freezing: Trocar Cryosurgery (Figs. 147, 150)

The efficiency of freezing is increased considerably when the cryoprobe is pushed directly into the depth of the tumor. Following are the advantages of this technique over surface freezing:

1. The entire tumor can be frozen to very low temperatures. This is essential in the treatment of carcinoma; cells are destroyed for certain only at temperatures below −80°C. The base of the tumor is not sufficiently frozen by surface freezing if its distance from the freezing surface is more than 0.5 cm.
2. As many frozen areas as necessary can be produced within the tumor. They thaw slowly with the natural warmth of the body after the heated probe has been separated from the frozen tissue.
3. Necroses remain in the depth of the tumor below the mucosa, thus avoiding the complications of wound infection. Necrotic tissue antigens provoke the formation of antibodies so that immunologic rejection is begun (Ablin).
4. Postoperative progress is surprisingly good when cryosurgery is performed extraurethrally (perineally and suprapubically).
5. The effects of radiation therapy (e.g., cobalt) are potentiated by cryosurgery. We start radiation therapy as early as possible — one to four days postoperatively.

For central freezing we have constructed the trocar cryoprobe (p. 175) and have found three different ways of approaching the prostate and bladder.

Perineal Access (Fig. 151)

For perineal access the skin is incised lateral to the anus. The trocar probe is then introduced as in lithotomy, guiding the tip of the probe parallel to the rectum by rectal palpation. Thus far we have seen no rectal injuries. When the tip of the probe enters the prostate or the bladder floor, palpation of the control knob helps with orientation. At the same time we can observe by suprapubic trocar cystoscopy the bladder floor or wall where the tip is moving beneath the mucosa (Fig. 151).

Perineal trocar cryosurgery is indicated in the following cases:

1. Prostatic cancer growing pericapsularly or encircling the rectum. These can be frozen.
2. In large prostatic adenomas, the median and lateral lobes can be frozen separately as a supplement to surface cryosurgery.
3. In tumors of the bladder floor, the bases can be frozen more effectively (Fig. 175).
4. In difficult urethral strictures, transurethral passage of the probe through the stricture can be avoided (compare perineal trocar cystoscopy).
5. Rectal cancer.

The Transurethral Approach

With experience, the trocar cryoprobe can be introduced transurethrally into the bladder without using a protective cover on the tip. Earlier, we armed the point with a cut-off plastic catheter tip secured by a thread. Today we ensure the proper passage by means of rectal palpation and endoscopy similar to the technique used for treatment of the urethra with a bougie (see Fig. 122, i). We have developed two modifications of the transurethral approach:

1. The tip of the probe is introduced transurethrally to the apex and then is pushed into the prostate as in accidental perforation of the urethra (see Fig. 36). Under rectal and endoscopic control, the probe is pushed into the center of the tumor (e.g., lateral lobe or carcinomatous infiltration). The control knob of the probe shows the depth of introduction (Figs. 147, 148).
2. The probe is introduced into the bladder through the urethra and there under endoscopic vision (trocar cystoscopy) pushed into the median lobe or a bladder tumor, for instance (Figs. 148, 175).

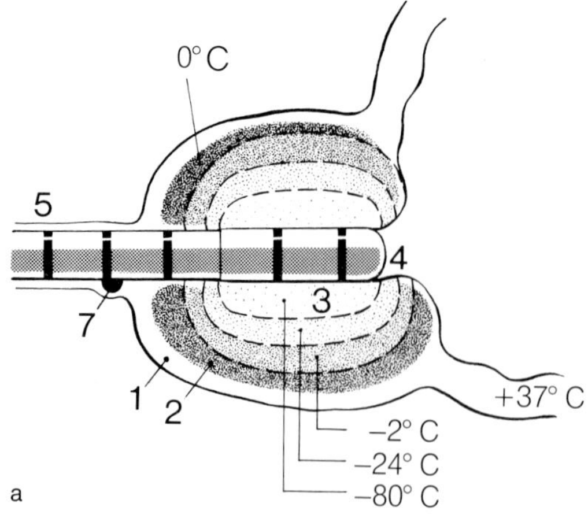

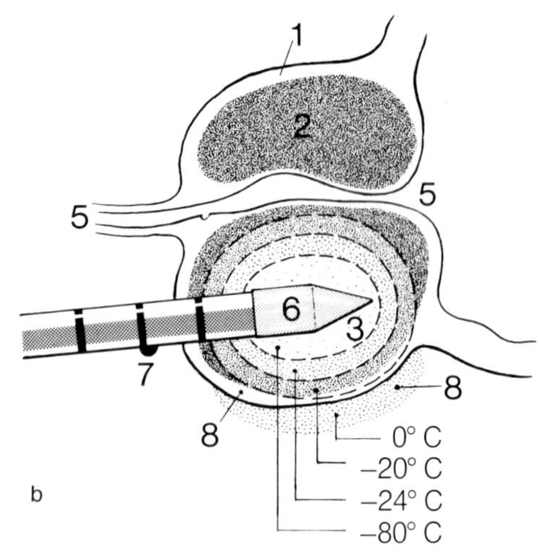

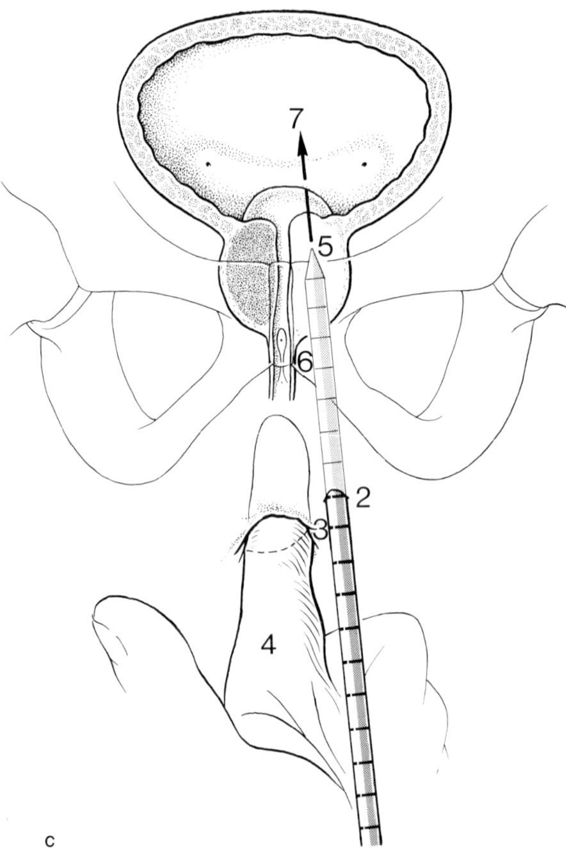

Fig. 147, a–c Transurethral and perineal technique of cryosurgery.

(a) Surface technique; transurethrally introduced probe; freezing zones 0° to −80° C.

(b) Central freezing technique with cryoprobe introduced perineally (trocar cryosurgery); freezing of the peripheral base of the tumor (compare Figs. 148, 172). 1 = Capsule; 2 = unfrozen adenoma; 3 = temperature zones within the frozen area; 4 = "Special" cryoprobe; 5 = urethra; 6 = trocar cryoprobe; 7 = control knob; 8 = infiltrated capsule; the frozen area extends into the periprostatic tissue.

(c) Perineal trocar cryosurgery (horizontal section through prostate and bladder). Closed technique: The cryoprobe (1) is pushed into the perineum (2) after a stab incision of the skin beside the anus (3). The finger in the rectum (4) controls the introduction of the probe between the rectum and pelvic wall; this approach was already known for lithotomy procedures in the middle ages. The tip of the cryoprobe is then pushed into the prostate (5). The control knob (6) is set onto the rim of the capsule at the apex. Now the lateral lobe can be frozen centrally. When necessary, the tip is made to perforate the bladder (7) or is positioned in whatever location in or beside the prostate is found to be desirable (compare Fig. 172).

Open technique: The perineum is incised (as in radical prostatectomy) in an arch, and the prostate is exposed. Now the trocar cryoprobe is pushed into the tumorous infiltrate, which is frozen. This may be repeated several times.

Fig. 148, a and b Approaches for trocar cryosurgery (central freezing with the trocar cryoprobe).

(a) 1 = Transurethral introduction of the trocar cryoprobe (endoscopic control by trocar cystoscopy; compare Figs. 145 and 175, c); 2 = transperineal introduction of the trocar probe (directed by trocar cystoscopy; compare Figs. 150, 151, 172); 3 = suprapubic introduction of the trocar probe (controlled by cystoscopy; see p. 184); 4 = bladder tumor; 5 = adenoma; 6 = finger in rectum (on the control knob).

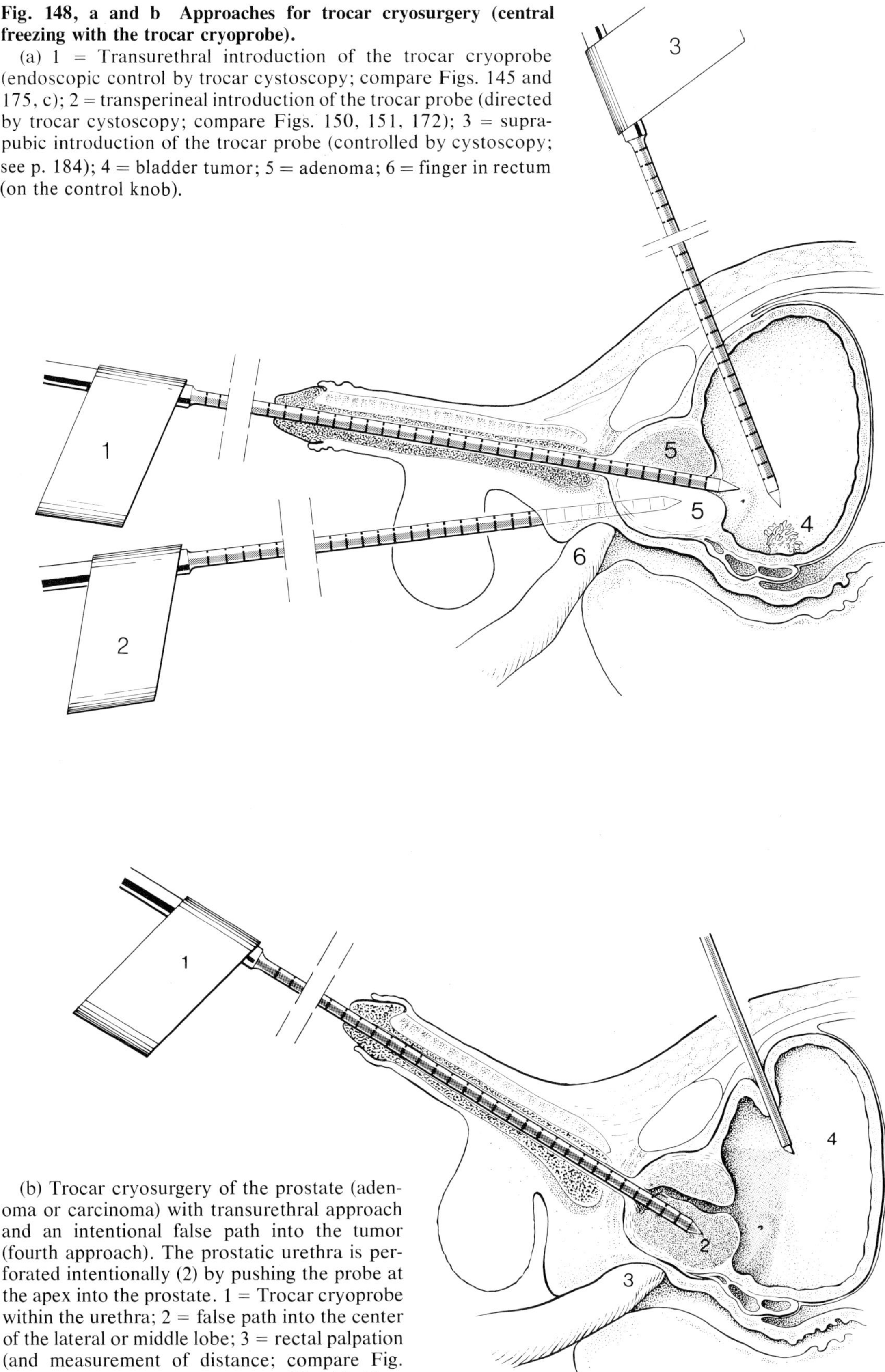

(b) Trocar cryosurgery of the prostate (adenoma or carcinoma) with transurethral approach and an intentional false path into the tumor (fourth approach). The prostatic urethra is perforated intentionally (2) by pushing the probe at the apex into the prostate. 1 = Trocar cryoprobe within the urethra; 2 = false path into the center of the lateral or middle lobe; 3 = rectal palpation (and measurement of distance; compare Fig. 145); 4 = trocar cystoscopy; gas-filled bladder.

Suprapubic Approach (Fig. 148)

The trocar probe is introduced into the bladder using the same technique as for trocar cystoscopy (see p. 31). This is controlled by routine cystoscopy (see Fig. 125). There are two modifications:

1. Intravesical trocar cryosurgery can be used to freeze bladder tumors that are difficult to reach transurethrally (lateral wall of the bladder, bladder floor; see the film on cryosurgery presented at the AUA, New York, 1972).

2. Perivesical trocar cryosurgery. The cryoprobe remains outside the bladder wall in order to freeze perivesical infiltrations at the base. The movement of the tip of the probe under the bladder mucosa can be controlled easily by endoscopy, suprapubic trocar cystoscopy or transurethral cystoscopy.

Open Technique of Cryosurgery

The prostate or bladder is approached by open perineal or suprapubic surgery. The exposed tumor is frozen as described above with a surface or trocar cryoprobe.

Freezing with open cryoprobes is much more effective than with probes utilizing closed circuits. In open probes, liquid nitrogen is evaporated in open tubes. This technique is difficult to control; therefore, we do not employ it.

Cryosurgery and TUR as a Combined Technique

These techniques complement each other in many ways:

(a) Freezing reduces the hemorrhage that occurs immediately after TUR and prevents extravasation of irrigants.

(b) TUR removes the destroyed tissue and completes the operation.

(c) Partial TUR can be completed with cryosurgery.

By 1968 we had performed successfully over a hundred combined operations. Other authors have confirmed our results (Fiedler; McDonald). The new concept of TURP with low pressure irrigation and continuous aspiration of irrigant (see p. 25) has made cryosurgery before TUR superfluous. Indications for cryosurgery are restricted to prostatic carcinoma, prostatic adenoma of the poor-risk patient and bladder tumors.

SPECIAL TECHNIQUES OF ENDOSCOPIC CRYOSURGERY

Prostatic Hypertrophy (Cryoprostatectomy)

Cryosurgery in one session achieves total or subtotal prostatectomy in only about 20 per cent of cases — i.e., adenomas less than 4 cm in diameter. In the majority of cases, only partial prostatectomy is achieved. The success of this operation is relatively good. There is an effect of induration of the tissue after freezing. The indication for cryosurgery of the prostatic adenoma depends on several factors. The most important are the operative risk of the patient (see p. 6) and the size of the adenoma. We only perform cryosurgery in patients of risk-degree II to IV. Life expectancy should not be more than five years; hence, most patients are over 70 years old. Exceptions to this rule are a few patients with a small adenoma, prostatitis or sphincter sclerosis. Here, the results of cryosurgery are often better than those of TUR or open prostatectomy. After freezing there is almost no stricture formation (below 0.6 per cent; see Table 13).

The length of the diameter of the adenoma is measured with the aid of the graduated cryoprobe. The control knob of the probe is set exactly at the rim of the apex by the rectal palpation; then the length is measured as the distance of the control knob from the tip of the probe minus the length of the probe-tip protruding into the bladder (trocar cystoscopy).

1. The small adenoma (up to 4 cm in diameter) is easily frozen. The "Special" cryoprobe (28 Fr) is the most useful. Total or subtotal prostatectomy is possible in most cases.

2. The medium-large adenoma (5 to 6 cm in diameter) is frozen with the "Standard" cryoprobe (see Fig. 162). Total cryoprostatectomy is not always possible in one session, although in about 90 per cent a good result is obtained. The trocar cryoprobe is used as an adjunct if there is a large median or lateral lobe (Figs. 149, 167).

The effective "Special" cryoprobe (28 Fr) is used when the adenoma is situated mainly subvesically. The apical and proximal halves of the adenoma are frozen in two sections.

For patients who do not live nearby or who are poor operative risks, it is recommended that a suprapubic bladder fistula be created and maintained for two to three months in order to facilitate home care. This also helps to prevent pyelonephritis, since urinary retention does not occur.

If the first session of cryosurgery does not produce satisfactory results, it is repeated after two or three months. Or TURP may be performed (in about 10 per cent of cases; see Table 13, p. 238).

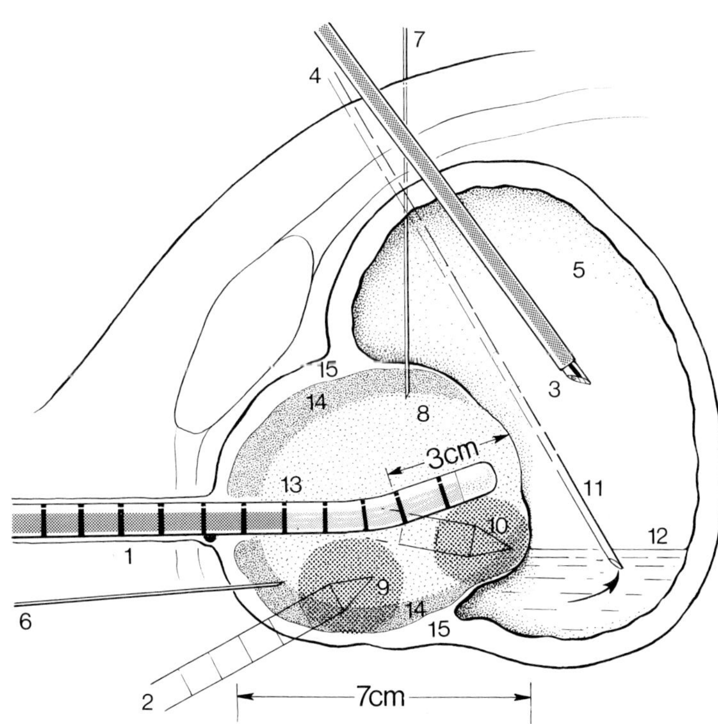

Fig. 149 Endoscopic cryosurgery of a giant adenoma: 7 cm long with a large endovesical component (3 cm).

Correct application of the long cryoprobe ("Standard"; 24 Fr; 4.5-cm freezing element). The newer probe — "Erbe" — is 28 Fr and has no insulated tip. Freezing is repeated to prevent necroses (compare Fig. 163). 1 = Correct positioning of the "Standard" cryoprobe; 2 = trocar cryosurgery completes freezing of the adenoma (see pp. 100–101) transperineally (9) and transurethrally (10); 3 = endoscopic control (trocar cystoscopy); 4 = suprapubic aspiration of urine to dry the bladder floor (compare Fig. 161); 5 = gas filling of the bladder (with helium or nitrous oxide) to prevent fogging; 6 = needle for rectal measurement of the distance between the external sphincter (apex) and the frozen area and for aspiration biopsy (compare Figs. 145, b and c); 7 = needle for suprapubic measurement of distance, meeting the frozen area (8); 8 = frozen tissue around the "Standard" cryoprobe (within the adenoma), which was introduced transurethrally; 9 = frozen tissue around the trocar cryoprobe (at the apex), transperineally introduced; 10 = frozen tissue around the trocar cryoprobe (in the middle lobe), introduced transurethrally; 11 = cannula (3 mm diameter); 12 = level of urine pool; 13 = rim of the freezing element (graduated in centimeters); 14 = unfrozen shell of the adenoma; 15 = capsule.

3. The giant adenoma (over 6 cm in diameter) presents difficulties in cryosurgery just as it does in TUR. We proceed as follows:

(a) Repeated freezing of the lateral lobes and, if necessary, of the median lobe with the trocar cryoprobe (Fig. 149).

(b) Repeated freezing of the prostatic urethra with the long cryoprobe ("Standard").

(c) Bladder fistula.

The suprapubic catheter (18 Fr) in combination with the transurethral catheter allows continuous irrigation of the bladder. After a few days the transurethral catheter is removed. The patient is now ambulatory and can be dismissed one to two weeks postoperatively. He should always carry a urinal to keep his bladder empty. Two to four weeks later the suprapubic catheter is closed intermittently during the day to make the patient void the necroses. Six weeks postoperatively an ambulant suprapubic cystoscopy is performed in the air-filled bladder. The necroses have by now been almost totally expelled, and a crater has formed at the bladder neck within the residual adenoma.

If urination is satisfactory, we do not repeat cryosurgery. In the few cases when a second session is undertaken after two to three months, the patient can be discharged a few days later. If the patient is in good general condition, a final TURP can be performed. TURP is easy then; little hemorrhage occurs owing to induration, and the patient tolerates the procedure well.

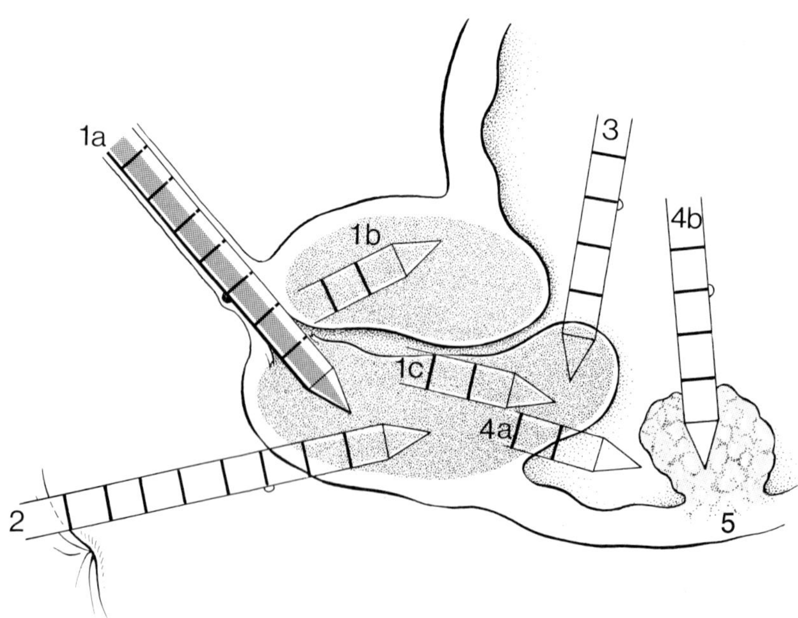

Fig. 150 Trocar cryosurgery of the prostate (1–3) and bladder (5).
1, a–c = Transurethral approach; 2 = perineal approach; 3 = suprapubic approach; 4, a = perineal and transurethral approach; 4, b = suprapubic (transvesical and perivesical) approach; 5 = bladder tumor.

Fig. 151, a and b Transperineal trocar cryosurgery of the peripheral prostatic carcinoma.

Explanation of the endoscopic photographs (Fig. 172, b): 1 = bladder neck; 2 = catheter in the urethra, surrounded by internal sphincter and adenoma; 3 = trigone with ureteral ostia; 4 = tip of the trocar cryoprobe introduced transperineally; 5 = intravesical part of the periprostatic tumorous infiltration (prostatic cancer); 6 = urethra; 7 = rectum; 8 = trocar cystoscope showing angle of view.

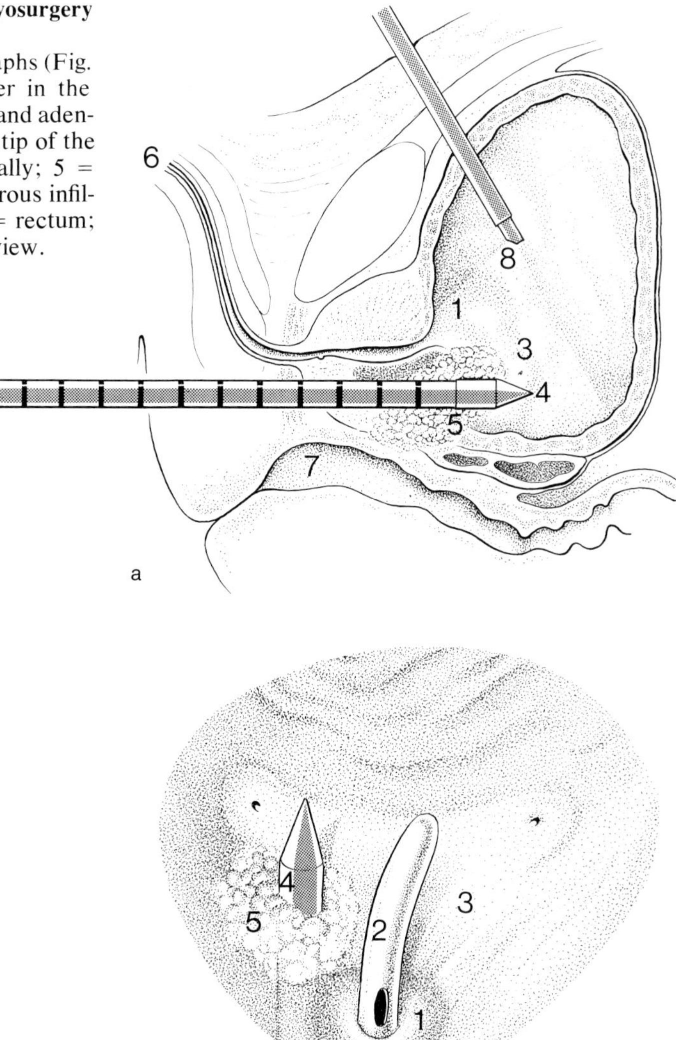

Prostatic Carcinoma (Figs. 171–173)

Cryosurgery of prostatic carcinoma achieves impressive results in about 40 per cent of cases. Most of the patients have cancer in stage T_3, where treatment is mostly palliative. It is often possible to keep the carcinoma under control until the patient dies of other reasons (about 70 per cent). Cobalt radiation therapy is an important aid in the treatment of progressive carcinoma after cryosurgery.

The advantages of cryosurgery over other operative procedures in prostatic carcinoma (radical TUR, open prostatectomy) are the following:

1. The technique is easy and is well tolerated by the patient.
2. It can be repeated several times; cryoimmunologic processes are induced.
3. Prostatic and endovesical infiltrations are frozen easily.
4. The effect of radiation therapy is potentiated.
5. During remission, repeated cryosurgery requires only a few days' stay in the hospital and no ambulatory treatment by permanent catheter.
6. Lymphadenectomy (with or without implantation of radioactive iodine) is performed independently of cryosurgery and is better tolerated.

Simultaneously estrogen therapy is begun (chlorotrianisene, polyestradiol phosphate) and orchiectomy is performed. Fosfestrol is given when the patient has bone pain because of metastases (10 ampules intravenously in five days). In the final stage, estramustine phosphate, a cytostatic agent, can be successful (reduction of pain, subjective amelioration of condition).

The technique of cryosurgery for cancer does not differ in principle from radical prostatectomy. We therefore repeat freezing of an infiltration as often as four times. The prostate is frozen until the rectal distance of the frozen area is reduced to 2 to 3 mm. The trocar cryoprobe is used as an adjunct for treatment of larger infiltrations.

Cryosurgery can be repeated several times at intervals of one to six months. Recurrences are often treated some years later with success. In these cases, we initiate cobalt radiation therapy.

Bladder Tumors (Figs. 174–180)

Cryosurgery of bladder tumors is as effective as TUR; in some cases, it is even superior (giant tumors, for example). Large papillomas (stage T_A) and papillary tumors (stage T_1) are the principal indications. Invasive tumors in stage T_{2-4} require additional treatment. Here, cryosurgery supplements TUR or is used as palliative treatment. It is likely that radiation therapy also is potentiated by cryosurgery, as we have noted in prostatic carcinoma.

Papillary Tumors (Stage T_A)

Giant papillomas are difficult to resect. Frequent hemorrhage, poor visibility and imminent perforation complicate TUR. Our largest resected papilloma was 455 gm (Fig. 1). Open surgery is contraindicated for the papilloma as a rule; cryosurgery, therefore, offers optimal treatment.

(1) Even the largest tumor can be clearly visualized by trocar cystoscopy because it is seen from the bird's eye view. An ordinary cystoscope or resectoscope can never provide this complete view.

(2) Filling of the bladder with gas (air, nitrous oxide, helium) avoids many of the disturbances seen with water cystoscopy — e.g., turbidity due to hemorrhage; flotation of the tumor. The tumor collapses over its base and is easier to locate.

(3) Freezing of the collapsed tumor in the well-filled bladder is as easy (for both surgeon and patient) as all other treatments are complicated. For giant tumors or large multiple papillomas, cryosurgery is performed in two or more sessions. The base of the tumor is excised after expulsion of necroses by TUR in order to gain material for histologic examination.

(4) Freezing the tumor prevents an implantation of tumor cells within the bladder and dissemination through the blood vessels.

(5) The postoperative recovery period is brief and uncomplicated because necroses are dissolved quickly and sloughs do not form. Eventually, a 20 Fr three-way Foley catheter is introduced transurethrally for permanent irrigation of the bladder with a cytostatic agent (see p. 59).

Malignant Tumors (Figs. 176–180)

Stage T_1. If a papillary tumor is suspected to be malignant, first the base in the bladder wall is frozen. Then TUR can be performed for staging and grading, either during the same session or after rejection of necroses, without danger of lymphatic dissemination of metastases. Subsequent sessions are possible at intervals of one and more weeks. The well-known rules for endoscopic or surgical treatment are also valid here.

On the other hand, the wound surface following TUR of a papilloma may be frozen secondarily if the histologic report shows invasive growth (T_2).

Stages T_2–T_4. The prognosis is not good. Neither operative nor physical therapy achieves a high rate of success. At least in the poor-risk patient, cryosurgery, perhaps in combination with TUR, is preferred over open surgery. Cryosurgery can also be performed as an adjunct to radiation therapy. In the recurrent tumor, cryosurgery (often as trocar cryosurgery) offers the final possibility for treatment.

Bladder Diverticula

In advanced prostatic hypertrophy, diverticula as large as the size of a walnut are not infrequent. The mouth of the diverticulum is resected transurethrally (see Fig. 181) to promote drainage. Cryosurgery of the diverticular mouth is easier than TUR and is without risk. The result is more reliable, because the mouth loses contractibility totally with induration. Freezing of tumors within diverticula is easier than electroresection. Large diverticula (over 3 cm in diameter) usually require surgical extirpation.

Strictures of the Bladder Neck

Strictures seldom occur after cryosurgery of prostatic hypertrophy (0.6 per cent). Therefore, we freeze all difficult strictures of the bladder neck. Scar tissue freezes more slowly than adenomatous tissue. The rim of the freezing surface of the "Special" cryoprobe therefore is positioned directly at the apex — not the rectal control knob as usual. Then the stricture is frozen for 10 to 60 seconds. The distance between the frozen area and the apex (external sphincter) is measured continuously. The freezing process is stopped when at least a distance of 2 mm has been reached (Fig. 182).

Radiation Cystitis (Fig. 183)

The bleeding of radiation cystitis is often life-threatening. It occurs frequently after radiation therapy of genital cancer.

TUR of the bleeding vessels must be meticulous and is not easy. We prefer the simpler freezing technique. The temperature, however, should not fall below −40° C because tissue damaged by irradiation is extremely sensitive to cold. Freezing time is reduced to a few seconds, because the bleeding vessels are situated at the surface of the mucosa and are easily destroyed. The hemorrhage is reduced after freezing and disappears slowly over the course of a few days. Seldom is a second session necessary. Success is assured when the mucosa in this region is replaced by scar tissue.

Vesical Ulcer

Ulcers and other pathologic processes can be treated by cryosurgery — e.g., ulcer simplex, irradiation ulcer, chemical cystitis, endometriosis, schistosomiasis and polypoid inflammation. Our own experience has not been extensive enough to offer recommendations here.

Text continued on page 196

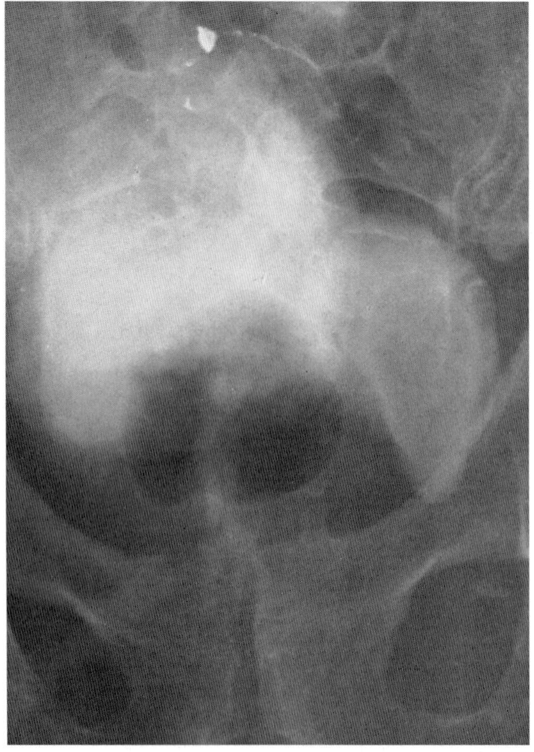

a

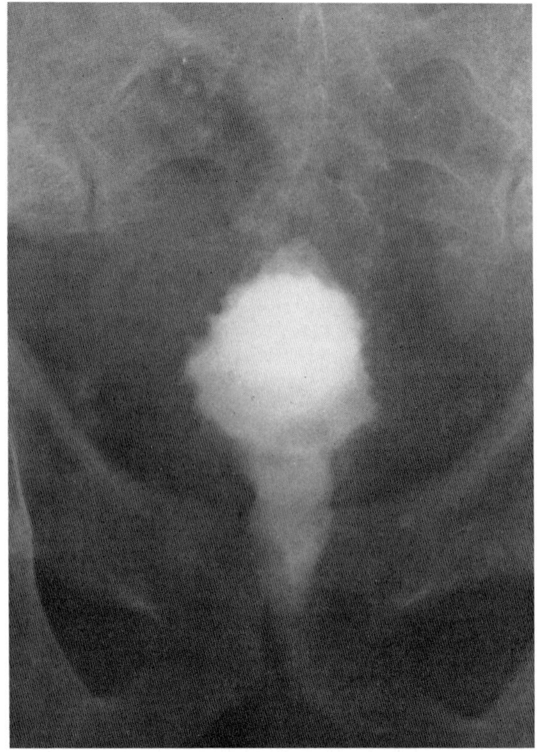

c

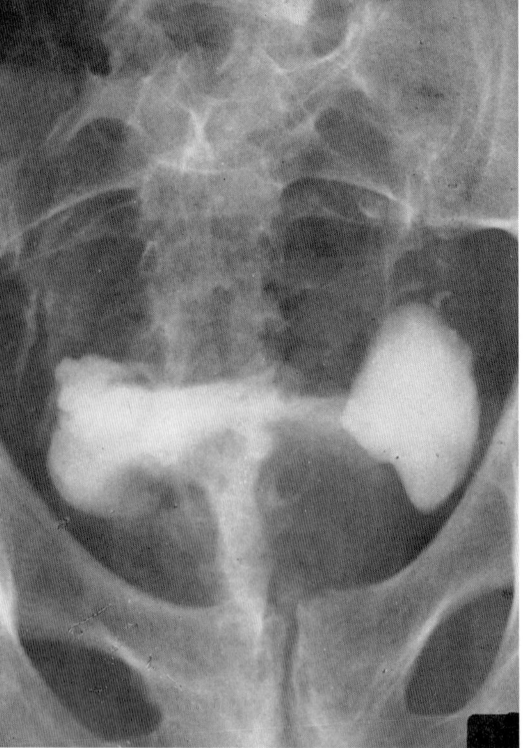

b

Fig. 152, a–f Palliative cryosurgery of poor-risk patients with prostatic hypertrophy.

(a) Preoperative cystogram (13 × 18 cm) of a giant prostatic adenoma. The atonic bladder has a large (about 7 cm wide) diverticulum at the right and a suprapubic fistula. The adenoma is 7 cm long; 70-year-old patient.

(b) Cystogram (13 × 18 cm; excretory urogram) one year after cryosurgery of the same patient. The bladder is well contracted but has irregular outlines. It lies in the shape of a sickle above the shadow of the adenoma. The bladder diverticulum is reduced to 4.5 cm in length. In the center of the middle lobe, a saber-shaped rigid tube is shown, corresponding to the prostatic urethra. The patient has no complaints about micturition; residual urine 6 years later is still below 50 cc.

(c) Cystogram (30 × 18 cm) 3 months after cryosurgery of a large adenoma 6 cm long. The bladder is almost empty. The prostatic urethra is pictured as a channel with a rigid wall within the adenomatous remainder. Good functional result in a 73-year-old patient.

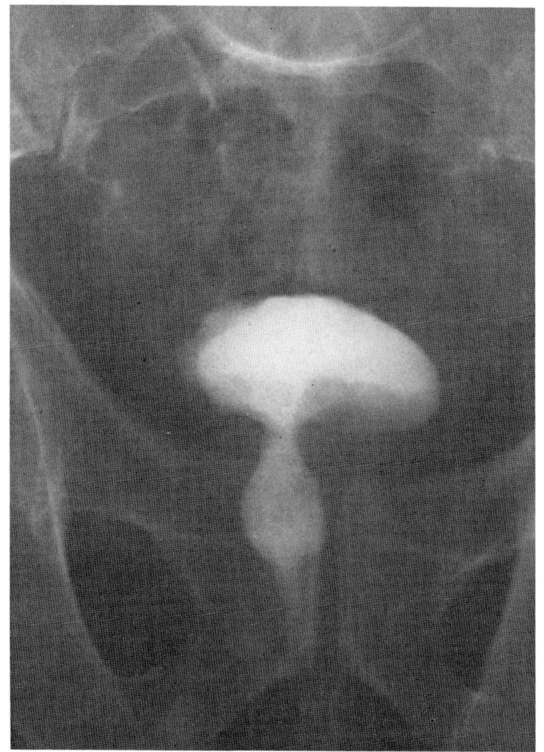

d

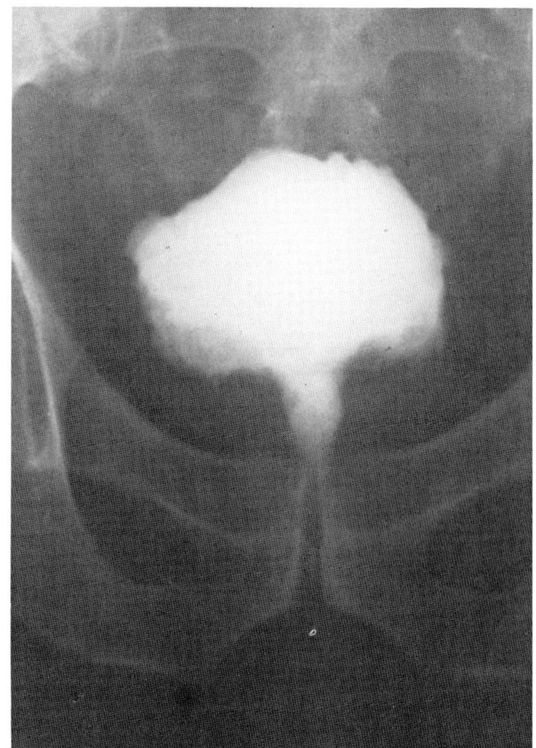

e

(d) Cystogram (13 × 18 cm) 6 months after cryosurgery of a prostatic adenoma about 5 cm long in a 82-year-old patient. A pear-shaped rigid cavity has been frozen into the prostatic urethra. The patient has no complaints and no residual urine.

(e) Cystogram (13 × 18 cm) 3 months after cryosurgery of a prostatic adenoma over 6 cm long in two sessions in an 80-year-old patient. The middle lobe of the adenoma is very much diminished; the prostatic urethra has the shape of a funnel (as after partial TUR). A good functional result was maintained until death at 90 years.

(f) Cystogram (13 × 18 cm; excretory urogram). Typical saber-shaped urethra after palliative cryosurgery in a 75-year-old poor-risk patient. The bladder neck is lifted by the remaining adenoma. In its center is the narrow, rigid channel, which corresponds to the prostatic urethra (compare Fig. 150). The patient is without urologic complaints 4 years later.

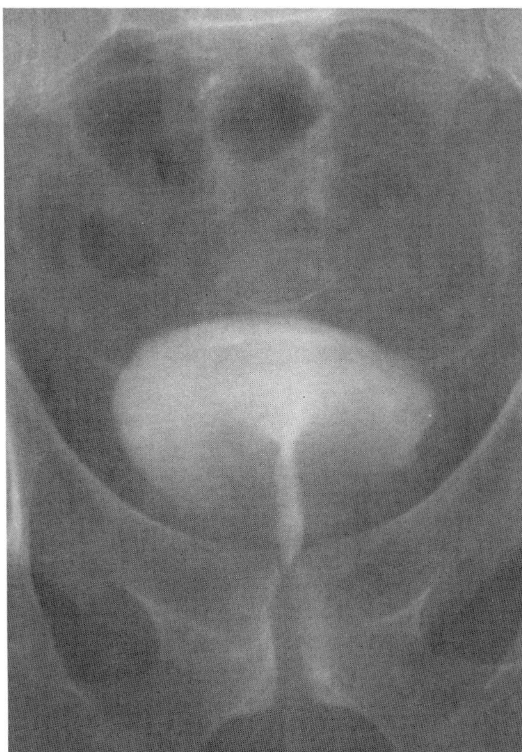

f

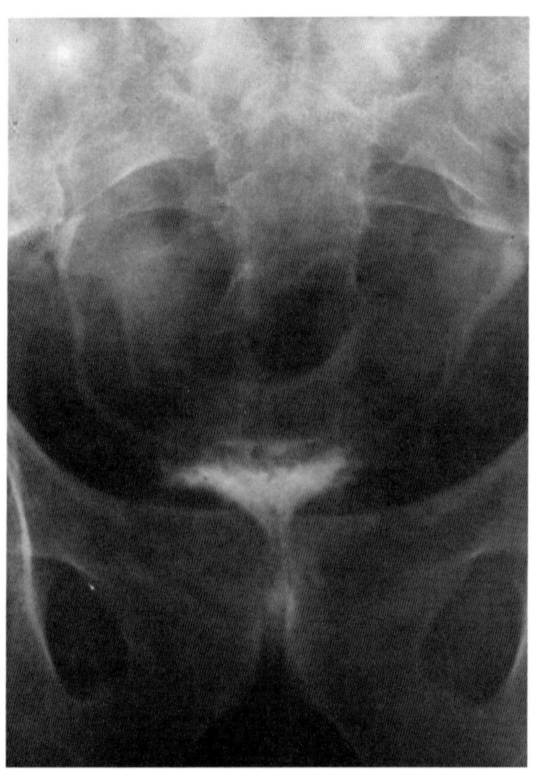

Fig. 153 Curative endoscopic cryosurgery of a prostatic carcinoma, stage $T_2N_0M_0G_2$.

Cystogram (13 × 18 cm; excretory urogam) 5 years after cryosurgery. The picture shows some remaining contrast medium in the emptied bladder and both ureters and a small prostatic fossa below the funnel-shaped bladder neck. This corresponds to normal findings; the 70-year-old patient is now clinically healthy.

Fig. 154, a and b Palliative cryosurgery of prostatic cancer with obstruction (13 × 18 cm).

Trocar cryosurgery of an advanced inoperable prostatic cancer, stage $T_4N_1M_0G_2$, in a 61-year-old patient.

(a) Cystogram (13 × 18 cm) before the operation. The bladder floor is irregularly elevated. Both ureters are kinked (excretory urogram 20 min after injection).

(b) Cystogram (13 × 18 cm) 3 months after trocar cryosurgery. The bladder was filled with 50 cc contrast medium through the indwelling catheter. Its wall is irregularly shaped. Left vesicoureteral reflux is demonstrated. The bladder neck is clearly distinguished from the prostatic fossa, which shows a rounded excavation to the left. The combination of orchiectomy, cobalt irradiation and estrogen therapy has prevented a "recurrence" of cancer for 5 years.

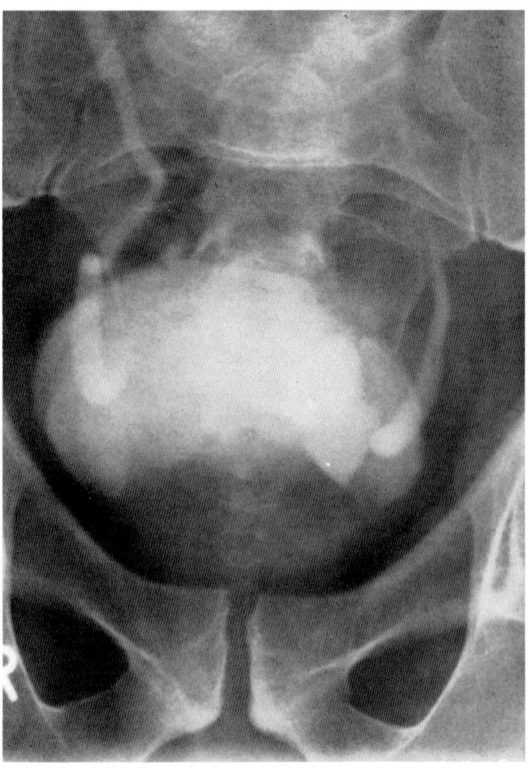

a

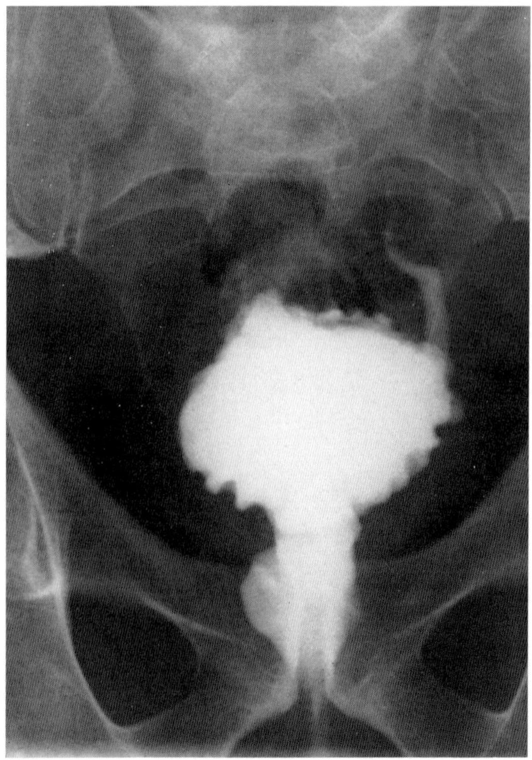

b

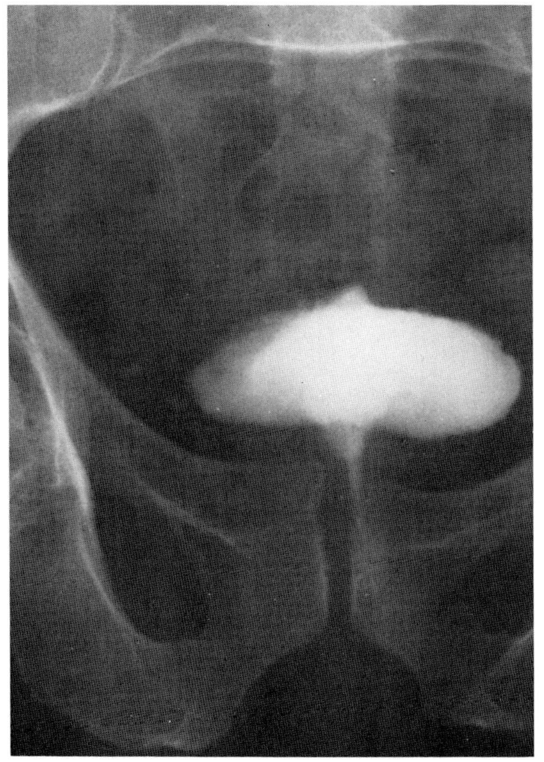
a

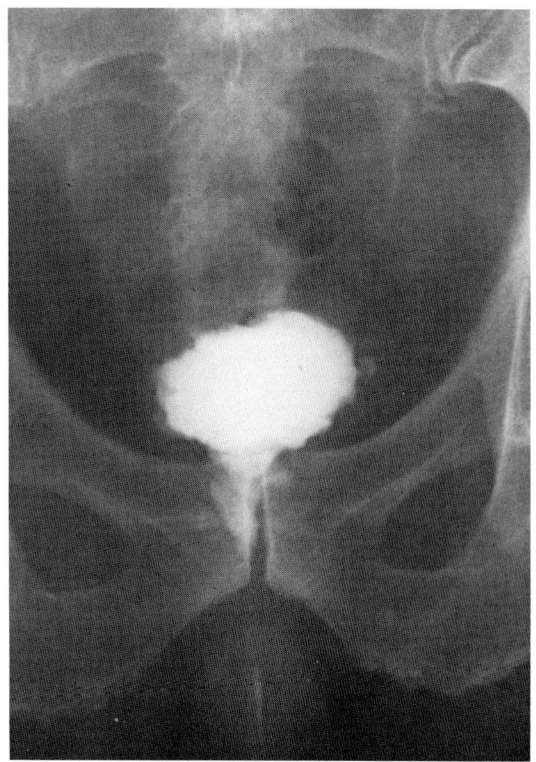
b

Fig. 155, a and b Palliative cryosurgery of a prostatic carcinoma, stage T_3.

(a) The cystogram (13 × 18 cm) demonstrates a cuneiform excavation below the bladder after cryosurgery, which corresponds to partial TUR (80-year-old patient). Stage $T_3N_xM_0G_3$; death occurred 5 years later, 10 months after one kidney was fistulated.

(b) The cystogram (13 × 18 cm) shows a small bladder with irregular outlines. A cuneiform prostatic fossa is seen below (81-year-old patient). At 78 years TURP had been performed; now, cryosurgery (stage $T_4N_xM_0G_3$). Death followed two years later.

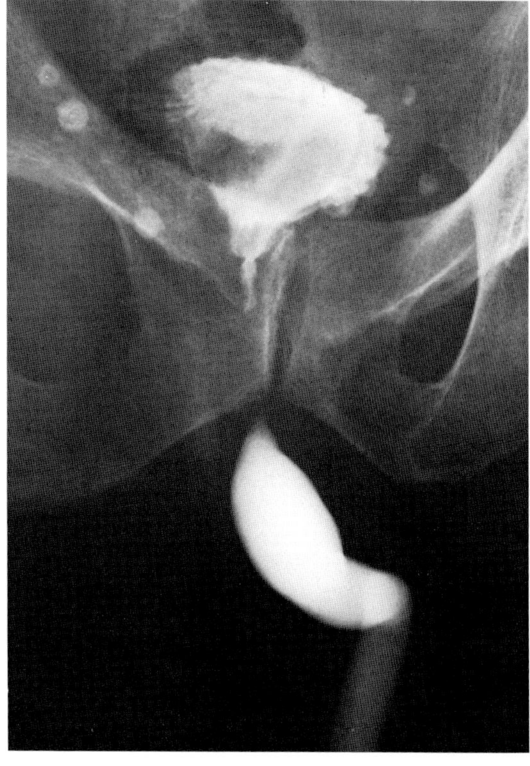

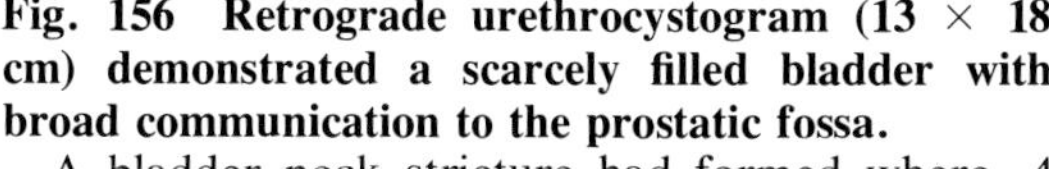

Fig. 156 Retrograde urethrocystogram (13 × 18 cm) demonstrated a scarcely filled bladder with broad communication to the prostatic fossa.

A bladder neck stricture had formed where, 4 years previously, radical TUR had been performed. The stricture was frozen. 60-year-old patient; stage $T_4N_xM_0G_3$ with bladder neck stricture. Death followed 2 years after cryosurgery.

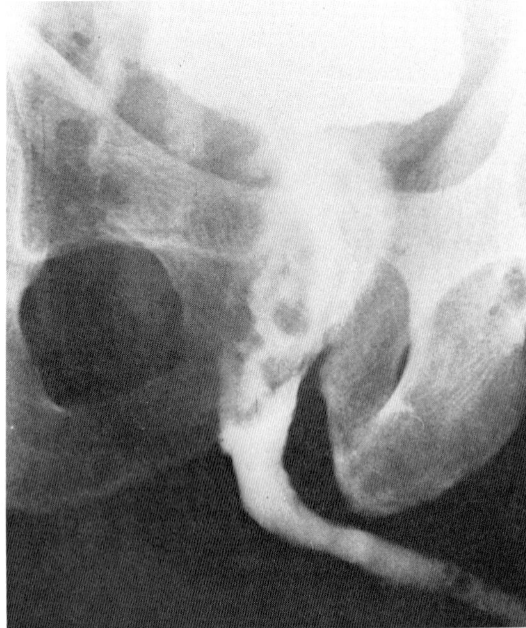

Fig. 157 Blind cryosurgery (Opelt Homburg, 1969).
The cryoprobe was positioned incorrectly owing to insufficient control of the freezing process. Thus, the entire bulbous urethra, including the external sphincter, was frozen. Complete incontinence was the consequence.

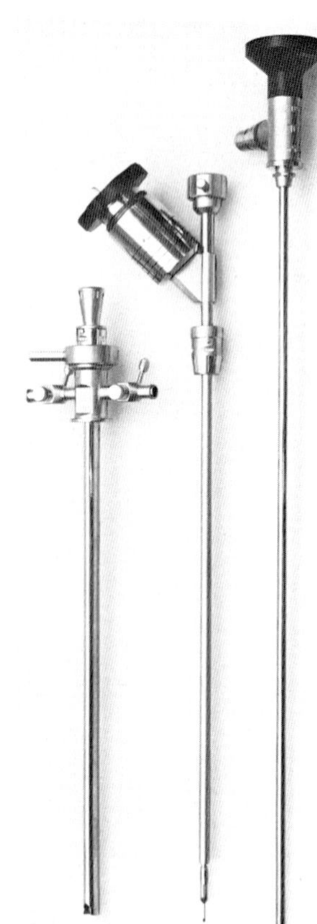

Fig. 158 Teflon injector ("Koblenz" model).
Instruments for transurethral submucosal injection of Teflon (after Politano) for treatment of urinary incontinence (R. Wolf).

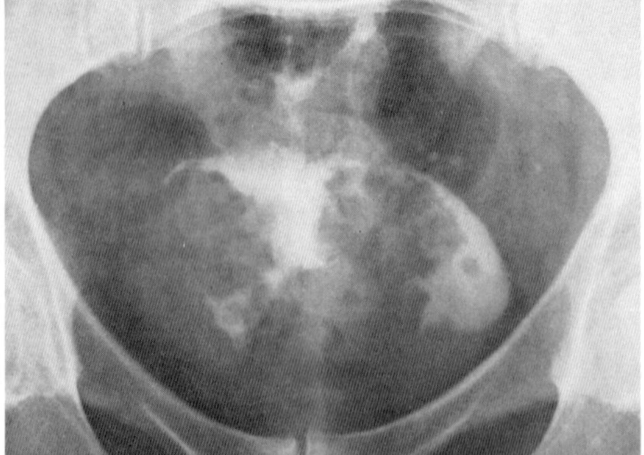

Fig. 159 Preoperative cystogram (13 × 18 cm) of a giant papillary bladder cancer.
The bladder is almost filled by a divided tumor (6 × 10 cm diameter). Stage $T_2N_xM_xG_1$; 72-year-old female patient; TUR of the base of the tumor two weeks after cryosurgery. Five years later there had been no recurrence; no further follow-up.

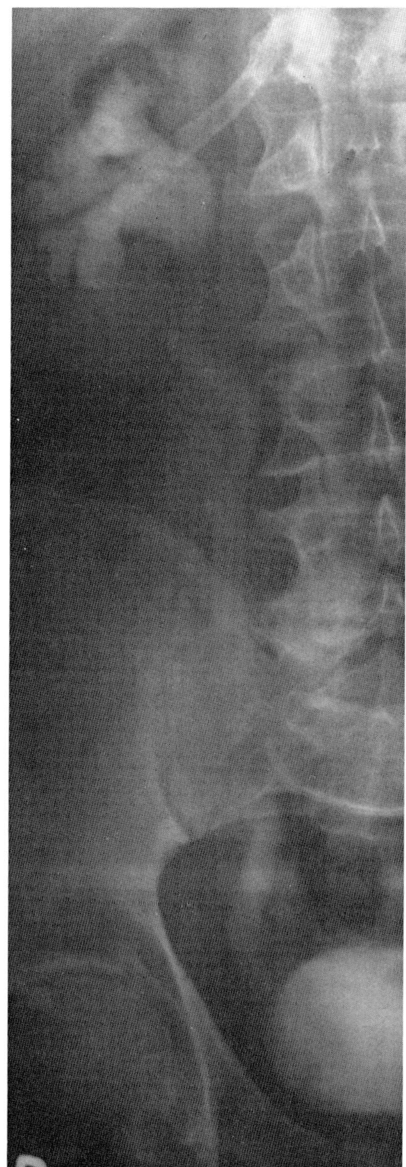

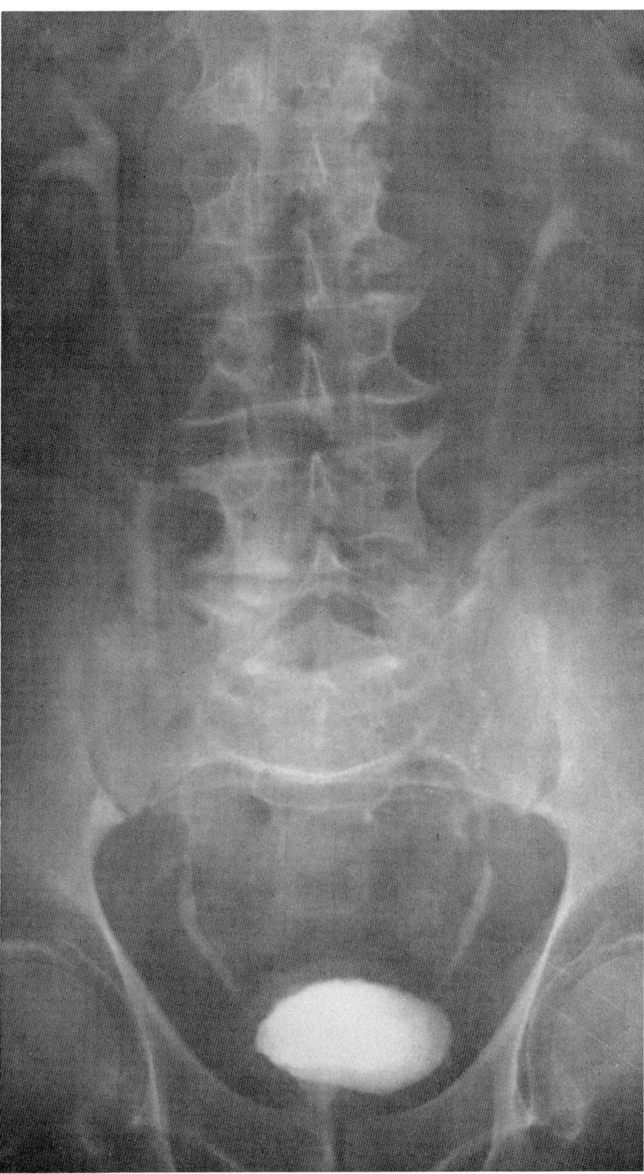

a b

Fig. 160, a and b Endoscopic cryosurgery of an inoperable bladder tumor (stage T_3) with obstruction of the right ureter.

(a) Preoperative excretory urogram (film 15 × 40 cm, 45 min after injection). The right half of the bladder is partially obscured by an irregular bladder tumor 2.5 × 5 cm in diameter. The right ureter and renal calyces are significantly dilated.

(b) Excretory urogram (35 × 40 cm) 2 years after cryosurgery. The bladder is well contracted and of regular shape. A slight double contour surrounds the right half. Both ureters are tender. The prostatic urethra leaves the bladder neck at the right and has the shape of a funnel (71-year-old patient); stage $T_3N_xM_0G_2$. There was no recurrence. Death occurred 5 years later.

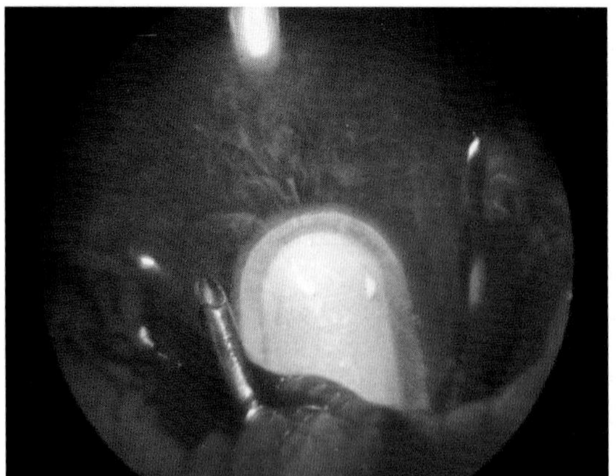
161 a

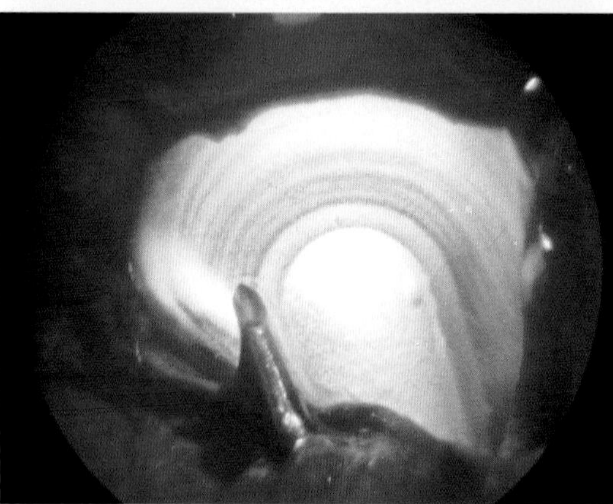
161 b

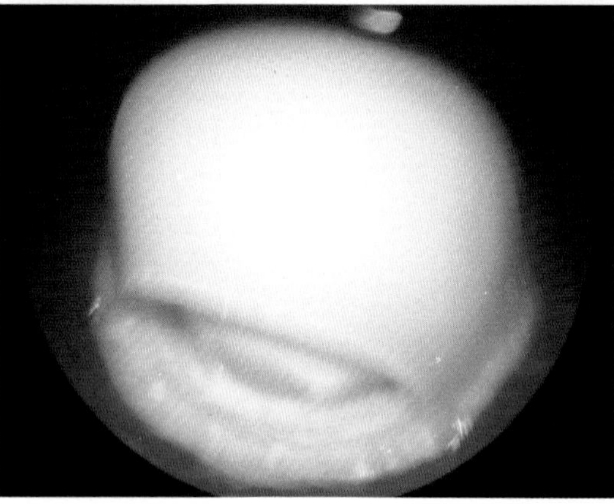
161 c

Uncontrolled Freezing of the Bladder Floor

Complications of blind cryosurgery and their prevention and control by endoscopy (suprapubic trocar cystoscopy with aspiration; see Figs. 169, a–e, 173, d).

Fig. 161, a Urine covering the bladder floor.
The tip of the "Special" cryoprobe projects into the bladder about 1.5 cm. The control knob of the cryoprobe is positioned at the apex of the prostate by rectal palpation (compare Fig. 145, a). Consequently, a pool of urine has collected on the floor of the gas-filled bladder (compare Fig. 162, a). The cryoprobe is half-immersed in urine. Since the probe is already freezing, an ice shell forms around the tip at the bladder floor. At the lower margin of the picture the ventral bladder wall is perforated by an injection needle, the point of which dips into the urine pool. The needle was inserted suprapubically to aspirate urine from the bladder floor and to maintain clear vision of the operating field. The flash bulb of the photo trocar cystoscope is reflected at 12 o'clock by the surface of this pool.

Fig. 161, b Freezing of the trigone.
A stratified frozen area has formed around the tip of the cryoprobe in the urine pool after one minute of freezing. The rectal aspiration needle meets solid ice. The ureteral orifices are at risk.

Fig. 161, c Dried bladder floor.
A large globe of ice has formed around the tip of the cryoprobe, jutting into the bladder. Below, the round frozen bladder neck is visible. Whether the back of the bladder is frozen can be proved by moving the handle of the cryoprobe up and down. The urine around the ice was aspirated suprapubically. Once the ice has thawed, the urine is aspirated again, and freezing is repeated.

Endoscopic Cryoprostatectomy of an Adenoma 5.5 cm Long (Suprapubic Trocarcystoscopy)

The "Special" cryoprobe (28 Fr; 2.5 cm long freezing element) is applied. The bladder is filled with 350 cc of helium. Peridural anesthesia. High-risk patient, 67 years old, with permanent catheter. The adenoma is frozen in two steps: (1) The endovesical part is frozen twice for 4 min under endoscopic control. (2) Then the apex is frozen twice for 3 min (repeated freezing). The cryoprobe is positioned at the apex by rectal palpation of the control knob. Rectal distance measurement: The frozen area is 5 mm away from the rectal mucosa (see p. 179). Cytology obtained by fine needle aspiration biopsy reveals group I (Pap.). Ten days of postoperative hospital care; indwelling catheter for 4 weeks, then voiding without residual urine. Three months later the urine is normal; nycturia occurred once. One year later the patient died of bronchial cancer.

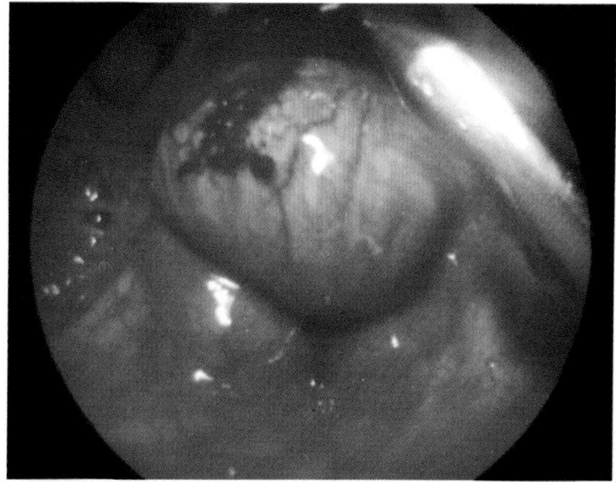

162 a

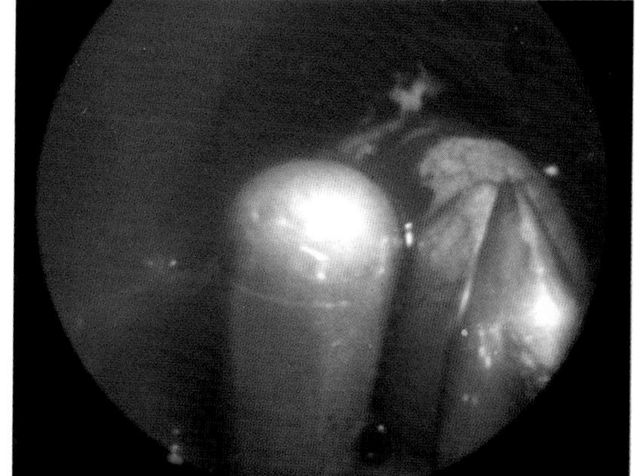

162 b

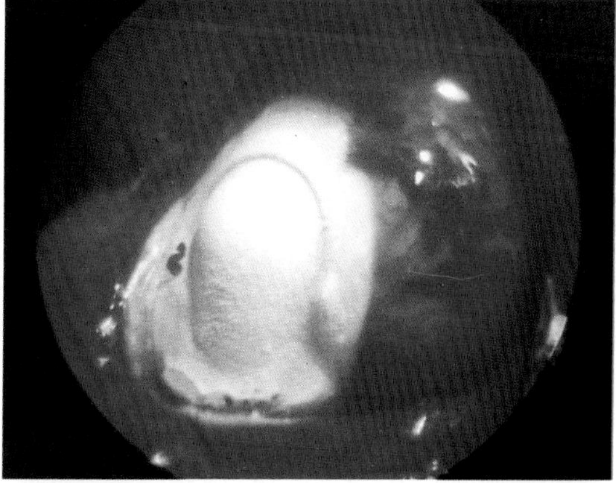

162 c

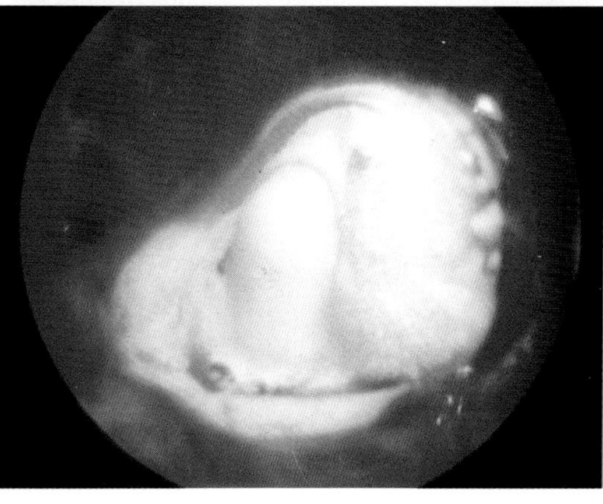

162 d

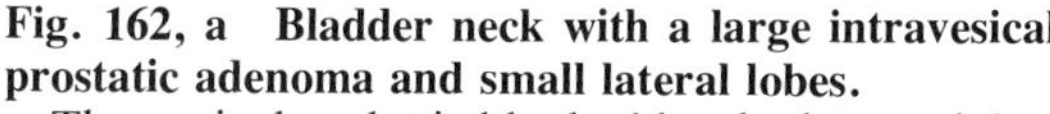

Fig. 162, a Bladder neck with a large intravesical prostatic adenoma and small lateral lobes.
The vesical outlet is blocked by the large, globular middle lobe of the adenoma. The bladder floor is dry; however, some urine foam remains. The mucosa covering the adenoma shows distinct alteration of vessels due to overdistention. The tip of a trocar at the upper right served as additional light source for filming.

Fig. 162, b Position of the probe for freezing.
The "Special" cryoprobe is positioned on the median lobe under endoscopic control. It is pressed firmly against the adenoma with the aid of the finger in the rectum.

Fig. 162, c Freezing.
After 30 seconds the tissue is frozen hard to a depth of several millimeters. The small lateral lobes have disappeared in the ice. More and more urine collects on the bladder floor.

Fig. 162, d Frozen area after three minutes.
The endovesical adenoma has been turned into ice. The diameter of the globe of ice is about 4 cm. Behind the adenoma (upper margin of the picture), fluid from diuresis has collected on the trigone (compare Fig. 161, a and b). After 4 minutes of freezing, the area is thawed for 8 min. Then freezing is repeated.

Endosopic Cryoprostatectomy of a Giant Adenoma (7.5 cm long)

For these lesions, the "Standard" cryoprobe (24 Fr; freezing element 4.5 cm long; insulated tip 1 cm long) is of suitable size. 77-year-old high-risk patient with a bladder fistula; two sessions with an interval of 3 months (without permanent transurethral catheter) were necessary. Freezing was done in two steps (compare Fig. 162), each of 4 min; 3 mm distance from frozen area to rectal mucosa; intravenous short-acting anesthetic. The bladder fistula was closed two months after the second session. Postoperatively, progress was monitored by suprapubic cystoscopy. Nine years later rectal palpation showed no abnormal findings (total removal of adenoma); the urine was normal. The efficiency of surface cryoprobes may be increased by additional central freezing with the trocar cryoprobe (compare Fig. 172, a) and with the cryocaustic unit (see p. 174).

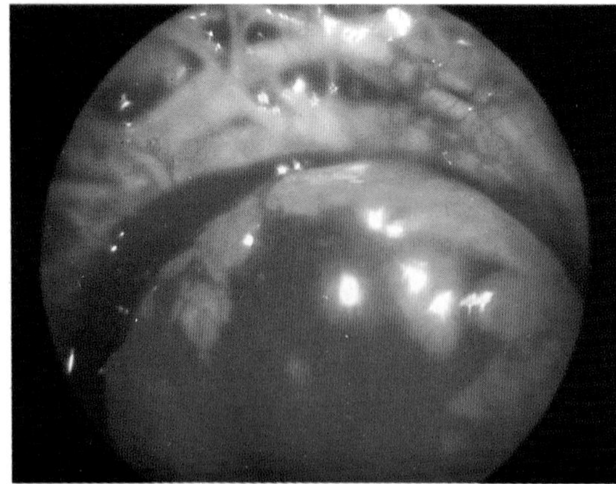

163 a

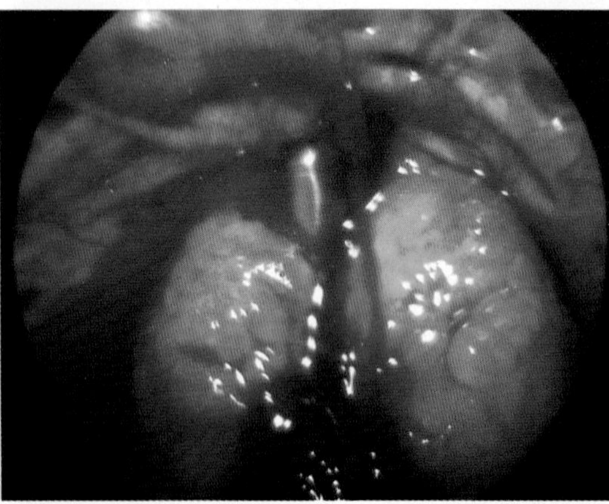

163 b

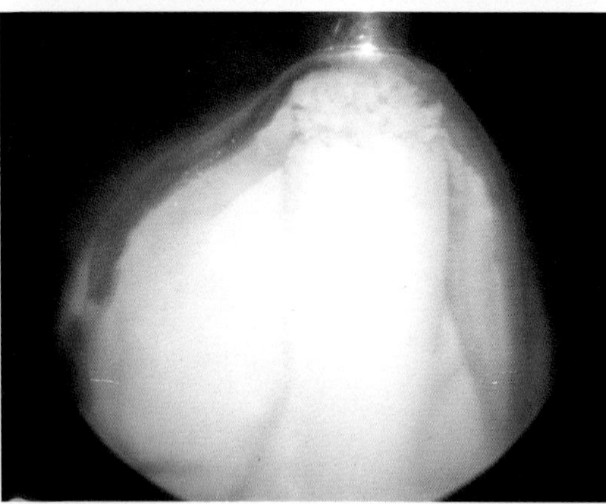

163 c

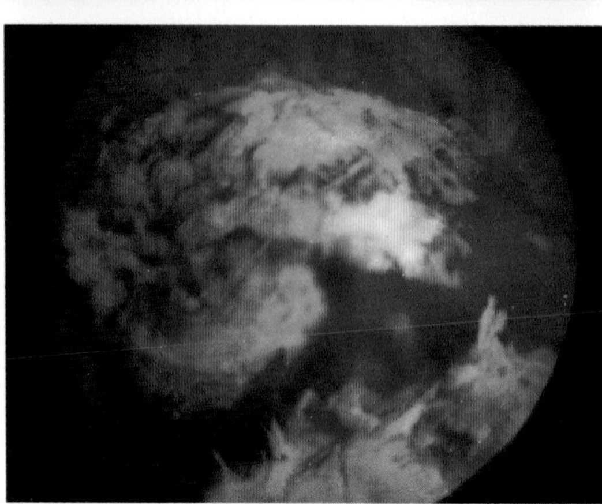

163 d

Fig. 163, a Giant endovesical median lobe; trabeculated bladder.
The trocar cystoscope is introduced first in order to control the passage of the probe through the prostatic urethra.

Fig. 163, b Cryoprobe in position.
The cryoprobe is introduced into the bladder. The freezing element of the probe is now placed on the center of the adenomatous node and is pressed hard, dividing the middle lobe into halves like a cushion. The extracorporal handle of the probe is elevated, and the finger in the rectum is used to move the bladder floor and the adenoma upward against the probe. This ensures the best contact between probe and tissue.

Fig. 163, c Frozen giant median lobe after four minutes freezing.
The tip of the probe already has thawed. Its insulation is not complete. Therefore, it may freeze the bladder wall (same case as Fig. 164).

Fig. 163, d Cryonecrosis after five days.
As the mucosa decomposes, its surface looks rough and gray. The trace of blood coming from the prostatic urethra was caused by a previous catheterization. Trocar cystoscopy is performed with the bladder filled with water; therefore, light is not reflected by the mucosa. Necrotic tissue still adheres to the tissue of the bladder neck; complete decomposition requires one to two months.

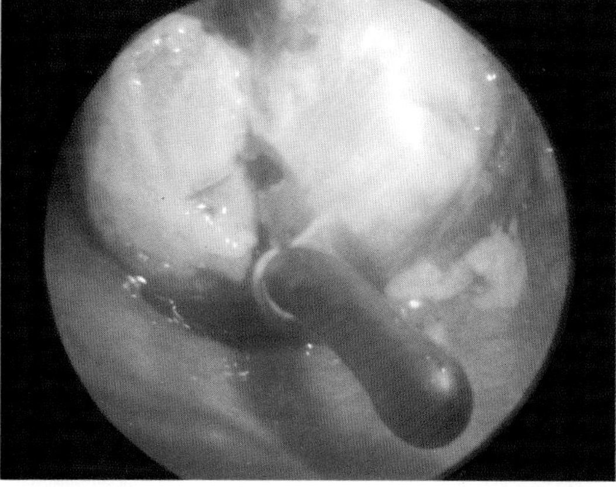

163 e

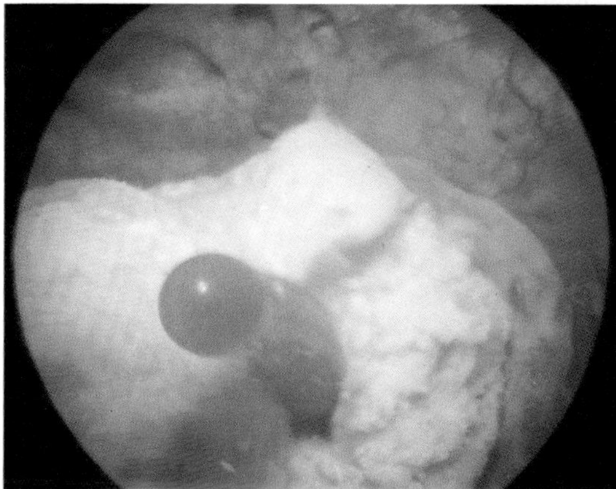

163 f

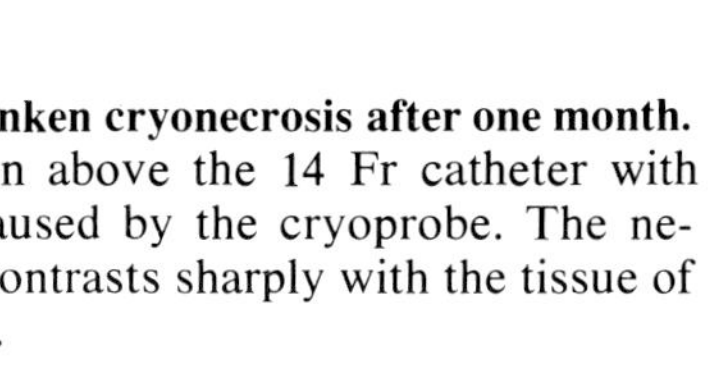

Fig. 163, e Shrunken cryonecrosis after one month. The indentation above the 14 Fr catheter with green tip was caused by the cryoprobe. The necrotic adenoma contrasts sharply with the tissue of the bladder neck.

Fig. 163, f Cryonecrosis in disintegration. Six weeks after cryosurgery the necrosis has decomposed almost completely. Its surface is rough and crusty owing to the intake of salts. The trabeculated posterior bladder wall has a tender mucosa. The orange catheter was introduced for orientation.

Fig. 163, g Adenomatous remnant. Eight weeks after cryosurgery the necrotic tissue has mostly disintegrated. Two white lumps remain at the bladder neck. Well-vascularized nodules of the subvesical adenoma remain around the orange tip of the catheter. The giant middle lobe has disappeared almost completely.

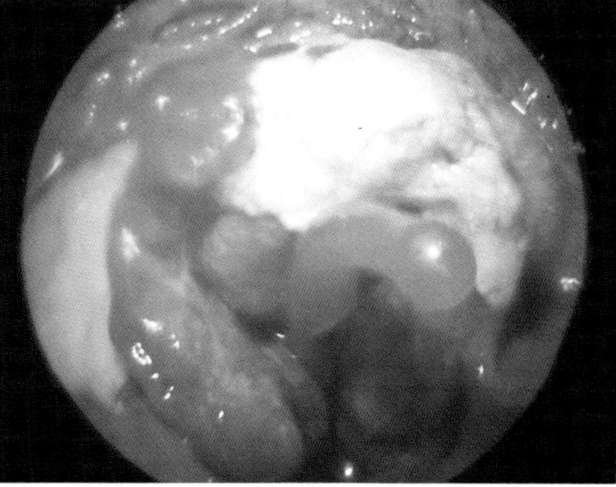

163 g

Second Session Two Months After Cryosurgery of a Giant Adenoma 13 cm Long

This 74-year-old high-risk patient has suffered 5 pulmonic emboli due to leg vein thrombosis and cardiac insufficiency. A permanent catheter is in place. Eight urologists had refused treatment. In four sessions 14 ice globes (freezing time 2–4 min; rectal distance 2 cm) were frozen into the adenoma and three bladder stones (diameter up to 4 cm) were crushed by trocar litholapaxy (compare Fig. 126). Two months later the chronic phlebitis has healed; voiding leaves no residual urine (postoperative follow-up of the remaining large adenoma continued for 6 years).

Fig. 164, a Nodular remnant of the median lobe after partial cryoprostatectomy.
Two months after cryosurgery, a deformed endovesical residual nodule is visible over the trigone. The yellow tip of a catheter lies in a fold between the middle and right lobes of the remaining adenoma. The base of the large node is at the bladder neck; its mass is free above the bladder floor.

Fig. 164, b Surface cryosurgery of the node.
The short "Special" cryoprobe is pressed against the residual middle lobe, which is frozen under endoscopic control. After a few seconds the 2.5 cm long freezing element is covered with ice. The frozen tissue is well delineated from the surrounding tissue. Freezing is repeated several times (4 min). The node is surrounded by a small urine pool (above).

Today we prefer to use the trocar cryoprobe for cryosurgery of giant adenomas, since central freezing is more effective (compare Fig. 172).

Partial Cryoprostatectomy with the "Standard" Cryoprobe. The Instrument is Not Suitable for the Medium Large Adenoma Because of Excessive Size.

The "Special" cryoprobe now optimal for adenomas 3 to 5 cm long (compare Fig. 162) had not yet been constructed.

Fig. 165, a Results following inadequate blind cryosurgery.
The adenoma has shrunk from 7 cm to 4.5 cm long. The remaining adenoma obstructs the opening of the scabbard-shaped prostatic urethra. The graduated scale on the probe allows measurement of the length of the prostatic urethra with the control knob at the apex. After a second session of endoscopic cryosurgery (repeated freezing: 5 and 3.5 min) and 6 weeks' treatment with a permanent catheter, the bladder is free of residual urine after voiding. Nine years later this good result is unchanged: there is no residual urine; the urine is normal; nycturia has occurred twice. The patient was then 78 years old.

Fig. 165, b Excessive length of the "Standard" cryoprobe.
The "Standard" cryoprobe was the wrong choice; it juts into the bladder an excessive length of 2.5 cm. For this adenoma the useful length is only 2 cm. The insulated tip is covered by ice crystals formed of condensed humidity. Around the cryoprobe a ring of frozen tissue with a radius of about 1 cm has formed at the bladder neck (radius of the probe; 4 mm). The background is veiled by haze.

Fig. 165, c Endoscopic control protects the left ureteral orifice.
The extent of the frozen area is monitored. The entire endovesical part of the adenoma, including the trigone, is already frozen. Between the light reflections (right) on the interureteral crest, small helium gas bubbles leave the left ureteral orifice — reflux due to lithopyelonephrosis. Eleven years later, this 79-year-old patient had no urologic complaints and no residual urine; nycturia had occurred once. The excretory urogram showed the bladder floor lifted by 2 cm.

Fig. 165, d Thawing of frozen bladder neck.
The heated cryoprobe (Fig. 165, a) has already been removed. Above is the interurethral crest with the two orifices. Thawing may be controlled with a needle (compare Fig. 161, a): it meets the hard frozen tissue below the mucosa (distance measurement; compare Fig. 146).

Fig. 165, e Bladder neck ten weeks later.
The cryonecrosis has sloughed completely. However, some small parts of adenoma still remain in the oval prostatic fossa. The urethra has been transformed into an indurated open tube without elasticity and contractability. This explains the good functional result of cryosurgery. With additional cryocaustic therapy, necroses are shed more quickly.

Fig. 165, f Final result.
The internal sphincter encloses a stiff channel within the adenomatous remnant. When the lateral lobes are indurated down to the verumontanum, function is secured for 5 years (compare Figs. 170, c and d).

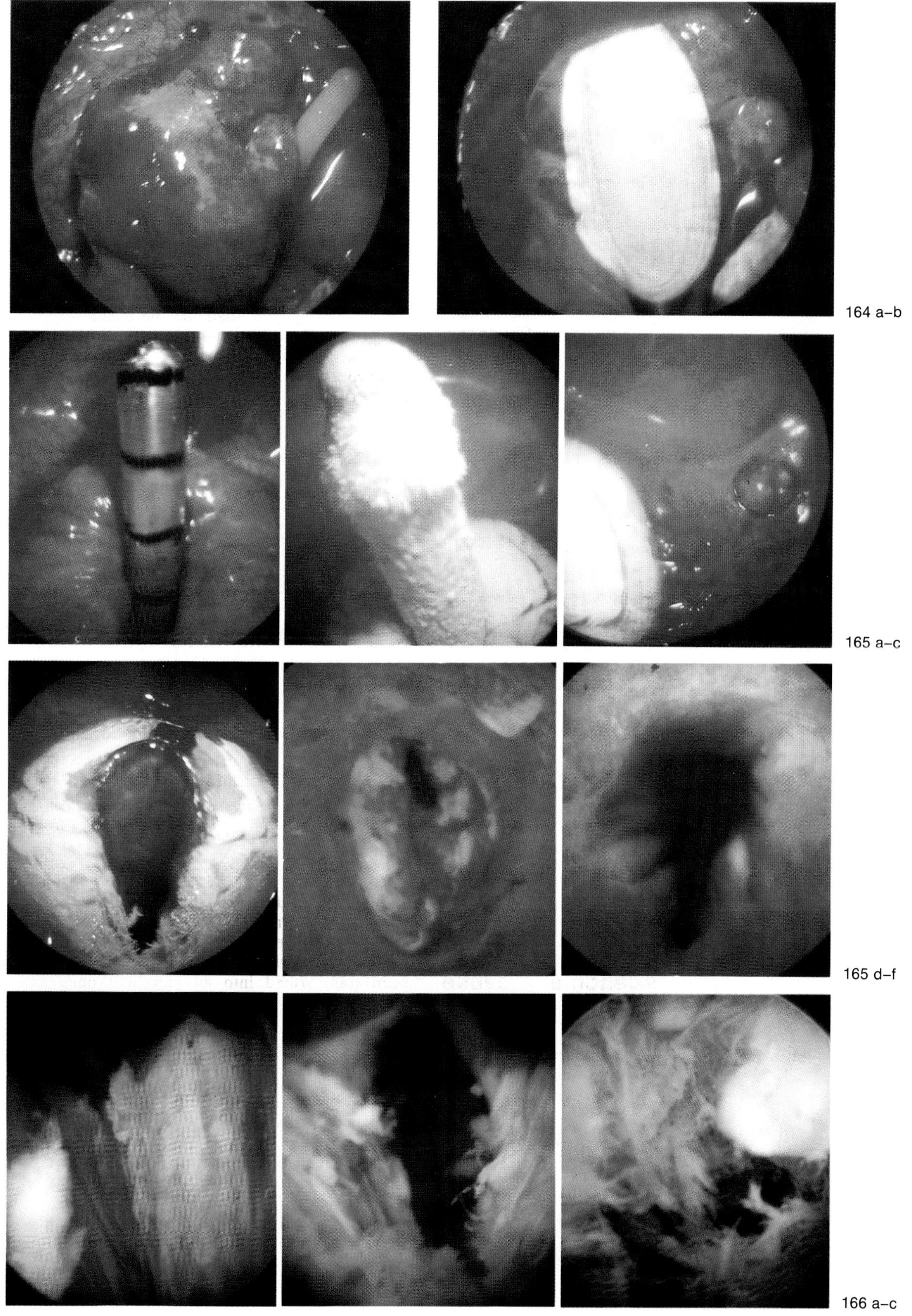

164 a–b

165 a–c

165 d–f

166 a–c

Disintegration of Cryonecrosis (Urethroscopy)

Fig. 166, a Necrotic median lobe of the adenoma.
The structure of the urethral surface disintegrates after two weeks.

Fig. 166, b Prostatic urethra with oval lumen three weeks later.
The necrotic adenomatous tissue has begun to disintegrate; it becomes pale. Above, the mucosa still remains untouched.

Fig. 166, c Destroyed necrosis after five weeks.
With correct technique (repeated freezing with freezing times of 2 to 4 min) usually no sloughs are formed. They usually develop from tissue that was not frozen quickly down to very low temperatures and when freezing times are prolonged over 5 min (compare Fig. 163, e). By heating up to 200° C after thawing (cryocaustic) this complication is prevented.

Partial and Total Cryoprostatectomy

Any adenoma can be frozen totally. With lengths over 4 cm, two or more sessions often are necessary. Here, central freezing (trocar cryosurgery; see Fig. 172) is helpful. A satisfactory result following the first partial cryosurgery often makes a planned second session unnecessary (15.9 per cent secondary operations; see p. 238). Unlike TURP, cryoprostatectomy leaves the internal sphincter rigid and wide open (compare Fig. 107, e).

Fig. 167, a Partial prostatectomy.
Three months after combined cryosurgery (trocar cryoprobe and "Standard" cryoprobe) the bladder neck is free of adenoma. Beyond the large round opening, a funnel is frozen into the prostatic urethra. The 20 Fr catheter was introduced for demonstration. (Sixty-three-year-old high-risk patient with two myocardial infarctions and a 6.5 cm adenoma). The median lobe and the lateral lobes were first frozen centrally with the trocar cryoprobe (twice for 4 min) and then frozen superficially with the "Standard" cryoprobe (4 min each; compare Fig. 164, a).

Rectal distance measurement showed that only 5 mm of unfrozen tissue remained between the rectum and the frozen area. A bladder fistula was maintained over 3 months. Acute pyelonephritis occurred 5 weeks later owing to insufficient fluid intake. Eight weeks after freezing, there was free micturition; 3 months later the urine was normal. Five years later a slightly enlarged prostate was palpated rectally. Nycturia occurred once; maximal urinary flow about 20 cc/sec. The planned second session was canceled.

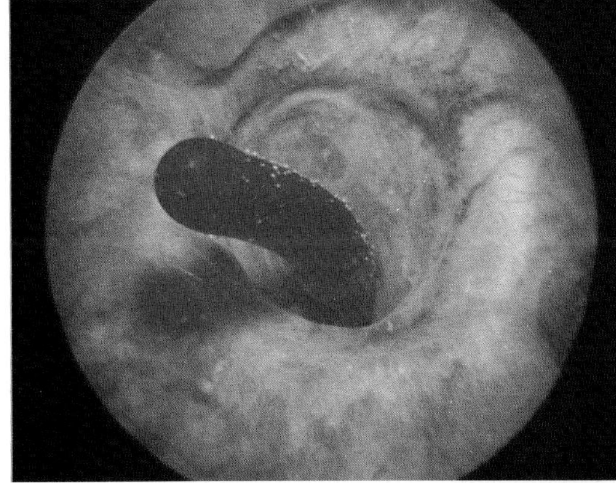

167 a

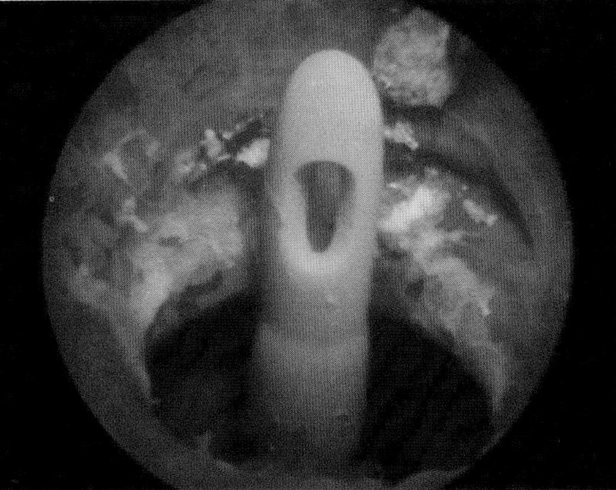

167 b

Fig. 167, b Total cryoprostatectomy six weeks after a first session.
A 20 Fr balloon catheter is introduced into the large, round prostatic fossa. Its diameter is about 2.5 cm. Above right, a necrotic particle lies on the bladder floor. For technical reasons, total destruction of the adenoma in one session is possible only to a length of 4 cm. Endoscopic and rectal controls of repeated freezing must be performed correctly (trocar cystoscopy, rectal distance measurement, etc.) In this 69-year-old high-risk patient with a urate stone (3.5 cm diameter) and an indwelling catheter, the adenoma (5 cm long) was frozen twice for 4 min. Rectal distance to the frozen area: 3 mm. Trocar litholapaxy (compare Fig. 126). Postoperative bladder fistula for 2 months. Eight years later all urologic findings are normal.

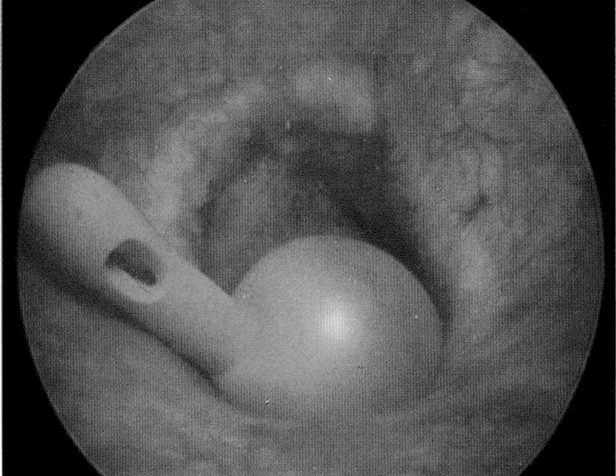

167 c

Fig. 167, c Total cryoprostatectomy; result after three months.
The spherical prostatic fossa is wide open. The balloon of the catheter is filled with 5 cc water. Freezing of the 4 cm long adenoma was stopped when rectal distance measurement showed the frozen area to be 2 mm away (freezing twice for 3 min). Cytology revealed group II (Pap.). One week of hospital care and 3 weeks of permanent catheter were necessary. Seven years later, all urologic findings were normal.

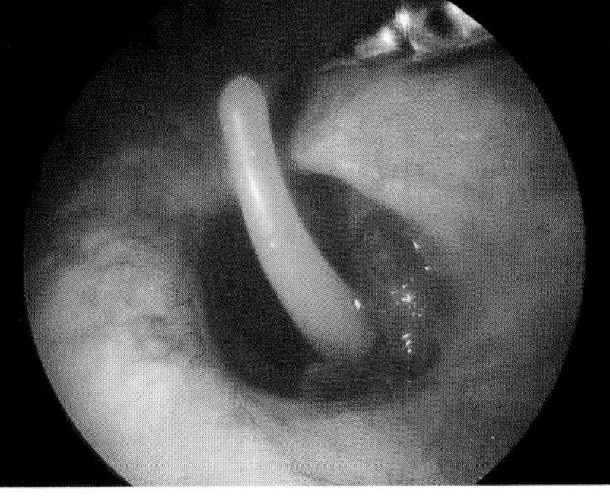

167 d

Fig. 167, d Result after cryosurgery and TURP.
The bladder neck and the wide-open prostatic fossa are pictured one year after cryosurgery and TURP. At the right, a small node has remained (compare Fig. 168, d). Above the catheter are the trigone and the tip of a small trocar cystoscope (12 Fr for children). In this 66-year-old high-risk patient, a 6 cm long adenoma was frozen; one month later, 60 gm net were resected because a large papilloma was detected (at the time, a cryoprobe suitable for bladder tumors had not yet been constructed; compare Fig. 174, a). Nine years later all urologic findings are normal; no nycturia. Today, with continuous low pressure irrigation, freezing before TURP has become unnecessary (compare Fig. 25).

168 a–c

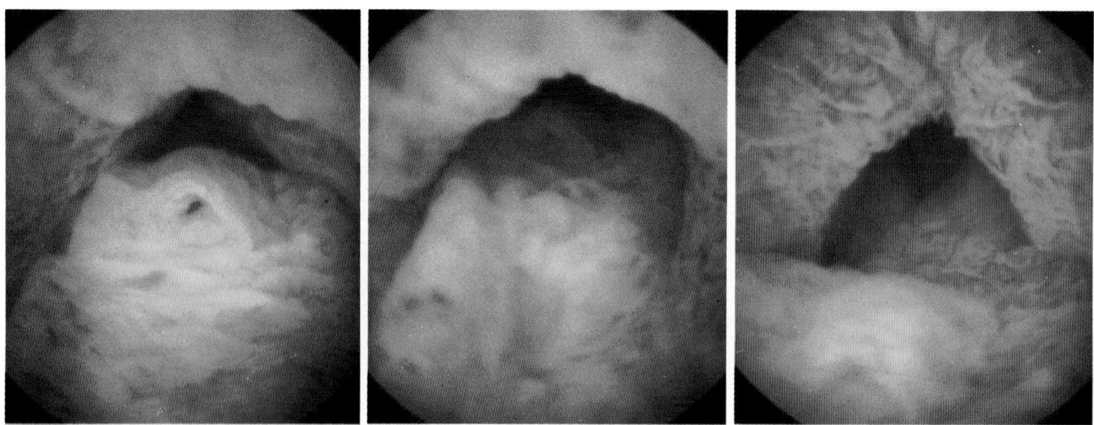

Prostatic Urethra After Cryoprostatectomy (Urethroscopy)

This 67-year-old high-risk patient had a permanent catheter following several strokes and cardiac insufficiency. Cryosurgery was performed for a 3 cm long adenoma with sphincter bar (freezing time: 1 min under intravenous short-acting anesthesia). Five weeks later micturition left no residual urine. Further strokes followed without urologic complications. The patient died 3 years later.

Fig. 168, a External sphincter with utricle.
The floor of the middle urethra is lifted. Beyond the verumontanum (with utricle), the black lumen of the prostatic urethra opens. The mucosa at the apex is altered by inflammation (*E. coli* infection).

Fig. 168, b Opening of the external sphincter.
Irrigation unfolds the urethra and pushes the verumontanum upward.

Fig. 168, c Prostatic apex.
The external sphincter is almost open. The transition to the apex is marked by its oblique bulge, which carries the flat verumontanum. Typical longitudinal folds run from here to the trigone.

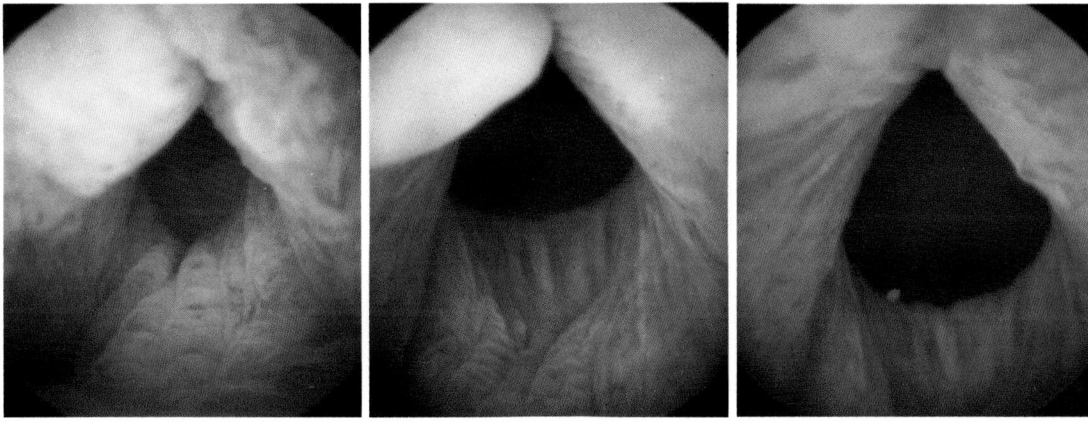

168 d–f

Fig. 168, d Prostatic urethra.
The entire prostatic urethra is not shown here. The longitudinal folds are seen running upward from the (hidden) verumontanum to the trigone. The lateral walls meet above, like a tent. Here, in the middle of the urethra, a small adenomatous node remains (insulating effect of an air bubble caused by incorrect technique without repeated freezing).

Fig. 168, e Internal sphincter.
The prostatic urethra opens into the bladder. The internal sphincter is pictured in the sector near the trigone. Its upper circumference is covered by the lateral walls of the urethra and a white adenomatous remnant.

Fig. 168, f Bladder neck and lateral walls of the urethra.
The lateral walls and floor of the urethra are now even more distinct from each other. The adenomatous node is now behind the optical window.

169 a–c

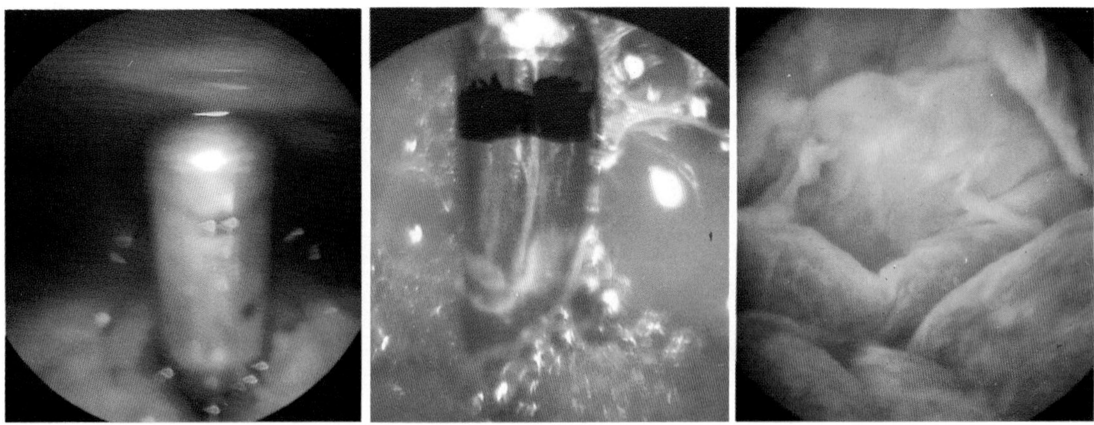

Incorrect Technique of Cryoprostatectomy (Trocar Cystoscopy)

The control knob of the cryoprobe and rectal palpation do not provide sufficient control for positioning the probe and regulating freezing. Precise cryosurgery can be controlled only by endoscopy, rectal distance measurement and aspiration of urine. These measures protect the sound tissue (ureteral orifices, bladder wall, prostatic capsule and external sphincter). Total cryoprostatectomy — comparable to TURP — is the desired result. It may be obtained with meticulous technique (Figs. 103, 107, 167).

Fig. 169, a Sphincter bar (sclerosis); prostatitis.
The control knob of the "Special" cryoprobe is correctly positioned at the apex. However, trocar cystoscopy reveals that the entire freezing surface projects into the bladder because the prostatic urethra is only 2 cm long. Blind freezing here would be without useful effect. The probe is drawn back 1.5 cm into the urethra. Its tip now juts only 0.5 cm into the bladder (graduated scale): the control knob is felt 1.5 cm distal to the apex. Freezing is stopped when the hard surface of the frozen tissue reaches a distance of 2 mm from the external sphincter (apex) or the rectal mucosa. This 48-year-old patient had chronic prostatitis and sexual neurosis, bloody discharge, urinary infection and prostatic stones. Repeated freezing twice for 2 min; permanent catheter for 2 weeks after the operation. For the next 7 years the patient had no complaints and urologic findings were normal. Nycturia occurred three times; sexual potency was maintained for 5 years after cryosurgery.

Fig. 169, b Flooded bladder neck.
The "Standard" cryoprobe juts far into the bladder. The adenoma and bladder floor are covered by urine. Freezing of the bladder neck cannot be controlled: the bladder floor and ureteral orifices are damaged. For correction: (1) the "Standard" cryoprobe must be replaced by the shorter "Special" cryoprobe; (2) the urine must be aspirated (compare Fig. 161, a); (3) the handle of the cryoprobe is lowered until the projecting tip of the probe stands free without touching sound tissue (compare Figs. 162, b; 165, a and b).

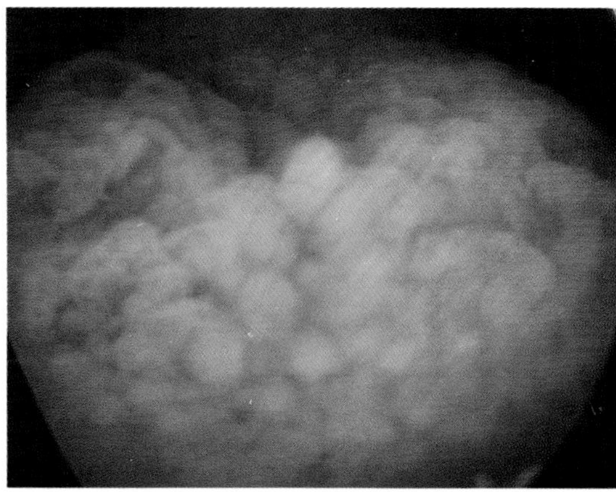

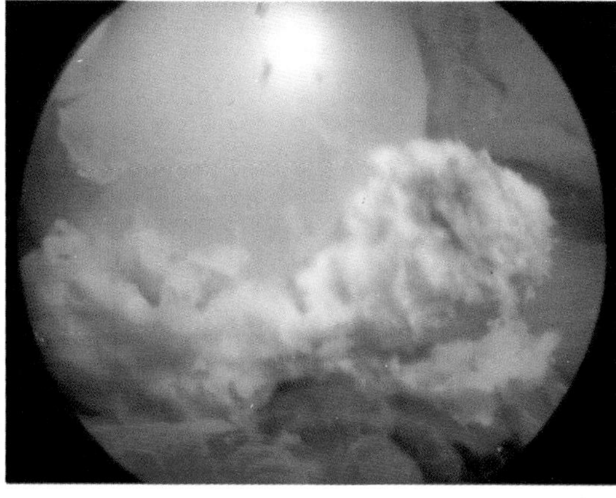

169 d–e

Fig. 169, c Necrosis of the posterior bladder wall (necrotizing cystitis).
This is the result one week after blind cryosurgery of the prostate. The cryoprobe had projected into the bladder, and the urine was not completely aspirated. The bladder floor, the ureteral orifices and the posterior wall are damaged (compare Fig. 161, d). Only at the left above is there untouched mucosa. Blind cryosurgery for 5 min and subsequent TURP (25 gm net) were performed in one session. On the third postoperative day, the patient suffered transient right renal colic. Four months later there was acute urinary retention due to cryonecrosis. This was removed under endoscopic control (trocar cystoscopy and forceps). Two years later chronic obstruction of the right kidney was revealed, but there were no other complaints.

Fig. 169, d Granulating infiltrative cystitis after cryonecrosis of the bladder wall.
Six weeks after cryosurgery the necrotic mucosa is shed (Fig. 169, c) and new epithelium grows.

Fig. 169, e Cryonecrosis five weeks after total cryoprostatectomy; two blind sessions.
Between the bladder neck (below) and the inflated balloon of the catheter there is whitish-gray cryonecrosis. In the background (right), the posterior wall of the bladder appears diffusely reddened and trabeculated. This 77-year-old high-risk patient had overflow incontinence (2900 cc) and uremia. After 5 months' treatment with a permanent catheter, cryosurgery was performed under intravenous short-acting anesthesia (5 min); there was a second session (4 min) 6 weeks later. One year later the right kidney was normal, the left was hyposthenuric. Normal urine; no residual urine. After 10 years, the 87-year-old patient is well.

170 a–b

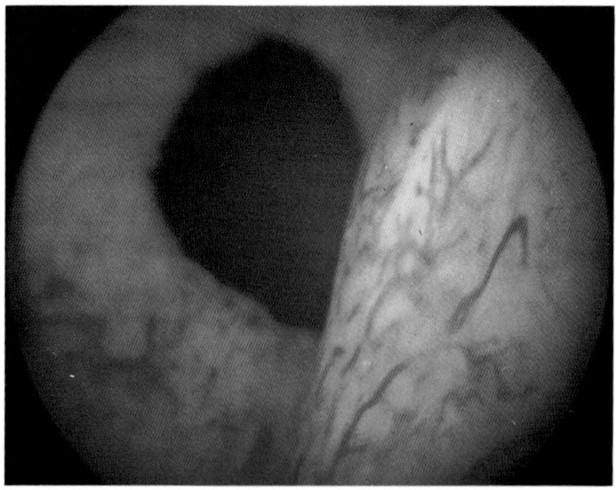

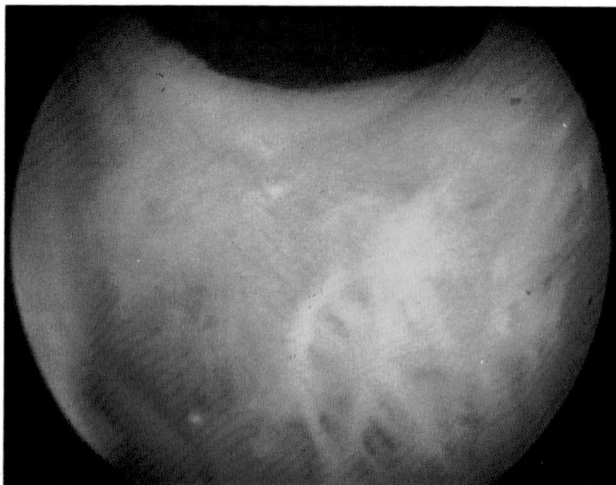

Postoperative Result Following Inadequate Technique of Cryoprostatectomy (Urethroscopy)

Single freezing with long freezing times and an inadequate cryoprobe produce unsatisfactory results. The technique of endoscopic cryosurgery with control of subvesical expansion of the frozen area (distance measurement, suprapubic aspiration, repeated freezing) avoids complications and gives consistently good results.

Fig. 170, a Adenomatous remnant in the prostatic urethra five months after cryosurgery.
A white adenomatous node shines through the regenerating mucosa at the right. The rest of the prostatic fossa is free of adenoma. Its concave wall forms a hollow sphere, connected through the open circle of the internal sphincter with the bladder (compare Fig. 167, b). The indurated node does not necessarily keep growing. In this 65-year-old high-risk patient with renal insufficiency and a permanent catheter, the adenoma was frozen only once for 4 min. The scheduled second session was not necessary. Ten years later the patient is without urologic complaints. Normal urine; nycturia twice. Rectally, a markedly enlarged prostate can be felt. The excretory urogram shows much better renal function than at the time of cryosurgery.

Fig. 170, b Prostatic capsule after total cryoprostatectomy and sloughing of a large cryonecrosis.
The prostatic urethra is pictured with a column of the lateral lobe at the apex (left) and the internal sphincter (above). One year after cryosurgery, the prostatic fossa is covered with thin regenerating mucosa. The structure of the deep capsule can be seen below the mucosa as a net of fibers (compare Figs. 106, c; 113, a). The endovesical prostatic adenoma was frozen for only 2 min under intravenous short-acting anesthesia. Postoperatively, the entire median lobe and the small lateral lobes, including the capsule, became necrotic. Ten years postoperatively, urologic findings are normal.

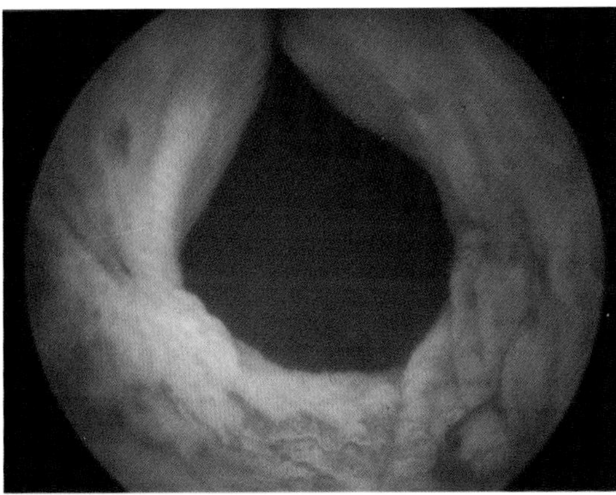

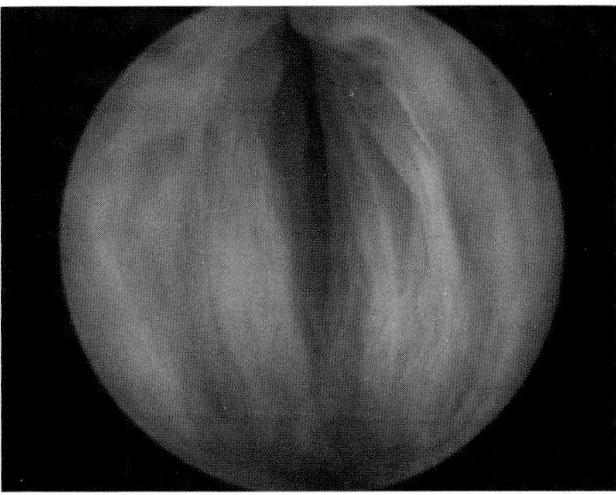

170 c–d

Fig. 170, c Indurated freezing channel with large subvesical adenoma.
The lumen of the prostatic urethra is unfolded widely by irrigation. Above, the remnants of the lateral lobes meet in a fold (Fig. 83, b). The convex cushions of the adenomatous lobes are frozen away to form a concave tube within the adenoma. The mucosa is altered by chronic inflammation and in part by scars. In this 83-year-old extreme high-risk patient (cerebrovascular accidents; permanent catheter), partial cryoprostatectomy was performed in two sessions with a freezing time of 2.5 min, using the "Standard" cryoprobe under local anesthesia. Three months later at a second session the freezing time was 3 min. Postoperative hospital care was one week following each session. Voiding of the bladder left no residual urine despite further strokes until the patient's death 3 years later. Normal urine; the excretory urogram showed a small remaining adenoma.

Fig. 170, d Indurated frozen channel at the apex (same patient).
Even when the irrigation is stopped, the lumen of the prostatic urethra remains open. Below, the verumontanum is just covered by the endoscope. At both sides, the apex and columns of the lateral lobes are seen. At the bladder neck the internal sphincter has contracted and closed the opening into the bladder (compare Fig. 165, f).

171 a–c
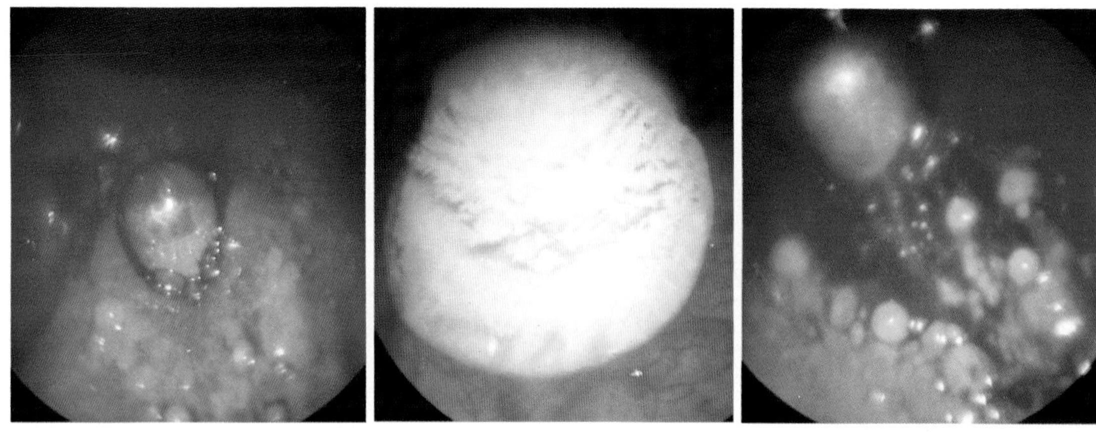

Radical and Palliative Cryosurgery of Prostatic Cancer (Trocar Cystoscopy)

Cancer cells are killed only at temperatures below −40° C by repeated freezing and thawing. This requires high efficiency of the freezing unit (see p. 174). Freezing may be controlled by thermocouples. With these, the position and depth of the needle tip within the tissue must be known, and therefore they are furnished with plastic tubes or balls for measurement. More important, however, is rectal distance measurement—the only effective means of controlling the subvesical progression of the frozen area. The correctness of this measurement in combination with endoscopy and aspiration of urine determines the quality of cryosurgery (see p. 177).

Fig. 171, a Bladder neck infiltrated by carcinoma.
A yellow tongue-shaped infiltrate extends from the urethra to the anterior bladder wall (below). Beyond the interureteral crest (above) the beginning of the dark bladder recess can be seen. It is covered with urine, reflecting light. In this 64-year-old patient, risk-degree O, stage $T_3N_0M_0G_2$, aspiration biopsy revealed carcinoma, grade IV (Pap.). The prostatic urethra was 4.5 cm long. The "Special" cryoprobe was applied twice for 3 min under intravenous short-acting anesthesia. Rectally, a minimal distance of 2 mm was measured between the frozen area and rectum. Postoperatively, estrogens were administered. Two years later a recurrent node was detected at the left of the prostatic fossa. Cryosurgery was again performed (twice for 30 sec), together with orchiectomy. Seven years later no recurrence; normal urine; normal excretory urogram. Nycturia occurred once. A hard plate was palpated rectally.

Fig. 171, b Frozen bladder neck.
The hood of the globe of ice covers the bladder neck. In the deeper tissues it is extended farther. Note the well-defined border between frozen and well-vascularized tissue (compare Figs. 162, c and d). This makes possible precise endoscopic control of freezing.

Fig. 171, c Thawing interval after radical freezing.
The tip of the "Special" cryoprobe protrudes 0.5 cm. The granular mucosa is swollen with edema; the arrangement of the granules has changed. After suprapubic aspiration of the bloody melted ice (compare Fig. 161, a), freezing is repeated; expansion occurs faster owing to the edema. The 28-Fr "Special" cryoprobe is more effective than the "Standard" cryoprobe (24 Fr) because of its larger diameter.

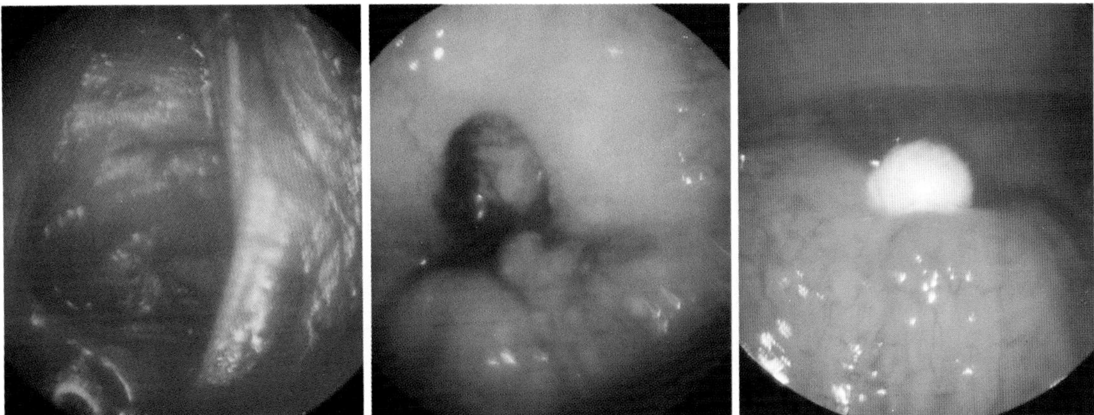

171 d–f

Fig. 171, d Channel of the suprapubic fistula as seen through the trocar cystoscope during extraction of the scope.

The deeper part of the channel has contracted where the defect in the bladder wall has closed. The abdominal rectus muscle delimits the opening at both sides. When trocar cystoscopy is unsuccessful, only yellow fat is seen through the cystoscope. Cystoscopy of the bladder roof then can verify the position of the trocar tip and correct it (compare Fig. 125).

Fig. 171, e Palliative cryosurgery of recurrent prostatic carcinoma.

The nodular tumorous infiltrate at the anterior bladder wall is seen here below the hollow prostatic fossa (after TURP) and the smooth bladder neck. This 79-year-old patient had TURP (110 gm net) of a giant adenoma with carcinomatous infiltrates three years previously. Now repeated freezing (2 min twice) and cobalt irradiation were given. Two years later, a sudden growth of metastases caused death.

Fig. 171, f Freezing of recurrent prostatic cancer; close-up.

The same carcinomatous infiltration (Fig. 171, e) looks like a hill from a different angle (the trocar cystoscope had been turned). The yellowish cancer (T_4G_2) shines through the reflecting mucosa. Its most prominent part is about 4 cm from the prostatic apex; the tip of the "Special" cryoprobe has begun freezing (white spot).

Trocar Cryosurgery for Central Freezing (Prostatic Carcinoma)

Surface freezing with the "Special" and "Standard" cryoprobes has an efficient range of 2 cm (radius) at the most. Carcinomas in the periphery and the prostatic capsule and large bladder tumors therefore cannot be frozen from the urethra or the bladder. Thus, we constructed the trocar cryoprobe to freeze tumors beyond the surface of the urinary system directly (J Urol *107*:389, 1972).

Fig. 172, a Trocar cryoprobe.
The trocar cryoprobe is graduated (black marks at a centimeter's distance) to measure the tumor's size. The diameter of the probe is 21 or 24 Fr. Its freezing element is 1.5 or 2 cm long. The larger probe was constructed to increase the efficiency of freezing. The control knob is 2 cm behind the rim of the freezing element and may be palpated rectally. It is pushed into the center of the tumor (median or lateral lobes of large adenomas, bladder tumor) or into the periphery (lateral prostatic infiltrations). Three routes of access are feasible (suprapubic, perineal, transurethral; see p. 182). Flocks first has applied trocar cryosurgery through the opened perineum. Surface cryosurgery usually is also applied.

Fig. 172, b Transperineal trocar cryosurgery of the peripheral prostatic carcinoma (stage $T_3N_xM_0G_3$).
Here, a recurrent tumor in the peripheral prostatic capsule is radically frozen. At the left, below, the yellow tip of a transurethral catheter juts into the bladder. About 2 cm away, the trocar tip perforates the carcinomatous infiltration on the bladder floor. The trocar cryoprobe was pushed through a skin incision in the left perineum and guided rectally beside the rectum and urethra through the prostate into the bladder (same access used in medieval lithotomy!). Suprapubic trocar cystoscopy controls and corrects the point of perforation of the tip into the bladder. (The bladder floor was folded before perforation.)

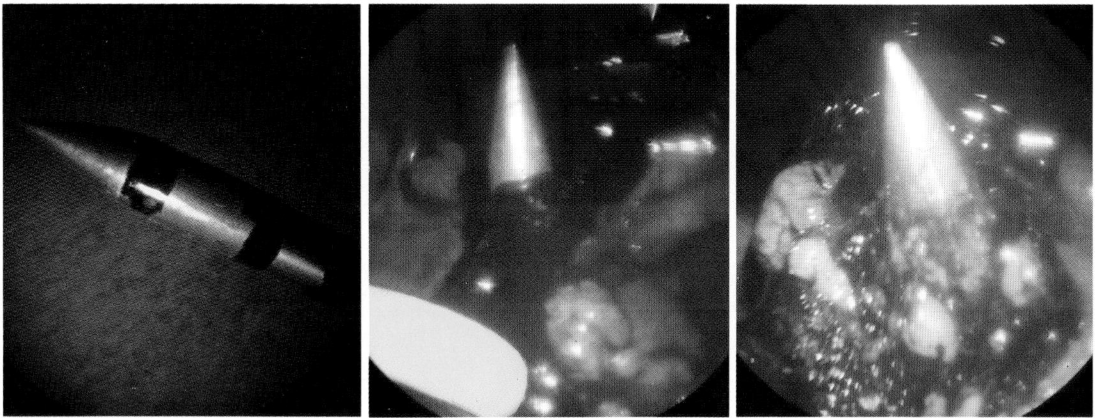

172 a–c

Fig. 172, c Close-up of the trocar tip.

After thawing, the probe is retracted slightly and refrozen. The tumorous infiltrate now is swollen with edema. This situation is explained by the schematic diagram in Fig. 151. This 82-year-old patient was treated for prostatic cancer 3 years previously with circular infiltration of the bladder neck (stage $T_3N_xM_0G_3$—group V Pap., freezing time twice—3.5 and 2 min). Now the tumor in the peripheral capsule and on the bladder floor is frozen four times from the inside at different sites for 3 min each. Then, in addition, the tumor surface is frozen transurethrally with the "Standard" cryoprobe (28 Fr) twice for 3 min. Two weeks after cryosurgery the patient was dismissed without a catheter. Five months later, all findings were normal. Five years later, at the age of 87, the patient had no complaints and no recurrence.

Palliative Cryosurgery of Prostatic Cancer (Urethroscopy)

Indications are: (1) lower urinary tract obstruction (permanent catheter); (2) upper urinary tract obstruction; (3) enhancement of the effect of radiation therapy; (4) pain from metastatic disease.

Fig. 173, a Prostatic fossa four months after freezing.
The remnants of the accompanying prostatic adenoma project into the large cavity, allowing a view of the internal sphincter only in the region of the trigone (the half-moon below is the result of incorrect positioning of the optical system within the sheath). In this 60-year-old high-risk patient (60 IU insulin) with permanent catheter (cancer stage $T_4N_2M_1G_3$), the prostatic cancer was frozen for 5 min with the obsolete blind technique of cryosurgery under intravenous short-acting anesthesia. Two years later micturition left no residual urine. Then cryosurgery was repeated: twice for 4 min: distance of freezing from the rectum, 2 mm. Two years after the second session, the patient died of uremia but had not needed a catheter.

Fig. 173, b External sphincter six months after cryosurgery.
Below can be seen the verumontanum and part of the external sphincter (left). In the center the remnants of the lateral lobes form a slit-shaped entrance into the prostatic fossa. 76-year-old high-risk patient; cancer stage $T_4N_xM_xG_3$. The frozen area has reached a distance of only 5 mm from the rectum. Blind cryosurgery for 6 min. Six months later floating infiltrates at the bladder neck (Fig. 173, c) were resected transurethrally. Histology revealed a tumor more like bladder cancer than prostatic cancer. Sixteen months later, the patient died of marasmus (no complaints about micturition; normal urine).

Fig. 173, c Carcinomatous nodes on the bladder neck.
The two sections show the lateral walls of the prostatic fossa that form a smooth tube free of tumor. At the point of transition into the bladder, however, a garland of fungiform tumors is found; these do not infiltrate the bladder or the fossa (Fig. 173, b).

Fig. 173, d Injured verumontanum three months after blind cryosurgery.
The whitish verumontanum rests upon the oblique fibers of the external sphincter. It is separated into halves by freezing (insufficient insulation of the probe) and has paled owing to degeneration of its blood vessels. The left top points to the lumen of the prostatic urethra, which is surrounded by adenomatous remnants at the apex. This 70-year-old low-risk patient has a cancer, stage T_4G_2, and a shrinking bladder with renal obstruction. It is frozen for 4 min under intravenous short-acting anesthesia. Rectal distance of the frozen area was 3 mm. Three months later TUR (30 gm net) was performed. No further follow-up.

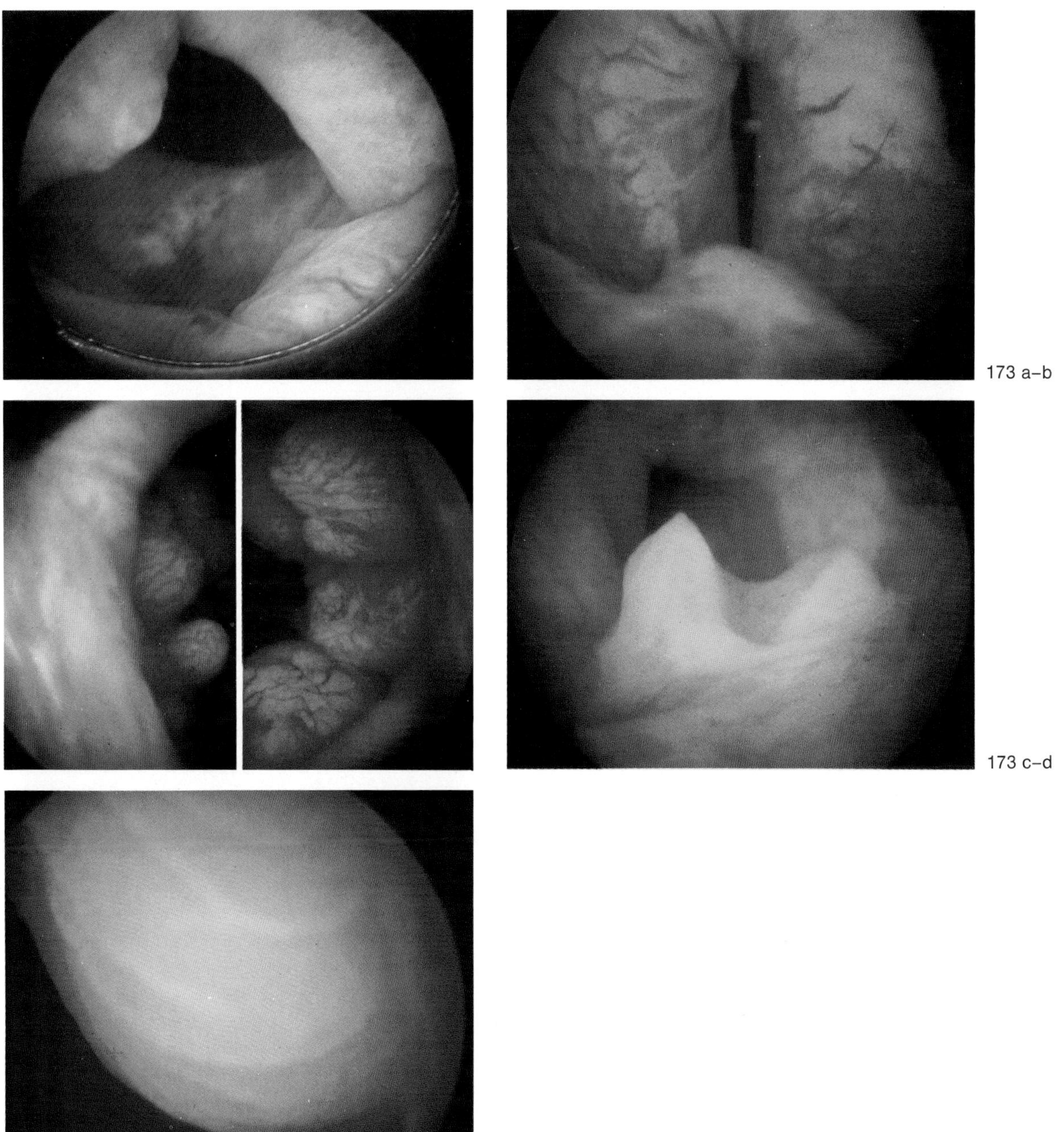

173 a–b

173 c–d

173 e

Fig. 173, e Typical edema of the rectal mucosa after cryosurgery of the prostate (proctoscopy in water). Just inside the anus the obliquely folded mucosa bulges into the lumen. The edema has changed its color and consistency (compare Figs. 116, e; 117). With the aid of rectal distance measurement, the freezing process can be controlled exactly (see p. 176). Here, the progression of the frozen area was stopped at a distance of 2 mm from the rectal mucosa. In this 70-year-old high-risk patient with carcinoma stage $T_4N_xM_1G_3$, the 5-cm prostate was frozen for 4 min under peridural anesthesia. There was significant relief of bone pain for the next 3 months; death followed 6 months later.

174 a–b

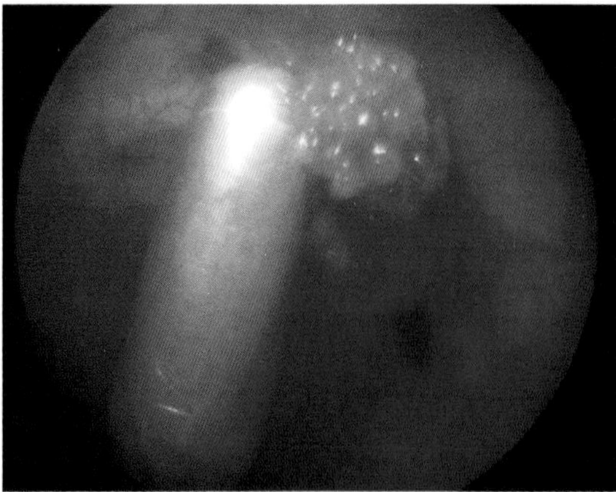

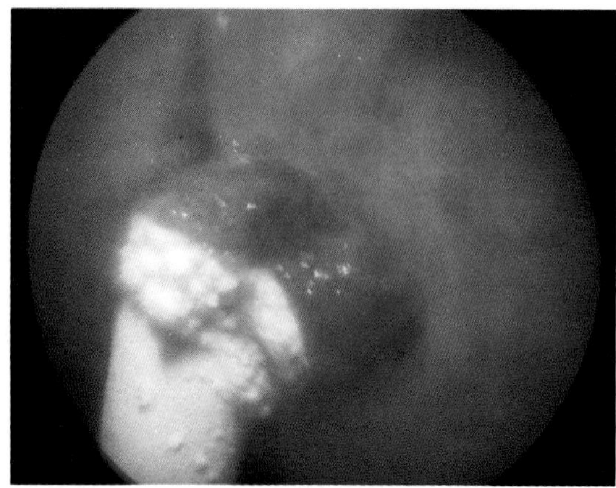

Cryosurgery of Bladder Papilloma, Stage T_A (Trocar Cystoscopy)

Bladder tumors may be destroyed by cold cryosurgery as well as by electric current (TUR). Cryosurgery, however, is easier technically, and there is no danger of perforation or hemorrhage. Filling the bladder with gas reduces the risk of seeding tumor cells within the bladder, unlike irrigation with water. For histologic examination a forceps biopsy is taken after cryosurgery. In addition, the voided necrotic tissue particles are examined histologically.

Figure 174, a Endoscopic cryosurgery of a small tumor on the lateral bladder wall (about 1.5 cm diameter).
The tumor is pushed aside with the tip of the "Special" cryoprobe to freeze the pedicle and the base in the bladder wall first. This is done to block seeding of tumor cells through the circulating blood and lymph. In this 71-year-old high-risk patient, the tumor was frozen twice for 30 sec; the coexisting prostatic adenoma was frozen twice for 2 min. Postoperatively, the bladder was continuously irrigated with a cytostatic drug (not a single concentrated instillation) through an indwelling 3-way catheter over 3 days. After 5 days the patient was dismissed; a permanent catheter was left in place for 5 weeks. Eight years later the patient had no urologic findings and no recurrence.

Fig. 174, b Freezing.
The anterior side of the tumor is half frozen here after 20 sec (counted from when the cryoprobe tip reached a temperature of −80° C). Its base and posterior half already are entirely frozen.

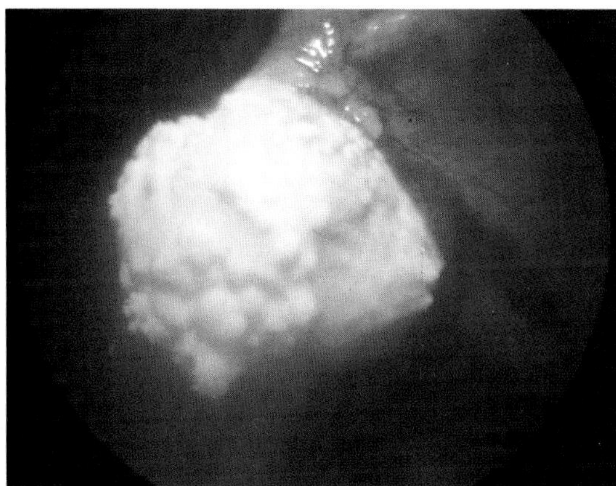

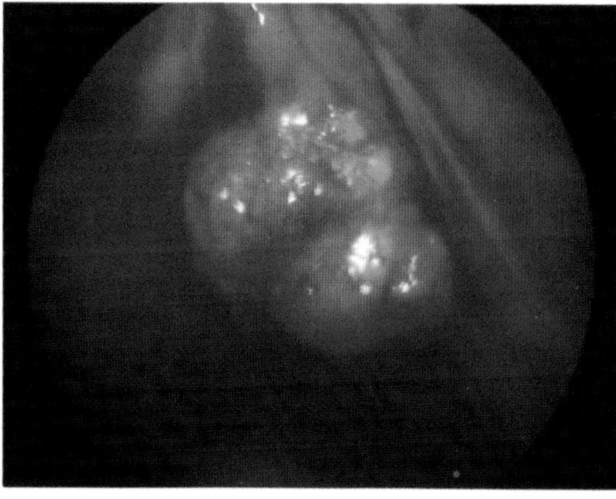

174 c–d

Fig. 174, c Frozen tumor.
After 30 sec the tumor is entirely frozen. The depth of the ice is controlled by the mobility of the bladder wall when it is tugged inside with the adherent probe, as demonstrated here, or by turning the tip. Another control is a suprapubically inserted needle pushed obliquely into the bladder wall (compare Fig. 161, a), which can measure the distance between mucosa and the peripheral base of the frozen area.

Fig. 174, d Thawed tumor.
After 10 minutes the tumor is passively thawed. The heated cryoprobe is removed immediately. The tumor is, like its surroundings, swollen with edema; it hangs down slackly. The mucosa is reactively inflamed.

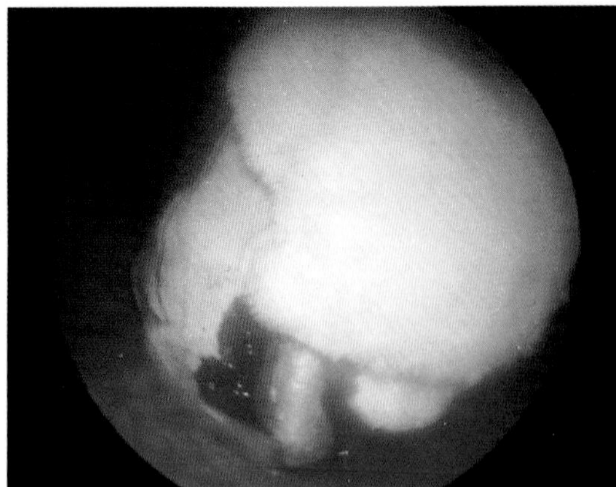
175 a

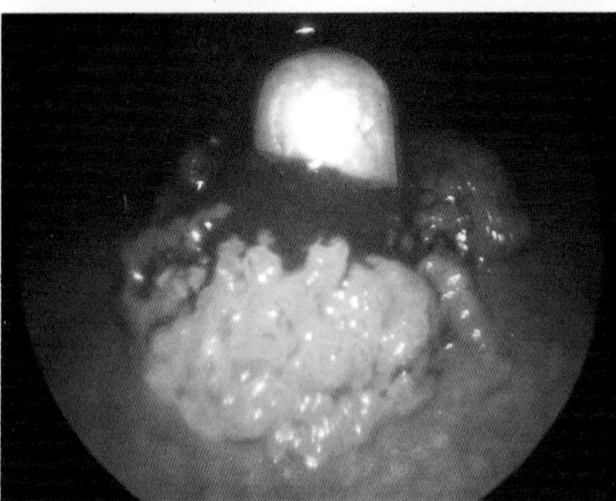
175 b

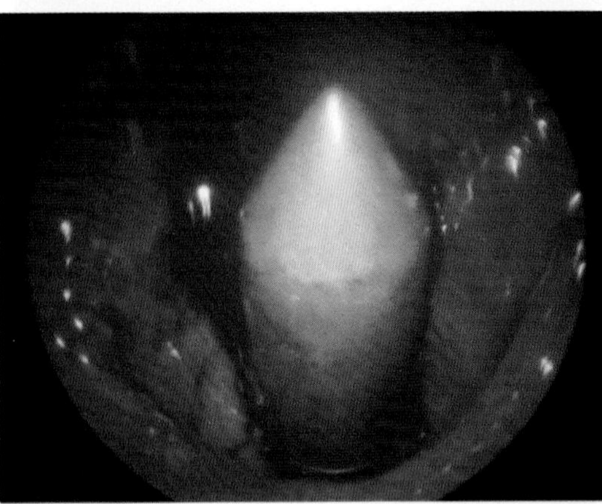
175 c

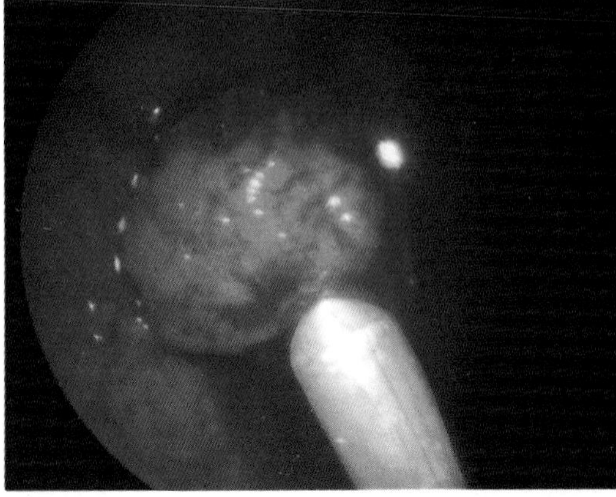
175 d

Trocar and Surface Cryosurgery of Larger Bladder Tumors, Stage T_A (Trocar Cystoscopy)

Here, cryosurgery is superior to TUR because the procedure is simple, easy to control (no hemorrhage) and carries very little risk. The necrosis is shed within a few days. Remnants of the base can be secondarily frozen or can be removed by TUR (sample excision for histology of the base). Our largest tumor (450 gm net) was laboriously resected (compare Fig. 131). Today, an operation of this kind is significantly facilitated by cryosurgery before secondary TUR of the remaining tumor.

Fig. 175, a Frozen bladder tumor.
The trocar cryoprobe has impaled the tumor, which has a diameter of 5 cm and is situated at the left bladder neck. The sheath of the probe is not frozen (metal below). The probe was introduced transurethrally. It is frozen three times for 1-2 min. The single functional (left) kidney was significantly obstructed by the tumor (T_A); a right pelvic kidney was useless. The patient was dismissed after 1 week; 2 weeks later the obstruction of the left kidney had cleared. The tumor was entirely rejected. No further follow-up.

Fig. 175, b Cryosurgery of a tumor (T_A) at the bladder neck.
This broad-based tumor has grown in a circle around the bladder neck and has a diameter of 3 cm. It is frozen, transurethrally together with the 4 cm long prostatic adenoma. After thawing, the villi of the tumor are edematous and there is some hemorrhage from the urethra. The "Special" cryoprobe is already heated and ready for repeated freezing. In this 55-year-old patient with no operative risk, the tumor was frozen several times for 20 to 25 sec; the prostate was frozen twice for 2 min after retraction of the probe; intravenous short-acting anesthesia. Further small recurrences of bladder tumor were resected at intervals of 2 to 20 months.

Fig. 175, c Trocar cryosurgery of a bladder tumor.
The trocar cryoprobe (24 Fr; short tip) was introduced transurethrally. It lies within the prostatic fossa, which was partially hollowed out by cryosurgery. Its mucosa, altered by inflammation, is bleeding (left). After secondary cryosurgery of the remaining adenoma, the bladder tumor is frozen (Fig. 175, d–f). The introduction of the probe through the urethra is not difficult because its tip is short and relatively blunt. Control by rectal palpation is necessary.

Fig. 175, d Positioning of the trocar cryoprobe.
The trocar cryoprobe (24 Fr; short tip) is introduced transurethrally and set on a tumor about 2 cm in diameter. Often a reduction of the bladder volume facilitates contacting the tumor.

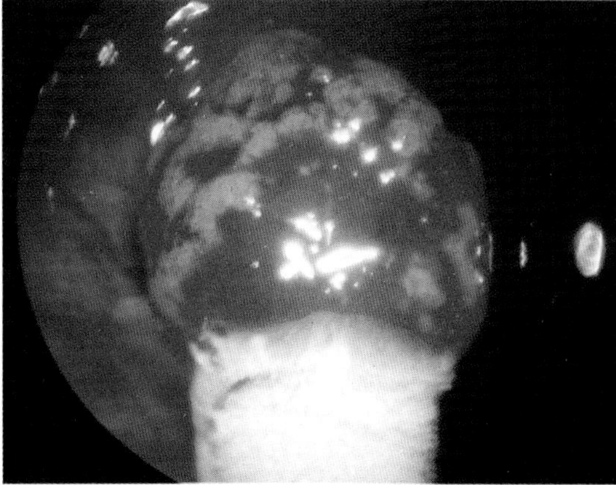

175 e

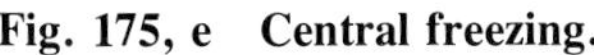

Fig. 175, e Central freezing.
The tumor is impaled and frozen centrally. Its surface becomes increasingly pale (30 sec time of freezing).

Fig. 175, f Thawing.
The frozen tumor thaws continuously. Below, the site where the probe was positioned and the tangentially frozen bladder wall are recognized. In this 59-year-old patient, a right nephrectomy was performed 3 years ago for a benign ureteral tumor (shrunken kidney); TUR of a large benign bladder tumor (10 gm net) also was performed. Then three tumors were frozen — each twice for 45 sec. Total cryonecrosis. Two years later an invasive tumor (T_2) was resected transurethrally. Five years later all urologic findings were normal.

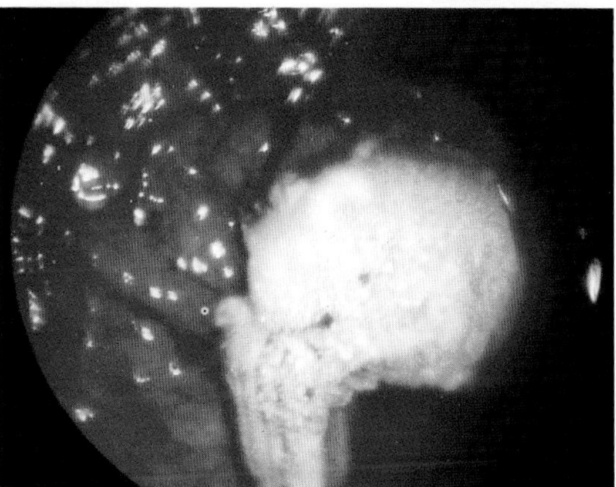

175 f

Fig 175, g Cryonecrosis one week after cryosurgery of a 3 × 4 cm large, broad-based bladder tumor, stage T_A.
A disintegrating necrosis adheres to the lateral wall of the bladder. It is scratched off with the cold loop. The base of the tumor is resected with electric current. Then electric litholapaxy of the bladder stone (right) was performed. Two years later the urologic findings in this 70-year-old patient were normal. An abdominal anus was created for cancer of the rectum.

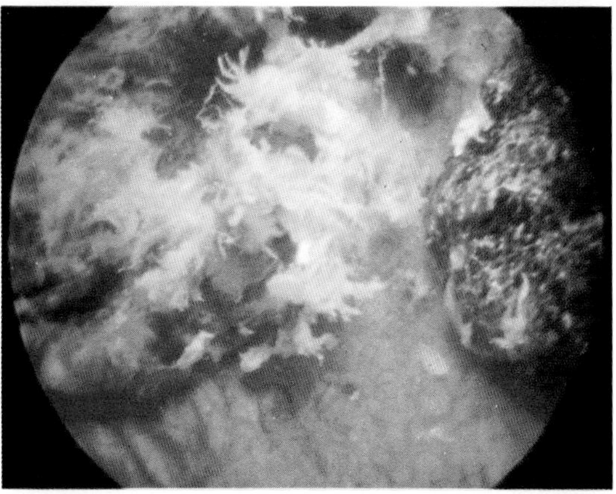

175 g

Fig. 175, h Scar in the lateral bladder wall.
Two months after cryosurgery of a large bladder tumor, a few small ulcerations of the mucosa still can be verified (below). Scar fibers radiate upward. Four weeks later, findings were normal. In this 66-year-old high-risk patient, a bladder tumor (T_A; 3 cm diameter) and a prostatic adenoma were frozen repeatedly under intravenous short-acting anesthesia with the "Special" cryoprobe for 2 min each. Biopsy from the base 4 weeks later (histology, P_0). Eight years later the patient had no abnormal urologic findings.

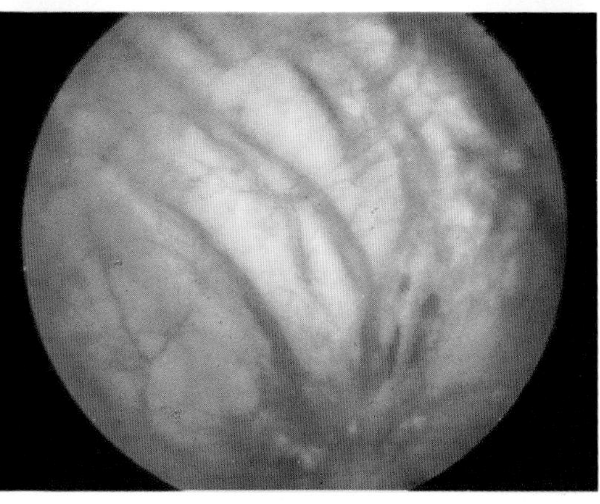

175 h

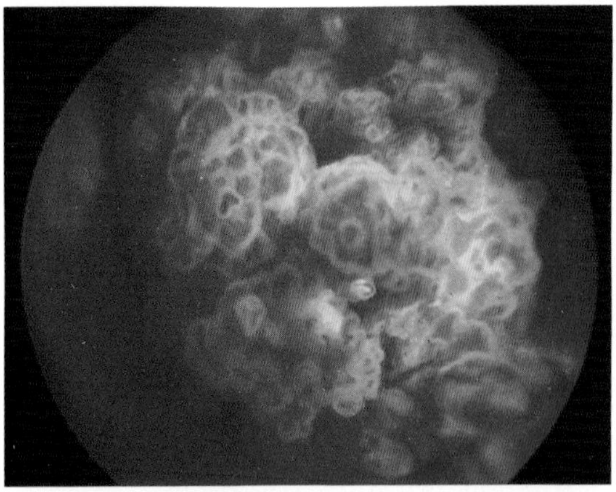

176 a

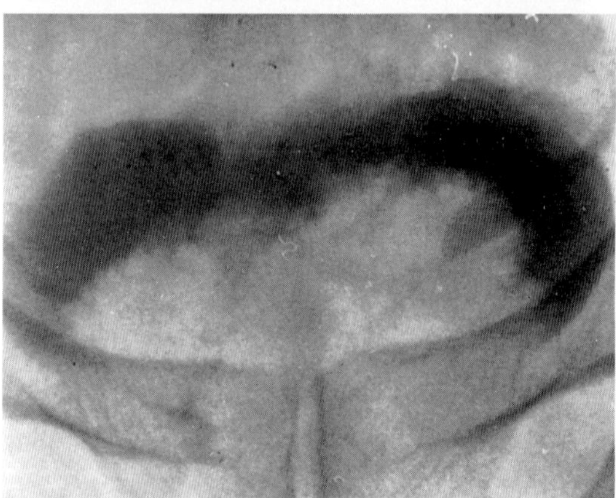

176 b

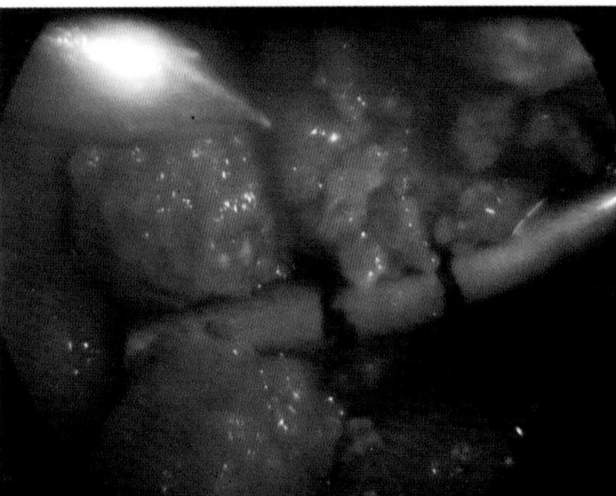

176 c

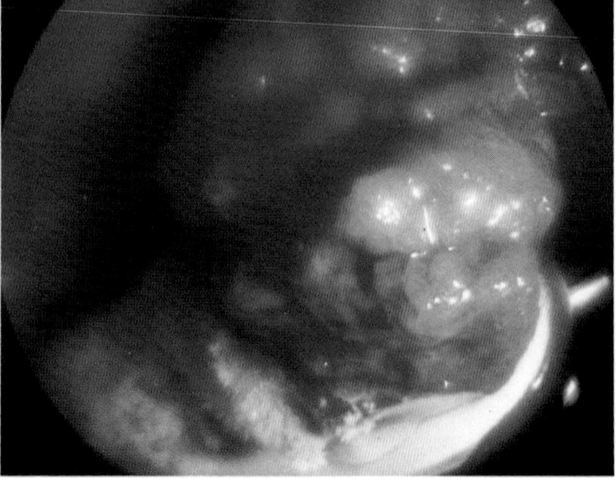

176 d

Cryosurgery of Invasive Bladder Tumors (Stages $T_{2\text{-}4}$ — Trocar Crystoscopy)

There are two possibilities: (1) the main mass of the tumor is frozen first and its base resected transurethrally later; (2) the tumor is resected first and its base is frozen immediately afterward (or only after unexpected positive histology). Both ways reduce the risk of perforation and hemorrhage. In addition, the effects of TUR and irradiation are potentiated. Additive therapy of all bladder tumors is possible: (a) cytostatic continuous irrigation (not instillation) of the bladder through an indwelling 3-way catheter or irrigation of the internal iliac artery (compare Fig. 140); (b) nonspecific stimulation of the immune system (plant or animal extracts combined with cytostatics), BCG inoculations, extracts of bacteria and others. Additional surgical operations such as partial or radical cystectomy, lymphadenectomy and so on always can be performed after cryosurgery.

Fig. 176, a Giant papillary bladder carcinoma stage $T_{3am}N_0M_0G_1$ (cystoscopy in water).
There are two large tumors (4 and 6 cm in diameter) on the bladder floor; several smaller papillomas lie beside them.

Fig. 176, b Bladder with extended space-occupying lesion in the cystogram (tumor 8 × 3 cm diameter).
This 72-year-old woman was refused an operation 3 years previously because of high-risk status. The left kidney is shrinking because of chronic obstruction.

Fig. 176, c Multiple tumors on the bladder floor.
The tumor covers the entire bladder floor. The freezing element of the cryoprobe is in place on the tumor. It was introduced through the urethra (meatus at the left) and into the bladder; it reaches the margin of the picture with its insulated tip at the right. In between is its 4.5-cm freezing element graduated in cm (black marks). At the left above is the tip of a trocar used to provide additional light (illumination over glass fibers for still photography and movies after Reuter).

Fig. 176, d Tumor after cryosurgery.
The tumor is swollen with edema (above) after several intervals of freezing and thawing. The lower part is still frozen. The cryoprobe (metal tip at the right), which is pressed deeply into the tumor, is now thawed for 3 min and frozen repeatedly. The freezing process is controlled by turning the probe, needle measurement of the distance to the vagina (2 mm distance) and trocar cystoscopy (peridural anesthesia).

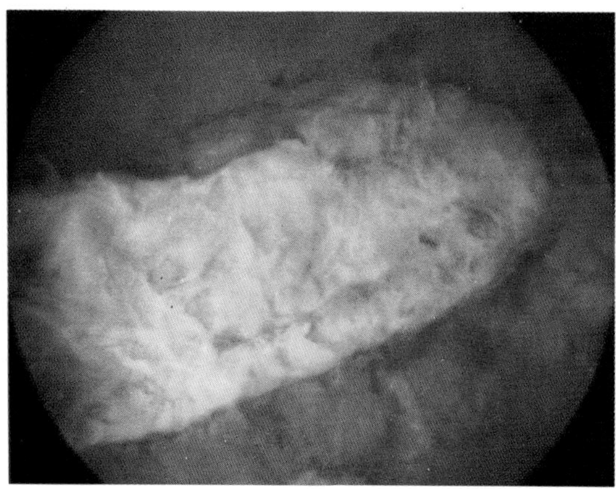

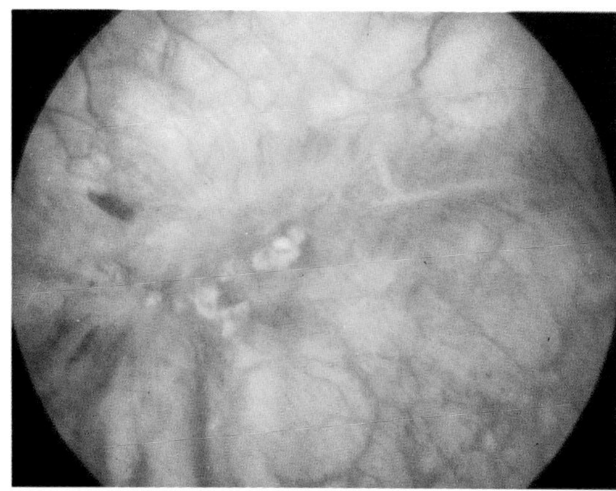

176 e–f

Fig. 176, e Cryonecrosis of the bladder wall.
Two weeks later, the entire tumor has been rejected (cystoscopy in water). The cryonecroses of the bladder wall lie obliquely on the bladder floor. The surrounding mucosa is reactively inflamed.

Fig. 176, f Scar after two months (cystoscopy).
The necrotic bladder wall has healed except for a small ulcer. A scar runs obliquely across the picture. The mucosa has grown pale and shows almost no irritation. In the following months, six more plum-sized tumors were frozen in three sessions. They had rapidly reformed at the bladder floor and on the anterior wall (freezing time 1 to 2 min with the "Special" cryoprobe under intravenous short-acting anesthesia). Subsequently, there was no further recurrence. Urologic findings remained normal until death occurred 8 years later at age 78 years.

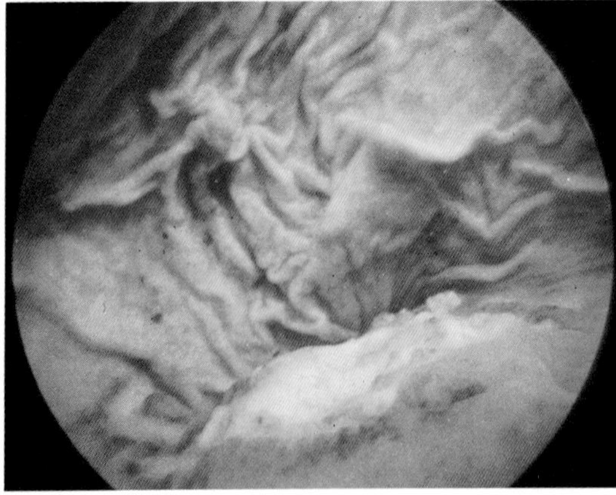

177

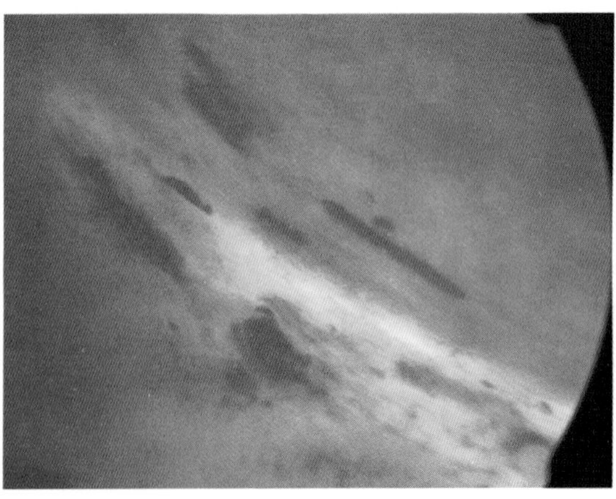

17

Fig. 177 TUR and cryosurgery of a bladder carcinoma (stage $T_2N_xM_xG_1$).
At the lower right, a flat cryonecrosis of the bladder floor is seen six weeks after cryosurgery. The ureteral orifice is at the right lower margin. The posterior wall of the bladder (above) is contracted by spasms; cystocele. In this 57-year-old woman a large 35-gm papilloma was resected. Histology revealed invasive growth. Therefore, the base of the resected tumor in the bladder wall was frozen one week after TUR ("Special" cryoprobe, twice for 1 min; vaginal distance of the frozen tissue 2 mm). Patient dismissed 2 days after cryosurgery. Three years later TUR of a small papilloma (T_1) was performed; 7 years later the urologic findings were normal.

Cryosurgery and Cobalt Irradiation of a Papillary Bladder Carcinoma (stage $T_{3a}N_xM_xG_1$)

In this 71-year-old patient without operative risk a 3-cm tumor was frozen repeatedly (1.5 and 2 min) with the "Special" cryoprobe. The coexisting prostatic adenoma also was frozen (2 and 2.5 min). Cobalt irradiation, 6000 R, followed. After 4 months the postoperative obstruction of the right kidney was relieved (Fig. 178, b). Five years later, urologic findings were normal.

Fig. 178, a Hemorrhagic irradiation cystitis.
The mucosa of the bladder is diffusely reddened. Below the mucosa of the right lateral wall (left), longish hemorrhagic infiltrations are embedded. The interureteral crest is continued beyond the ureteral orifice (at the right below) by a bright scar that runs toward the upper left.

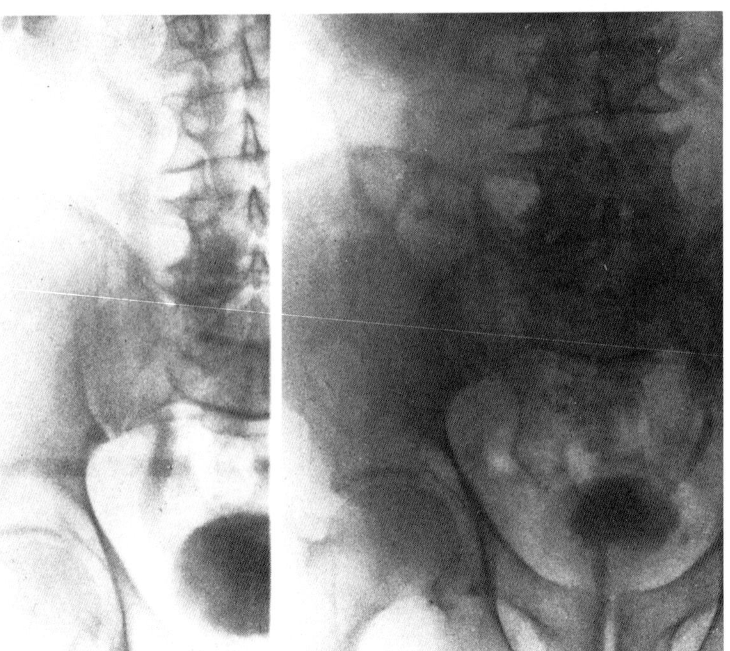

178 b

Fig. 178, b Excretory urogram: bladder cancer with unilateral ureteral obstruction (left section).
After cryosurgery the right ureter and kidney have become normal (right section). A saber-shaped urethra was formed in the adenomatous remnant by partial cryoprostatectomy.

Carcinoma in Situ (TiS) and Cryosurgery

Cryosurgery of preinvasive cancer is technically easy. However, treatment of these tumors is complicated by multifocal growths and high rates of recurrence. The prognosis following procedures intended to preserve the organs is therefore dubious.

This 48-year-old patient had cystitis with hematuria that resisted therapy for 1 year. Histologic examination of biopsy material revealed nonspecific infiltration of the bladder muscle. Four months later another histology report showed malignancy, and the infiltration was treated by cryosurgery. The planned cystectomy was refused by the consultant university hospital. Biopsy (TUR) one month and 2 years later showed nonspecific inflammation of mucosa and muscle, but no malignancy (Figs. 179, a–e).

Four years after the first cryosurgery, carcinoma developed within the right ureteral orifice. TUR, cryosurgery and cobalt irradiation (Fig. 179, d) were performed. Two years later, the patient died of generalized metastatic disease. Just before death a right nephrectomy was performed for transitional cell carcinoma.

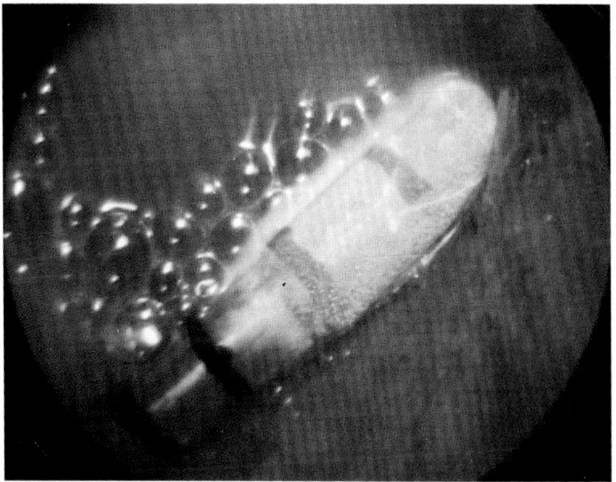
179 a

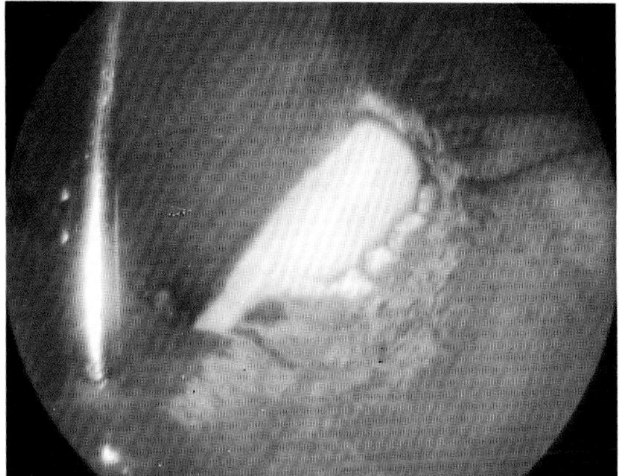
179 b

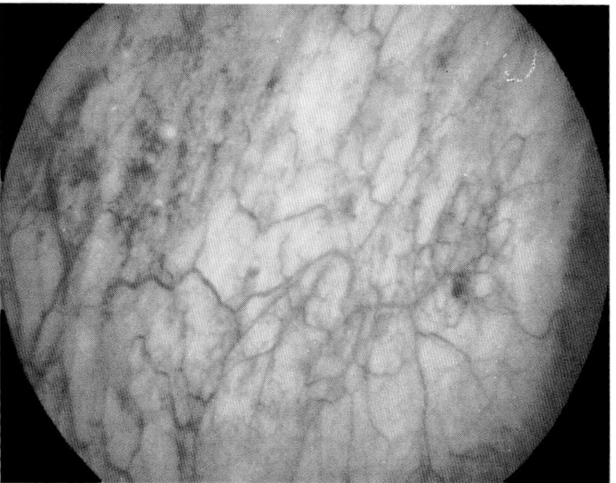
179 c

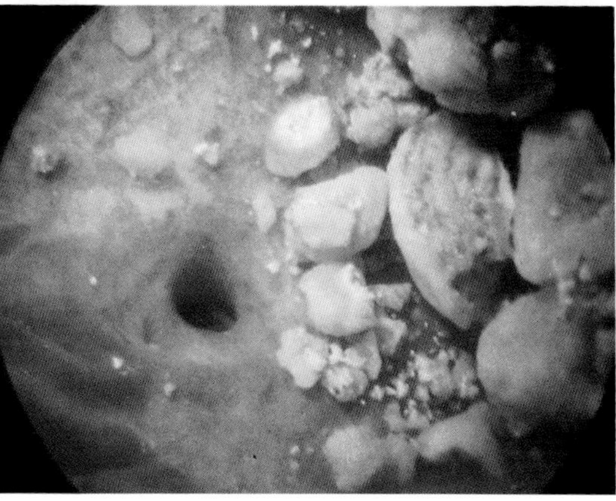
179 d

Fig. 179, a Cryosurgery of infiltrative cystitis.
The mucosa shows red spots in a well-defined region on the left lateral bladder wall, which is covered with small granules. The graduation of the cryoprobe in cm is clearly visible (freezing surface 2.5 cm; 28 Fr). At the left of the cryoprobe, water with small helium gas bubbles has collected on the bladder floor. Transurethral surface cryosurgery was repeated several times.

Fig. 179, b Cryosurgery and suprapubic aspiration.
After a freezing time of 20 sec the frozen area has advanced 2 to 3 mm deep into the tissue around the cryoprobe. The mucosa at the right is altered by edema; at the right above, hyperemic vessels are seen. At the left, an aspiration needle is introduced suprapubically to remove the collected urine (Figs. 161, a and b). The cryoprobe is turned on its axis to freeze a larger surface of the bladder wall.

Fig. 179, c Regenerated mucosa.
Six months later the bladder mucosa is pale (atrophic) and interlaced by atypical (regenerated) blood vessels. The small infiltration at the left above (granular cystitis) is caused by inflammation (histology: P_0). No recurrence after several years.

Fig. 179, d Regenerated right ureteral orifice.
The cryonecrosis sloughed after 3 months; its remnants are calcified. An invasive carcinoma (stage $T_2N_xM_xG_3$) in the right orifice was frozen. Mucosa and ostium have regenerated. There is neither reflex nor obstruction of the right ureter. The soft petrified necroses were treated by litholapaxy (endoscopic forceps).

180 a–c

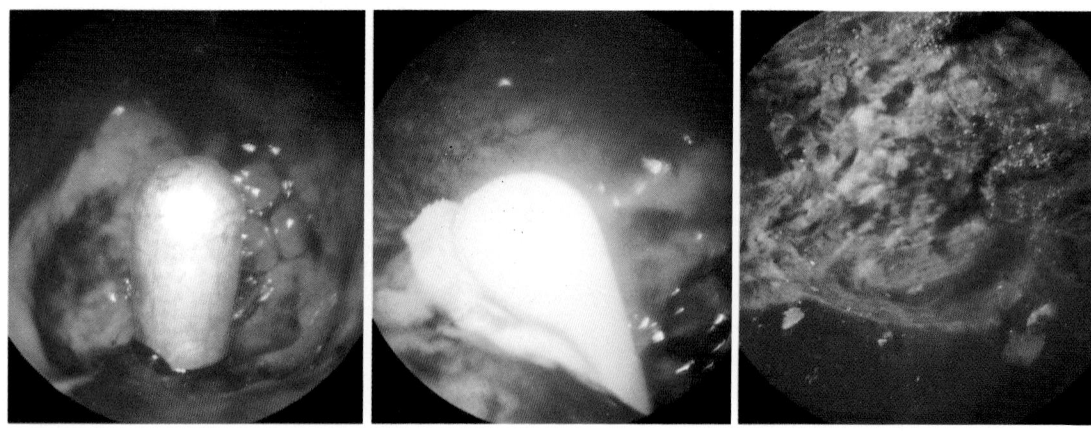

Cryosurgery of Bladder Neck and Prostate after TUR of an Infiltrating Bladder Carcinoma (Stage $T_{4a}N_XM_XG_2$).

In this 64-year-old patient an excretory urogram revealed obstruction of the left kidney. One week after TUR (12 gm net), cryosurgery was performed (freezing 4 times for 1 min; Figs. 180, a and b). The planned cystectomy was refused by the consulting university hospital because 3 months after cryosurgery there were no further pathologic findings. Cobalt irradiation was given. One year later, a tumor (stage $T_1N_XM_XG_0$; 2 cm diameter) was frozen repeatedly 3 times between 1 and 3 min. Two years later, multiple T_1 tumors were resected. After 3 years a left nephrectomy was performed because of pyelonephrosis. A biopsy perforated the left bladder neck into the peritoneum (compare Fig. 96, laparotomy). Five years after first treatment, the patient died of uremia.

Fig. 180, a Prostatic fossa with cryoprobe after TUR of bladder carcinoma (trocar cystoscopy in helium).
The tip of the "Standard" cryoprobe is introduced into the fossa. The freezing element is set on the base of the bladder cancer, which had been resected one week before and found to infiltrate the prostate. The wound surface is covered with necrosis; the surrounding mucosa of the bladder neck is reactively inflamed.

Fig. 180, b Freezing of the base of the tumor in the fossa.
The freezing surface of the probe is covered with ice and is surrounded by a margin of frozen tissue. Control by rectal distance measurement; repeated freezing of four different sectors of the fossa.

Fig. 180, c Extended lesion after TUR of cryonecrosis (diameter 5 cm).
Below the resected necrotic bladder wall, the red, inflamed mucosa on the bladder neck is seen. The entire depth of cryonecrosis could not be resected because of the danger of perforation. Exploratory TUR was performed one week after cryosurgery of a bleeding bladder tumor (stage $T_{3a}N_XM_{1c}G_3$) and three metastases on the bladder floor in this 50-year-old patient (freezing five times between 1 and 3 min). Cobalt irradiation followed. Five months later, the excretory urogram was normal. Cystoscopy revealed an irradiated bladder, but no tumor. Six months later the patient died of hemophilia due to metastatic disease of the bone marrow.

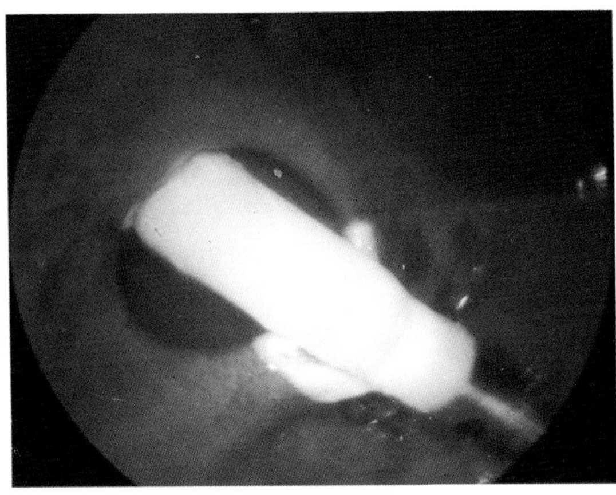

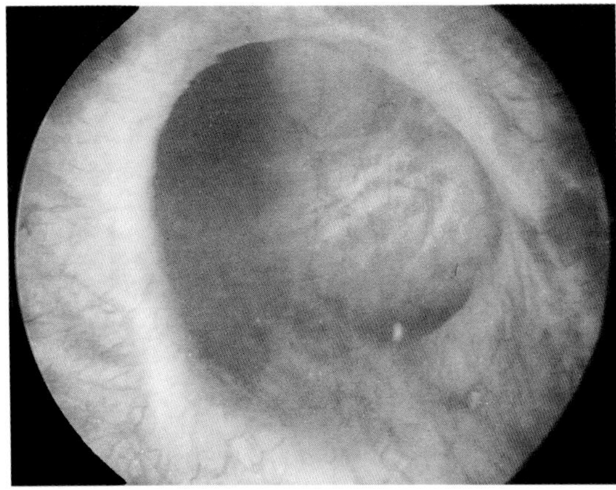

181 a–b

Cryosurgery on a Bladder Diverticulum

This 89-year-old patient had an *E. coli* infection. Two diverticula were frozen (30 sec each), and the coexisting prostatic adenoma was frozen twice for 2 min. Three months later urologic findings were normal. The patient died 2 years after treatment but had no urologic complaints.

Most bladder diverticula can be operated transurethrally because their diameter is less than 3 cm. Formerly, we destroyed the sphincter by TUR; today, we prefer cryosurgery because it is easier and carries less risk. The induration of the frozen mouth of the diverticulum guarantees a good long-term result.

Fig. 181, a Mouth of a diverticulum about 1.5 cm in diameter (trocar cystoscopy in helium).
The sphincter of the diverticulum is frozen with the "Special" cryoprobe at two sites. Then the probe is turned in order to freeze the rest of the rim.

Fig. 181, b Result (cystoscopy in water).
The diverticulum is transformed into a large cavity in the bladder wall. Above, a scarred portion of the mouth of the diverticulum has remained. Below, it flattens into the bladder lumen (still photo from the film, *Cryosurgery of the prostatic carcinoma*, shown at the AUA meeting, New York, 1973).

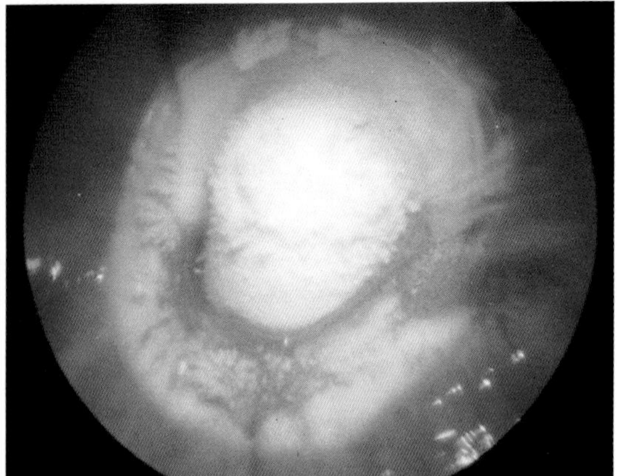

182 a

182 b

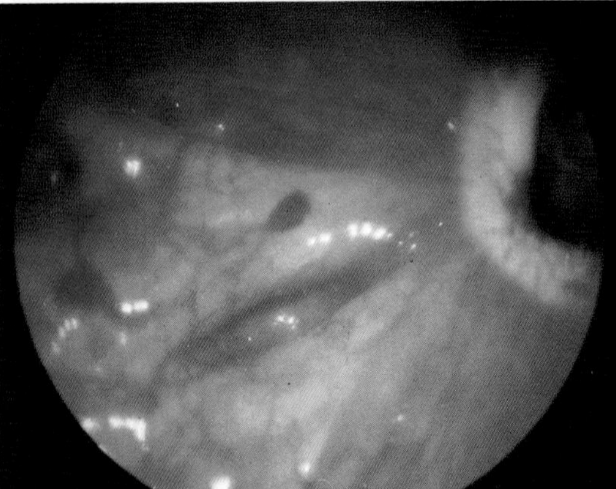

182 c

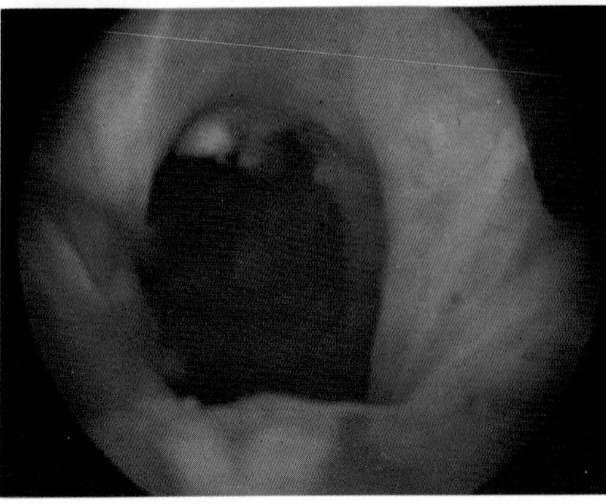

182 d

Cryosurgery of a Postoperative Bladder Neck Stricture (Trocar Cystoscopy)

Frozen tissue tends not to form scars. This explains the rare complications caused by scars, especially when compared with TUR (see p. 237).

Freezing extends more slowly in scarred tissue, which contains little water. The rectal distance between the frozen area and the external sphincter must be only 1 to 2 mm; otherwise, the operation may not be successful (as in Fig. 182, a). For this reason, the control knob is drawn 1 to 1.5 cm distal to the apex into the middle urethra.

Fig. 182, a Bladder neck stricture after partial TUR (25 gm).
The bladder neck is frozen at a radius of about 5 mm around the "Special" cryoprobe. Its tip protrudes about 1 cm into the bladder; its freezing element is about 1.5 cm deep within the prostatic urethra; the control knob is 1 cm distal to the apex. The unrepeated freezing time of 1 min was too brief, because the situation was incorrectly judged. Thus, 5 months later another TURP was necessary (12 gm net of adenoma).

Fig. 182, b Thawing.
The cryoprobe already has been removed to give a clear view into the prostatic fossa. The ice is thawing. Its margin with the unfrozen tissue is poorly defined.

Fig. 182, c Scarred contracture of the bladder neck.
After thawing, the remaining narrow zone of ice is surrounded by adenomatous mucosa. To the left, scarred fibers radiate through the bladder wall.

Fig. 182, d External sphincter after cryosurgery.
This is the result 6 weeks after cryosurgery of a bladder neck stricture. Urethroscopy shows small necrotic particles of tissue hanging around the prostatic fossa. Below, the flat sides of the external sphincter run distal to the verumontanum. Freezing was stopped at a distance of 3 mm from the apex (rectal measurement of distance). This 74-year-old patient had a stricture 6 years after partial TUR. After cryosurgery, the patient had transient incontinence for 1 month. Over the succeeding 7 years, no stricture recurred (no nycturia; no residual urine; compare Fig. 103, c).

Cryosurgery of Bleeding Irradiation Cystitis (Cystoscopy in Water)

This 46-year-old patient had combined x-ray and radium irradiation of a uterine carcinoma. Serious hemorrhages recurred for 2 years but ceased immediately after cryosurgery. The necrosis was resected transurethrally after 2 months. Since then, small necrotic stones are voided from time to time. Histologic examination of biopsy material from the remaining ulcer (Fig. 183, c) revealed nonspecific granulation. After biopsy the defect healed within a short time. Over the following 7 years there were no urologic complaints. The mucosa was without irritation and without degenerated vessels in the region of the scar of cryosurgery.

Degenerated mucosal vessels (in the sense of varicosis) caused the serious hemorrhages. These vessels lie superficially and are therefore easily frozen and destroyed. The technique is simple: in the gas-filled bladder the bleeding sites are easily verified. They should be frozen only for a few seconds at −40° C. Lower temperatures cause uncontrolled destruction because tissue damaged by irradiation is very sensitive to cold. This method is clearly superior to laborious TUR (compare Fig. 139).

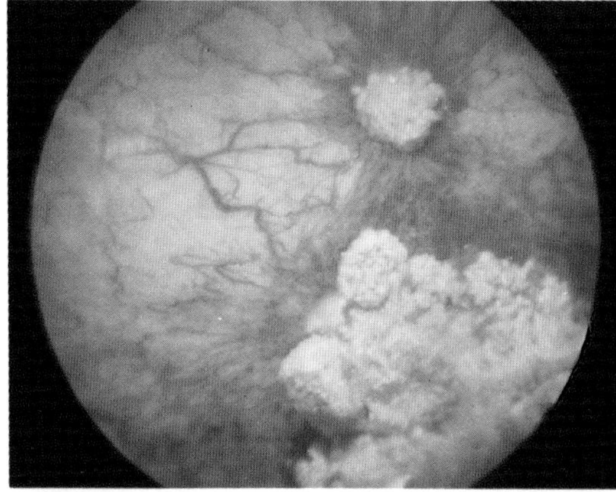

183 a

Fig. 183, a Cryonecrosis after 2 months.
The trigone, bladder floor and the posterior wall are covered by masses of gray necrotic tissue. The spot toward the top has a diameter of about 1 cm. Somewhat enlarged (but not pathologically altered) vessels extend from the necrosis (to the left).

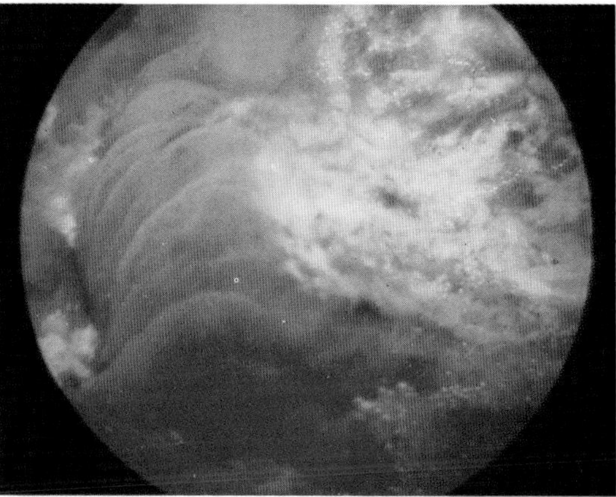

183 b

Fig. 183, b Bladder floor 2 weeks after TUR.
The cryonecrosis has been removed as much as possible. The rim of the wound is reactively inflamed and edematous.

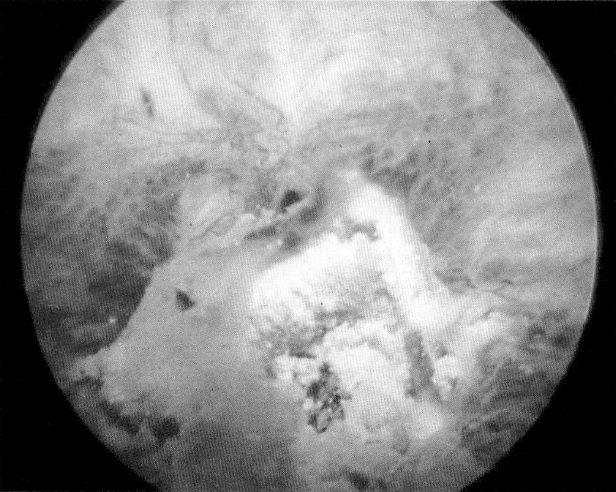

183 c

Fig. 183, c Late result.
The surface of the wound has now shrunk, except for this small ulcer (close-up). The regenerated mucosa is pale and poorly supplied with vessels. Fibrin flakes and small calcified necroses lie above the trigone (compare Fig. 179, c).

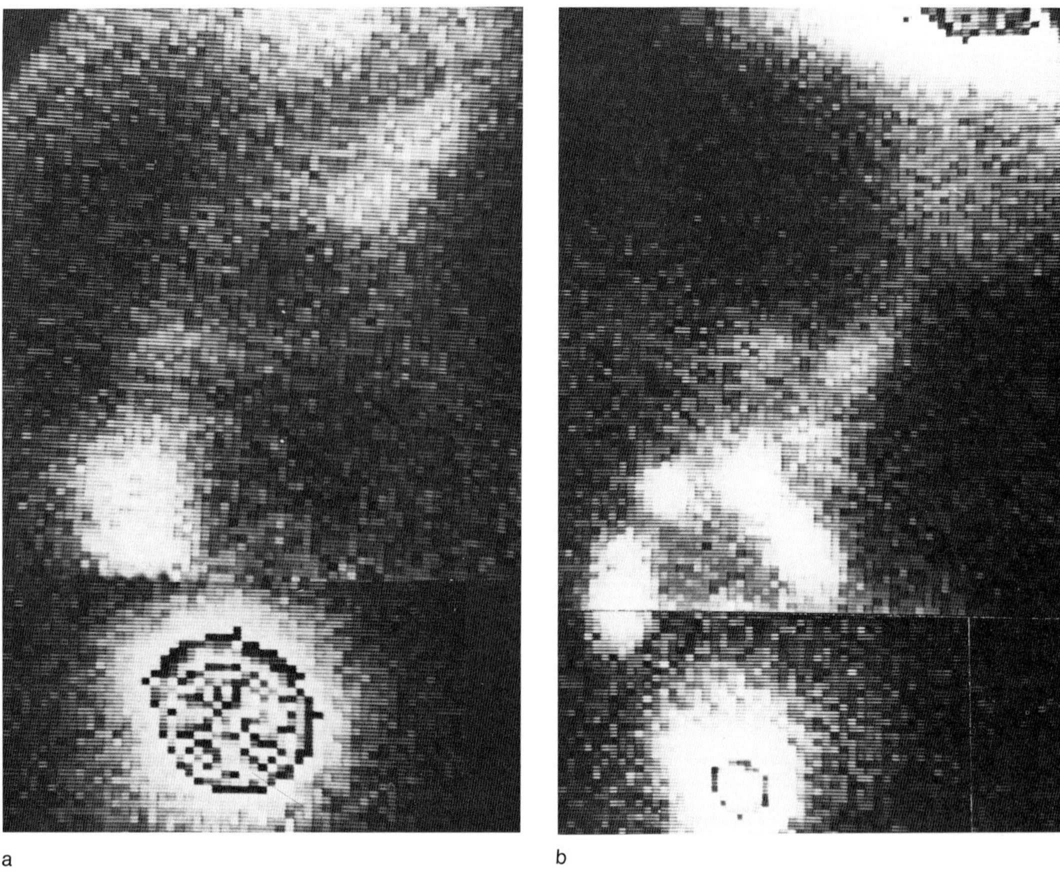

a b

Fig. 184, a and b First radionuclide scintigram of the regional lymph nodes of the prostate (Scientific exhibition at the AUA meeting, New York, May 1979; cancer stage $T_2N_2M_0G_1$).

Transrectal injection of 2 to 3 mCi ^{99m}Tc colloid bilaterally into the prostatic capsule. (Gamma camera with data system; Department of Nuclear Medicine, Urologic Hospital Professor Dr. Reuter, 1978.)

(a) AP exposure showing large deposit of radioactive material in the prostate. The right lymphatic chain is demonstrated up to level of the aorta; the left is not seen. External and internal iliac nodes project one onto the other.

(b) Lateral exposure of the right lymphatic chain. The iliac lymphatic channels are seen as a bifurcation of the external and internal. The prostate is at the lower rim of the composite picture; the liver is at the right. The external iliac lymph nodes are at the right of the prostate; the internal nodes are at the left. Above them, the para-aortic nodes may be seen.

By this method the right lymphatic chain can be demonstrated separately from the left; the side away from the camera is not visualized owing to the distance.

NEW PROSPECTS

The "Deutsche Forschungsgemeinschaft" (DFG, German Research Association) has charged ten urologic hospitals, including the eight most important German university hospitals, to test prostatic cryosurgery. The president of the DFG, Prof. Dr. H. Maier-Leibnitz, drew the following conclusion: " . . . Today scientists can declare that local application of extreme cold in the treatment of diseases of the bladder neck and the prostate opens new ways to an operation that causes little patient stress and that offers good results . . . Cryosurgical operative procedures offer, in the opinion of the participating scientists, an enrichment of urologic treatment methods, sparing many patients pain and increasing the longevity of many."

The efficiency of cryosurgery can still be improved. This is achieved by using the newer probes with thicker freezing elements that we have developed. In addition, the effects of cold eventually can be increased by ischemic tissue reactions (injection of vasoconstricting drugs) and subsequent local hyperthermia (with long-wave high frequency). Cryocaustic is hemostatic and necrolytic; it reduces the time that a permanent catheter must be left in place. Necrolysis can be speeded by instillation of enzymes (e.g., pancreatic), softening agents, etc. Septic complications are reduced by continuous irrigation (povidone-iodine solution 1:200 = 0.5%) or instillation of 10 per cent PVP-iodine compounds (povidone-iodine, 1:20). This prevents growth of bacteria in the necrotic tissue. We tend to perform more and more routine suprapubic stabcystostomies with a 18 Fr balloon catheter (ca. 95 per cent of patients); this provides a "security valve." A thin plastic tube (as used, for example, in disposable infusion sets) can be introduced through the sheath of the trocar cystoscope and drawn out blindly through the urethra with a forceps (similar to an endless renal fistula; it eventually can be cleaned by the patient himself!). Also, with the help of a guide rail, a 14 Fr balloon catheter can be drawn through the fistula into the bladder. A more convenient system is a semicircular guide sheath around the trocar (Figs. 49,b; 145,d) for insertion of a regular Foley catheter. The suprapubic fistula is removed only when all necroses have been sloughed and voided (control by suprapubic cystoscopy in air) and when micturition leaves no residual urine. If necessary, a second (or third) session of cryosurgery (or TURP) can be added—usually with only a short hospitalization (2 to 4 days). Calcified (stones) or residual slough can be removed with trocar litholapaxy (see Fig. 126) or by extraction under suprapubic vision with local anesthesia through the urethra or the fistula with the lithotriptor.

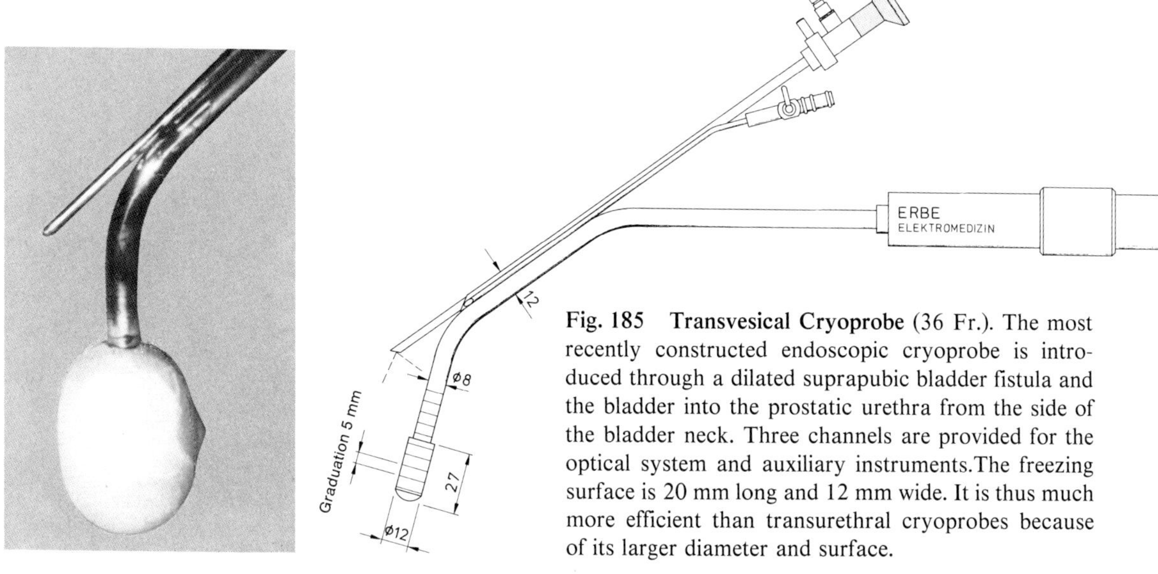

Fig. 185 Transvesical Cryoprobe (36 Fr.). The most recently constructed endoscopic cryoprobe is introduced through a dilated suprapubic bladder fistula and the bladder into the prostatic urethra from the side of the bladder neck. Three channels are provided for the optical system and auxiliary instruments.The freezing surface is 20 mm long and 12 mm wide. It is thus much more efficient than transurethral cryoprobes because of its larger diameter and surface.

Statistics

TUR

In the two decades since our hospital was established, 6121 TURs have been performed. Of these, 4536 were TUR of the prostate and 1446 were TUR of the bladder. Only 139 open prostatectomies were performed. Transurethral operations cause the least stress to the patient as well as the lowest risk. The nursing staff required and the expenses for material are significantly lower than for any other method.

Low Pressure TUR

Tables 1 through 10 document the influence of low pressure TUR on mortality rates, which were reduced from 1.2 to 0.3 per cent. The break-through came with the new technique of trocar TUR. Endoscopic cryosurgery affected the mortality rates of TUR insofar as adenomas in patients at high operative risk and about half the patients with prostatic carcinoma are now treated by cryosurgery, not by TUR. The best example of this effect is the reduction in number of patients aged over 80 years treated by TUR from 74 (Series 1) to 27 patients (Series 3, Table 1). The number of cases with adenomas weighing over 50 gm treated by TUR was reduced because many patients with giant adenomas are poor-risk patients and now are treated by cryosurgery. Postoperative hospitalization was reduced because there is a lower rate of complications after trocar TURP; more than half of the patients (Series 3) are at home after two weeks. Complications due to irrigant absorption (TUR syndrome) do not occur. Furthermore, there is no postoperative mortality due to pulmonary embolism in Series 3 (Series 1 and 2 together: 9 lethal emboli). Reduced cardiac stress is expressed by the numbers 2:4:1 of cardiac failure. The mortality after trocar TURP is reduced to almost one fourth (Tables 2 and 3).

There is a strikingly high rate of disturbance of sexual potency after TURP (58.7 per cent; Table 4, b). The causes, however, are still unknown. Reduced interest in active sex owing to the altered psychologic situation and increasing weakness of erection are of importance here. Most patients, however, are not amenable to a penile implant for correction of this problem.

In one patient an abnormally deep peritoneal recessus was opened by perforation of the posterior prostatic capsule. Laparotomy and suture were necessary.

Strictures were classified as pre- and postoperative. Among the latter, strictures of the bladder neck and prostatic urethra predominated (1.6 per cent). The anterior and middle urethra were less often affected (1.1 per cent; Table 7).

Cumulative Statistics

Table 8,a lists data obtained from the literature concerning the mortality rates of different prostatic operations. These data can be compared only with reservations, although it is evident that TUR produces significantly less postoperative mortality than do open operations.

How the data of individual authors differ is demonstrated in Table 8, b. We do not know why the cold punch technique has the highest mortality rate.

The rate of blood transfusions (Table 9) is — at least for transurethral prostatectomy — an indirect expression of intraoperative bleeding. Trocar TUR seldom requires a transfusion (1.6 per cent), in contrast to high pressure TUR, where almost half the patients require transfusion. In open surgical prostatectomy, most patients are transfused.

We can state conclusively that low pressure and trocar TUR has in our hands — for all concerned (patient, relatives, surgeon, trainees and personnel) — many advantages, making this method the most recommended and extending its indication also to large adenomas.

Prostatic Cancer

With trocar TUR, mortality of (sub)radical TUR was reduced from 3.3 per cent (280 patients) to 0.7 per cent (144 patients); such complications as perforation into the rectum (1.4 per cent) no longer occurred (see Table 21).

Table 1, a–c 3000 TURP with High and Low Pressure Irrigation
1000 patients each are included in:

Series 1:	6/1/1957 to 12/15/1964
Series 2:	12/16/1964 to 10/6/1970
Series 3:	10/7/1970 to 2/2/1977

Table 1, b Weight of the Adenoma (gm net; 18–48% loss of weight by diathermy)

Grams	Series 1 %	Series 3 %
up to 10	2.4	7.2
11–50	62.3	70.2
51–100	27.4	19.6
101–250	7.9	3.0
	100.0	100.0

Table 1, a Age Distribution

Age	Series 1 %	Series 3 %
up to 49	2.1	1.1
50–59	15.5	13.9
60–69	44.5	48.2
70–79	30.5	34.1
80–89	7.2	2.7
over 90	0.2	0.0
	100.0	100.0

Table 1, c Postoperative Hospital Care Required

Weeks	Series 1 %	Series 3 %
up to 2	27.6	55.1
up to 3	43.3	38.6
up to 4	21.4	4.9
over 4	7.7	1.4
	100.0	100.0

Table 2 Relation Between Mortality of TURP and Type of Irrigation (2 Series of 1000 Cases Each with High Pressure Irrigation; 1 Series of 1000 Cases with Continuous Low Pressure Irrigation)

Series	1000 Cases Each	Cm*	Deaths	Mortality %
1	High pressure TURP	80	11	1.15
2	High pressure TURP	80	12	
3	Low pressure TURP	30	3	0.3

*Mean height of water level in irrigating reservoir over the fossa.

Table 3 Causes of Death After High Pressure (Series 1 and 2; compare Table 2) and Low Pressure TURP (Series 3; compare Table 2)

	Series 1	Series 2	Series 3
Emboli	5	4	0
Uremia	3	2	1
Cardiac	2	4	1
Other failure	1	2	1*
Total deaths	11	12	3
Per cent	1.1	1.2	0.3

*Stroke.

Table 4, a and b Low Pressure TURP (1000 Cases of Series 3 (see Table 1): 440 Cases without Aspiration; 660 with Aspiration: Trocar-TURP)

Table 4, a Corresponding Data (Mean Values)

Age	67.3 years
Net weight of adenoma	39.2 gm
Weight of resected tissue per hr	56.1 gm
Secondary procedure (see Tab. 4, b)	1.4 %
Mean urinary flow	13.3 ml/sec*
Maximal flow	20.2 ml/sec*
Rate of survival (5 years)	78.7 %**
Mortality	0.3 %

*100 cases.
**225 cases.
Mean life expectancy (5 years) of the population: 81.9% at 65.2 years.

Table 4, b General Data (%)

Secondary coagulation (–4th week)	2.3
Blood transfusion (trocar TURP)	4.2*
Compression catheter – 50-cc balloon for sinus hemorrhage	0.6
Litholapaxy	8.4
TUR of mouth of the diverticulum	3.9
Coexisting bladder tumor	2.3
Transfer to other department (1 death)	0.9
Persistent stress incontinence after 8 months	3.5
Persistent urinary infection after 1 year	4.8
Residual urine more than 50 cc (0.7% after 6 months) after 1 year	0.3****
Postoperative stricture	3.0
Secondary TUR within 1st month	1.0
TURP for recurrency after 2–8 years	0.4***
Sexual potency impaired	58.7**
Laparotomy (intraperitoneal perforation of capsule)	0.1
Surgical drainage (extraperitoneal perforation)	0.0
Perforation of rectum or bladder	0.0
Incontinence (permanent)	0.0

*660 patients.
**256 patients; note: retrograde ejaculation ≈100%.
***Patients treated elsewhere are included, if known.
****2 patients underwent a secondary operation elsewhere (1 without success): 1 was not followed up.

Table 5 Net Weight of the Resected Adenoma and Net Weight of Tissue Resected per Hour in 1000 Patients Treated by Low Pressure TURP (see Table 1, Series 3)

Net Weight of Adenoma (gm)	%	Resected Net Weight (gm/hr)
below 10	3.4	20
10–29	37.4	40
30–59	40.5	48
60–99	14.9	72
100–250	3.8	81
Total	100.0	56.1

Table 6 Patients Requiring Transfusion Following:
(a) Low Pressure TURP with a Pressure of up to 30 cm water in the Prostatic Fossa without Trocar Aspiration
(b) Intermediate
(c) Trocar TURP with a Pressure of up to 10 cm water in the Prostatic Fossa with Trocar Aspiration

Method	Year	No. TURP Performed	Transfusions	%	Total Average (%)
(a)	1970	45	18	40.0	
	1971	171	66	38.6	35.8
	1972	128	39	30.5	
(b)	1973	155	42	27.1	27.1
(c)	1974	137	11	8.0	
	1975	176	9	5.1	
	1976	198	7	3.5	3.6
	1977	171	3	1.7	
	1978	160	2	1.3	

Table 7 Preoperative and Postoperative Strictures in 1000 TURPs*

Type of Stricture	No.	%
Preoperative	20	2.0
Postoperative (total)	30	3.0
Bladder neck	6	0.6
Posterior urethra	10	1.0
Middle and anterior urethra	11	1.1
Meatus	3	0.3

*See Table 1, Series 3.

Table 8, a and b Mortality Following Prostatic Operations (Review of Literature)

Table 8, a Mortality Rate by Method Used

Surgical Method	Cases	Deaths	%
Open surgical prostatectomy			
USA (1960–1972)	7799	260	3.3
German literature (1963–1978)	6329	268	4.2
TUR			
USA (1962–1970)	7763	94	1.2
Germany (1974–1978)	7457	113	1.5
Cryosurgery			
(1967–1973)	1181*	29	3.4

*Reuter (1974).

Table 8,b Postoperative Mortality of TUR as Reported by Individual Authors

Author	Mean Weight (gm)	Mean Age (yr)	Cases	Deaths	%
Frohmüller & Bülow (1978)	34.7*	70.9	1490	31	2.1
Thiel et al. (1977)	27.0**	66.8	100	2	2.0
Chilton et al. (1978)	†	–	1004	10	1.0
Mauermayer et al. (1980)	–	–	–	–	0.9††
Bandhauer (1978)	–	–	1011	7	0.7
Perrin, Barnes et al. (1976)	20.7**	–	270	2	0.7
Ignatoff & O'Conor (1977)	16**	–	632	2	0.3
Reuter (1977)	39.2**	67.3	1000	3	0.3

*Cold punch (total weight).
**TURP (net weight).
†70% below 20 gm.
††1–25 postoperative day only.

Table 9 Transfusion Requirements for Prostatic Surgery

Method	Cases	Transfusions	%
Suprapubic Prostatectomy (Eisenberger 1978)	767	572	74.6
TUR			
Cold punch TUR (Frohmüller & Bülow 1978)	1490*	702	47.1
High pressure TURP (Reuter 1970)	1000	449	44.9
Low pressure TUR (Thiel et al. 1977)	100	27	27.0
Trocar TUR (low pressure) (Reuter 1977/1978)	377*	6	1.6
Cryosurgery (Reuter 1978)	471*	49	10.4

*Includes carcinoma.

Table 10 Mortality Following Trocar TUR (Low Pressure) and Endoscopic Cryosurgery

Method	Cases	%	Deaths	Mortality (%)
TUR				
Adenoma	1252	74	5	0.36
Carcinoma	144			
Cryosurgery				
Adenoma	357	26	9	1.8
Carcinoma	143			
Total	1896	100	14	0.7

CRYOSURGERY

Since 1967, almost 1500 cryosurgical operations have been performed in 1203 patients. Most surgical interventions were performed in poor-risk patients with prostatic adenoma (644 patients) and in patients with prostatic cancer (283 patients). Bladder tumors were frozen in 167 patients. Further indications for cryosurgery were bladder neck strictures following prostatic operations, bladder diverticula in connection with cryoprostatectomy and dangerous bladder hemorrhage after radiation therapy (109 patients altogether; Table 11). Average mortality was 2.2 per cent.

Prostatic Adenoma

These were frozen blindly at first (113 patients; Table 12). The many failures of this procedure led us to search for new methods of control: (1) Endoscopy; (2) Rectal measurement of the frozen area (distance between the frozen area and the rectum or the external sphincter); (3) Temperature measurement with thermal needles marked by a knob 5 or 10 mm from the tip.

This so-called endoscopic cryosurgery was performed in 531 patients (Table 12), and 305 patients were followed for five years (Table 13, a). The average age of these patients was markedly higher (about 6 years) than in the TURP cases. Secondary procedures were necessary in 15.9 per cent; one tenth of these, however, represent a second session of a cryoprostatectomy. Here it should be noted that large adenomas (over 4 cm long) cannot be removed entirely in one session — even when large lateral or median lobes are also frozen with the trocar probe (6.9 per cent). Often, however, a scheduled second cryosurgical operation proves unnecessary because the functional result from the first procedure is good. Urinary flow is a good parameter; it is tested after filling the bladder with at least 200 cc through the suprapubic fistula. The rate of failure is low (3.6 per cent) in sequential treatment (1–3 sessions).

The "Special" cryoprobe (Table 13, b) is most often used (77.7 per cent) because of its greater efficiency. The "Standard" cryoprobe is too thin at 24 Fr and should be used only when modified to 28 Fr — and then only in adenomas over 5 cm long. The trocar cryoprobe is used mainly in combination with one of the other two probes. It increases the efficiency of freezing at the sides (centrally freezing of nodes; see above).

Apart from insignificant suppuration of suprapubic fistulas, we have seen only one instance of abscess formation by extravasation of urine due to abdominal straining with a plugged catheter (0.1 per cent). More often, gas is lost during the operation through the suprapubic stab wound in the bladder. It sometimes is recognized as crepitation under the skin. At first the gas lies extraperitoneally, where it cannot be palpated. This never caused complications. Postoperative hemorrhage almost always stopped spontaneously, because it is mucosal bleeding. Only when the cryoprobe is moved or turned forcefully does the frozen area break the mucosa, causing postoperative hemorrhage. As a rule, bladder stones are treated with trocar litholapaxy, which is superior to other methods, because trocar cystoscopy prevents all trauma of the bladder by the lithotriptor and the view in the gas-filled bladder is not obscured (see Fig. 126). Freezing of the mouth of a diverticulum is (unlike TUR) not dangerous: the contractile mouth becomes an indurated ring (see Fig. 181).

Incontinence after cryoprostatectomy is rare, because columns of the lateral lobes still remain when the rectal distance from the frozen area to the verumontanum is measured correctly. Perforation into the rectum also is prevented. Of these patients, 38.9 per cent died within five years — 8 per cent per year — mainly of cardiovascular disease and cancer (Tables 13, k and l).

Prostatic Cancer

Two hundred eighty-three patients with prostatic cancer were treated by cryosurgery — 124 of these by blind procedures (Table 14). One hundred sixteen patients were followed for five years (Table 15). Only about half of the deaths were due to the prostatic cancer. The "Special" cryoprobe was the preferred instrument in 84.5 per cent; in 15.5 per cent, the trocar cryoprobe was also applied for freezing peripheral infiltrations transperineally in 4.3 per cent).

Bladder Tumors

The mortality rates five years after TUR and cryosurgery are compared in Tables 16 through 19. Of 45 patients with TUR of benign papillomas (stage T_1), one died (not from tumor), whereas three papillomas became malignant. After cryosurgery of 32 papillomas, two patients died of the cancer and eight from other causes. The rate of recurrence after cryosurgery was significantly lower in the presented material than after TUR. Tumors recurred after TUR in 29 to 32 per cent per year. After cryosurgery, the rate of recurrence was 53 per cent in the first year; in the following four years, however, only between 4 and 21 per cent. Eleven patients died from the carcinoma (stage T_1 to T_4) within five years after TUR; 16 after cryosurgery. Comparison of these data is possible only when it is taken into consideration that TUR is preferred in younger patients (with lower risk) and in smaller tumors. Larger tumors (with a diameter of 2 to 10 cm) and cases with increased risk are treated by cryosurgery. With both methods, TUR and cryosurgery, we obtained comparable results. However, cryosurgery carries less risk of hemorrhage and perforation and is a simple technique. The rate of recurrence is significantly lower after cryotherapy than after TUR in the presented material. Postoperative mortality of both methods was zero.

Table 11 Experience With Cryosurgery (11/28/67–12/31/78)

Diagnosis	Cases	Total	Deaths	%
Prostatic adenoma	644		15	
Prostatic carcinoma	283	927	11	2.8
Bladder cancer (T_1)	75			
Bladder cancer ($T_{2\text{-}4}$)	92	167	0	0
Bladder neck stricture	60			
Bladder diverticulum	43			
Irradiation bladder	5	109	0	0
Vesical ulcer	1			
Total		1203	26	2.2

Table 12 Experience With Cryosurgery for Prostatic Adenoma (1/5/68–12/31/78)

Method	No. Cases
Blind cryosurgery	113
Endoscopic cryosurgery	531

Table 13 (a-m) Five-Year Follow-Up Data: Endoscopic Cryosurgery for Prostatic Adenoma (305 Patients; 12/17/69–12/7/73)

Table 13, a Clinical Data (Averages)

Patient age	73.2 years
Length of adenoma	4.4 cm
Freezing time	1–3 min twice
Second operation required*	15.9%
Permanent catheter in place**	4 weeks
Postoperative urinary flow, mean	12.6 cc/sec†
Maximum urinary flow	20.3 cc/sec†
Unsuccessful after 5 years (permanent catheter; uremia; high residual urine)	3.6%
Survival rate (5-year)	61.1%
Statistical survival rate of the population at mean age of 73	63.9%
Postoperative mortality (7 of 305)	2.3%

*Operation for recurrence, 5.2%; see Table 13, b.
**For bladder fistula, 6–8 weeks.
†100 patients.

Table 13, b Clinical Data (Percentages)

	%
Cryoprobe used: "Special" (28 Fr; 24-mm freezing element)	77.7
"Standard" (24 Fr; 45-mm freezing element)	15.4
Trocar (24 Fr; 28-mm freezing element)	6.9
Bladder fistula* (7% before operation; 0.1% complication: abscess)	12.8
Bladder fistula (1977–1978 in 200 cases)	52.5
Postoperative coagulation/TUR	0.3
Blood transfusion*	9.1
Bladder tumor	3.9
Litholapaxy (trocar)	11.2
Diverticulum (cryosurgery)	4.3
Transfer to other hospitals (for complications; no deaths)	0.3
Stress incontinence	0.9
Permanent incontinence	0.6
Postoperative urethral stricture (2.9% preoperative)	0.6
Urinary infection after 5 years	10.3
Urinary infection after 1 year	11.9
Residual urine after 5 years (bladder atony: 3 of 179)	1.1
Prostatic cancer (T_1)	1.6
Secondary TUR (after 1 year)	1.5**
Secondary cryosurgery (after 2 years)	8.6**
Operation for recurrence	5.2
Open surgical drainage of perivesical infiltration	0.3
Laparotomy; surgical prostatectomy, perforation of rectum or bladder	0.0

*352 cases.
**257 cases.

Table 13, c Age Distribution

Age	No. Patients	%
up to 49	2	0.6
50–59	14	4.6
60–69	78	25.6
70–79	146	47.9
80–89	62	20.3
over 90	3	1.0
Total	305	100.0

Table 13, d Operative Risk

Risk-Degree	No. Patients	%
0	8	2.6
I	45	14.7
II	121	39.7
III	124	40.7
IV	7	2.3
Total	305	100.0

Table 13, e Cryoprobe Used

Cryoprobe	Fr	Length of Freezing Element (cm)	No. Patients	%
"Special"	28	2.5	237	77.7
"Standard"	24	4.5	47	15.4
Trocar	24	1.8	21	6.9
Total			305	100.0

Table 13, f Complications (93 in 305 Patients)

	No. Patients	%
Surgical drainage	1	0.3
Postoperative hemorrhage	9	2.9
Temperature >38°C	72	23.6
Chills	11	3.6
Hemorrhage requiring coagulation and/or resection	0	0.0

Table 13, g Permanent Catheter (Postoperative, 206 Patients; No Data for 99 Cases)

Weeks	Patients	%
1–2	6	2.9
3–4	97	47.1
5–6	61	29.6
7–8	29	14.1
9–10	7	3.4
11–16	6	2.9
Total	206	100.0

Table 13, h Secondary Cryosurgery or TURP after Primary Cryosurgery (257 Patients; for 48, No Data)

	Patients			
Year	Cryosurgery	TUR	Total	%
1	22	4	26	10.1
2	8	1	9	3.5
3	1	3	4	1.5
4	1	–	1	0.4
5	1	–	1	0.4
Total	33	8	41	15.9

Table 13, i Urinary Infection 0.25 to 5 Years Postoperative (194 Patients; for 111, No Data)

Years	Infection	%	No Infection	%
After 1/4	71	36.6	123	63.4
After 1–3	13	6.7	181	93.3
After 4–5	20	10.3	174	88.7
Total	104	53.6		

Table 13, j Residual Urine 1 to 5 Years Postoperative (179 Patients; for 126, No Data)

Year	No. Patients	%
After 1st	8	4.5
After 2nd	1	0.6
After 5th	4*	2.2
Total	13	7.3

*1 cleared after TURP.

Table 13, k Mortality 1 to 5 Years After Cryosurgery (257 Patients; for 41, No Data)

Year	Cause: Adenoma	Cause: Other	Total	%
1st	3	19	22	8.6
2nd	2	23	25	9.7
3rd	—	18	18	7.0
4th	—	12	12	4.7
5th	1	22	23	8.9
Total	6	94	100	38.9

Table 13, l Causes of Death (100 of 257 Patients)

Cause	No. Patients
Adenoma (uremia)	6
Cardiac	36
Stroke	11
Lung (pneumonia, 3; embolism, 1)	4
Cancer	11
Miscellaneous (accident, asthma, liver, ileus, diabetes)	14
Old age	18
Total	100

Table 13, m Postoperative Deaths

Cause	No. Patients
Acute cardiac failure	3
Uremia	1
Pneumonia	2
Pulmonary embolism	1
Total	7

Table 14 Cryosurgery of Prostatic Carcinoma in 283 Patients (11/28/67–12/31/78)

Blind cryosurgery	124 patients
Endoscopic cryosurgery	159 patients

Table 15, a-i Five-Year Follow-Up after Endoscopic Cryosurgery of Prostatic Carcinoma (116 Patients, 12/22/69–8/9/73)

Table 15, a Significant Clinical Data (Average)

Age	72.1 yr
Length of adenoma	4.2 cm
Freezing time:	2–3 times for 2–3 min
Secondary operation	39.7 %
Permanent catheter for	ca 4 weeks
Five-year survival rate:	39.4 %
Corresponding population	66.3 %
Mortality from the carcinoma	31.7 %
Mortality from other causes	28.9 %
Total mortality	60.6 %
Postoperative mortality	2.5 %

Table 15, b General Clinical Data

	Patients	%
TURP 1–10 years before cryosurgery	12	10.3
Cancerous bladder neck stricture (preoperative)	13	11.2
Bladder fistula before cryosurgery	8	6.8
Cryoprobe: "Special" (28 Fr; 24-mm freezing element)	98	84.5
"Standard" (24 Fr; 45-mm freezing element)	13	11.2
Trocar (in combination with "Special" or "Standard")	18	15.5
(a) Introduced transurethrally	13	11.2
(b) Introduced transperineally	5	4.3
Postoperative hemorrhage (no operative coagulation)	3	2.6
Fever over 38° C (chills: 9 patients = 7.7%)	29	25.0
Bladder fistula (1977/78: 27 patients = 51.5%)	9	7.7
Renal fistula	1	0.9
Orchiectomy	10	9.3
Stricture (bladder neck, 2 patients; middle urethra, 1 patient)	3	2.6
Bladder stone	6	5.1
Bladder cancer	1	0.9
Urinary infection after 5 years (from 71 patients)	7	9.9
Incontinence (total)	2	1.9
Cobalt irradiation	13	12.1
Cytostatics (estramustine phosphate)	3	2.8
Transfer to another department (1 stroke; 1 encephalomalacia)	2	1.7
Secondary TUR after cryosurgery	1	0.9
Secondary cryosurgery in 1st to 5th year	38	35.5
Tertiary cryosurgery in 1st to 5th year	7	6.5
Laparotomy, surgical revision, perforation	0	0.0

Table 15, c Age Distribution

Age	No. Patients	%
up to 49	1	0.9
50–59	6	5.2
60–69	29	25.0
70–79	59	50.8
80–89	21	18.1
Total	116	100.0

Table 15, d Distribution by Risk-Degree and Stage

Risk-Degree	No. Patients	%	Stage	No. Patients	%
0	3	2.6	T_0	–	–
I	25	21.5	T_1	27	23.3
II	41	35.3	T_2	46	39.7
III	43	37.1	T_3	36	31.0
IV	4	3.5	T_4	7	6.0
Total	116	100.0	Total	116	100.0

Table 15, e Length of Prostate

Cm	No. Patients	%
Up to 2	3	2.6
2–3	57	49.1
3–4	20	17.2
4–5	27	23.3
Over 5	9	7.8
Total	116	100.0

Table 15, f Permanent Catheter (76 Patients)

Weeks	No. Patients	%
1–4	48	63.2
5–6	19	25.0
7–8	7	9.2
9–10	2	2.6
Total	76	100.0

Table 15, g Secondary Cryosurgery (38 of 116 Patients)

Year	No. Patients	%
1st	25	23.4
2nd	8	7.5
3rd	3	2.8
4th	1	0.9
5th	1	0.9
Total	38	35.5

Table 15, h Deaths in the 1st to 5th Year (63 of 104 Patients)

Year	No. Patients	%
1st	20	19.5
2nd	16	15.4
3rd	5	4.8
4th	13	12.5
5th	9	8.7
Total	63	60.9

Table 15, i Causes of Death

Time	Causes			No. Patients	%
Postoperative*	Cardiac; embolism; pneumonia			3	2.5
1st to 5th year**	Carcinoma			33	31.7
	Other causes: Total			30	28.9
	Cardiac disease	16	15.4		
	Age	5	4.8		
	Lung (2 embolisms; 1 fibrosis)	3	2.9		
	Stroke	3	2.9		
	Ileus; thrombosis; encephalomalacia	3	2.9		
Total				66	63.1

*Group of 116 cases; 9 not verified = 7.8 %.
**Group of 104 patients.

Table 16 Five-Year Follow-Up after TUR or Cryosurgery of Bladder Tumors (Postoperative Mortality = 0%)

Stage	TUR	Cryosurgery	Total	%
$T_A G_0$	45	32	77	53.5
T_1–T_4	33	34	67	46.5
Total	78	66	144	100.0

Table 17 Five-Year Follow-Up after TUR or Cryosurgery of Bladder Tumors: Operations and Deaths after 1–5 Years

Stage	Operation	No. Patients	Causes of Death CARCINOMA	Causes of Death OTHERS	No. Deaths	%
$T_A G_0$	TUR	45	–	1	1	2.2
	Cryosurgery	32	2	8	10	31.2
T_1–T_4	TUR	33	11	9	20	60.6
	Cryosurgery	34	16	7	23	67.6
Total	TUR (78) Cryosurgery (66)	144	29	25	54	37.5

Table 18 Age Distribution (78 Patients Had TUR; 66 Had Cryosurgery)

Age	TUR (%)	Cryosurgery (%)
Below 40	9.6	4.2
40–49	6.7	6.2
50–59	16.3	18.8
60–69	32.8	27.1
70–79	31.7	31.2
80–89	2.9	12.5
Total	100.0	100.0

Table 19 Risk (78 Patients Had TUR; 66 Had Cryosurgery)

Risk-Degree	TUR (%)	Cryosurgery (%)
0	26.9	16.7
I	47.1	37.5
II	22.2	31.2
III	3.8	14.6
IV	0.0	0.0
Total	100.0	100.0

Table 20 Temperature in the Frozen Area (In Water at 20° C)

Freezing Time	Distance of Thermoneedle from Cryoprobe (Thickness of Freezing)		
−196° C	0.5 CM	1 CM	1.5 CM
0 min	+ 20° C	+ 20° C	+ 20° C
1 min	− 20° C	− 5° C	+ 6° C
1.5 min	− 60° C	− 10° C	+ 5° C
2 min	− 68° C	− 14° C	+ 4° C
2.5 min	− 74° C	− 18° C	+ 2° C
3 min	− 76° C	− 20° C	± 0° C
3.5 min	− 78° C	− 22° C	− 1° C
4 min	− 80° C	− 24° C	− 2° C

TREATMENT OF PROSTATIC CANCER: COMPARISON OF CRYOSURGERY AND RADICAL TUR (Table 21)

A first series of patients was treated with TUR (high pressure irrigation). The complications caused by water intoxication were responsible for the relatively high postoperative mortality (3.1 per cent of 261 cases). The five-year survival was 43.2 per cent; however, only 34.4 per cent died from the carcinoma.

More recently, a second series of patients was treated with TUR and continuous low pressure irrigation by suprapubic trocar. Postoperative mortality here was zero. The survival is best in this group, where 60 per cent of the 62 patients were still alive after five years. Deaths due to the carcinoma occurred in 25.5 per cent; by other diseases, in 14.5 per cent. This group was also more intensively treated by such further measures as orchiectomy, cobalt irradiation and immunobiologic agents (extracts of viscera and viscum album).

A third group was treated by cryosurgery. Here, the average age and risk-degree were definitely higher due to selection: cryosurgery is preferred for patients with a higher risk-degree and more advanced stages of cancer. Postoperative mortality was 2.5 per cent. Of the 125 cases, 57.5 per cent were dead after five years; however, only 27.4 per cent died from the carcinoma. Repeated sessions of cryosurgery are recommended for poor-risk patients or as palliative measures — exceptionally for an early carcinoma stage $T_{1\text{-}2}$.

Radical TUR with trocar is preferred for stages $T_{1\text{-}3}$. The rate of complications is low, and the prognosis is definitely better. Additional therapy is necessary to improve the results.

Table 21 Prostatic Carcinoma: Comparison of Treatment by Cryosurgery and High Pressure or Low Pressure TUR

(A) Endoscopic cryosurgery: 125 cases (12/22/69 to 7/18/74)
(B) High pressure TUR: 261 cases (8/10/57 to 10/ 2/70)
(C) Low pressure TUR: 62 cases (12/16/70 to 8/12/74)

Group (in % Unless Otherwise Stated)	A	B	C
Average age (years)	72.1	70.6	66.9
Average weight of prostate (gm)	(45.5 est)	46.9	41.3
Postoperative hospitalization (days)	10.5	16.2	17.6
Five-year survival rate	42.5	43.2	60.0
Mortality: postoperative	2.5	3.1	0
within 5 years (from the cancer)	27.4	34.4	25.5
within 5 years (from other diseases)	30.1	22.4	14.5
Total	57.5	56.8	40.0
Previous TUR for benign adenoma	10.3	5.8	1.6
Preoperative bladder neck stricture	11.2	3.4	4.8
Simultaneous bladder stone	4.8	8.8	4.8
Simultaneous bladder tumor	0.8	2.3	0
Postoperative treatment			
Hemorrhage (treated)	2.4	3.1	3.2
Fever over 38° C	25.6	1.5	35.5
Stricture of urethra	0.9	1.2	0
Stricture of bladder neck with recurrent cancer	1.9	10.4	14.6
Incontinence	1.6	8.7	9.1
Incontinence 1 year postoperative	1.1	3.2	5.5
Secondary procedures:			
TUR within 1 year	0	3.6	1.8
TUR within 2–5 years	0.8	2.0	1.8
Cryosurgery within 1 year	23.3	0.8	3.6
Cryosurgery within 2–5 years	15.5	4.0	14.5
Total	39.7	10.4	21.7
Orchiectomy	9.3	10.4	23.6
Cobalt irradiation	12.1	10.8	20.0
Renal fistula	0.9	0.8	0
Preternatural anus	0	0.8	0
Surgical intervention for perforation	0	3.1	0
Cerebral vascular accident; encephalomalacia	1.7	0	0

References

Ablin, R. J.: Immunological aspects of the development and advances of cryosurgery of the prostate. In: Cryosurgery in Urology, hrsg. von H. J. Reuter. Thieme, Stuttgart 1974

Ablin, R. J., W. A. Soanes, M. J. Gonder: Elution of in vivo bound antiprostatic epithelial antibodies following multiple cryotherapy of the prostate. Urology 2 (1973) 276

Alvarez, J.: Persönl. Mitteilung

Ammon, J., J. H. Kartens, P. Rathert: Urologische Onkologie. Springer, Berlin 1978

Bandhauer, K.: Die transurethrale Prostatektomie. Med. Welt 29 (1978) 1199

Barnes, R. W.: Endoscopic Prostatic Surgery. Mosby, St. Louis 1943

Baumrucker, G. O.: TUR, 2. Aufl. Krieger, New York 1976

Bjerle, P.: Relationship between perivesical and intravesical urinary bladder pressures and intragastric pressures. Acta physiol. scand. 92 (1974) 465–473

Bjerle, P.: Transmural pressure of the urinary bladder wall. Acta physiol. scand. 92 (1974) 465–473, 474–475, 480–487

Bjerle, P., B. Sandström: Intra- und extraperitoneal pressures. Acta physiol. scand. 92 (1974) 447–475

Bouffioux, C.: Le cancer de la prostate. Acta urol. belg. 47 (1979) 414–421

Chilton, C. P., R. J. Morgan, H. R. England, A. M. I. Paris, J. P. Blandy: A critical evaluation of the results of transurethral resection of the prostate. Brit. J. Urol. 50 (1978) 542

Cifuentes Delatte, L.: Cirurgia urologica endoscopia. Editorial Paz Montalvo, Madrid 1961

Conger, K.: Transurethral Prostatic Surgery. Wiliams & Wilkins, Baltimore 1963

Dubois, P.: Über den Druck in der Harnblase. Dtsch. Arch. klin. Med. 17 (1876) 158–163

Eisenberger, F.: Offene Operationsverfahren beim Prostataadenom. Med. Welt 29 (1978) 1203

Emmet, J. L., S. N. Rous, L. F. Green u. Mitarb.: Preliminary internal urethrotomy in 1036 cases to prevent urethral stricture following TUR. J. Urol. (Baltimore) 89 (1963) 829–835

Fiedler, G. A. zit. bei Reuter 1974

Flocks, R. H.: Foreword. In: Cryosurgery in Urology, hsrg. von H. J. Reuter. Thieme, Stuttgart 1974

Flocks, R. H., D. A. Culp: Surgical Urology, 3. Aufl. Year Book Medical Publishers, Chicago. Deutsche Ausgabe hrsg. von K. M. Bauer. Schattauer, Stuttgart 1969

Flocks, R. H., C. M. Nelson, D. L. Boatman: Perineale Kryochirurgie des Prostata-Carcinoms. J. Urol. (Baltimore) 108 (1972) 933

Frohmüller, H., H. Bülow: Die transurethrale Stanzresektion der Prostata (cold punch). Med. Klin. 73 (1978) 715

Fürst, F., G. Conradi, E. Koranyi: Die Bedeutung der präoperativen akuten Pyelonephritis für die Entwicklung der postoperativen Komplikationen bei transvesicaler Adenomektomie. Z. Urol. 69 (1976) 635–638

Garrier, M.: Cryochirurgie en Cancerologie. Service du Prof. Agrégé J. Cuillerte, Lyon 1977

von Gerven, H.: Die technische Ausrüstung zur Kryokaustik. Techn. Med. 7 (1977) 102–104

Gil Vernet, S.: Morphology and Function of Vesico-Prostatourethral Musculature. Edizioni Canova, Treviso 1968

Gil Vernet, S.: Obstrucciones Prostato-Uretrales. Arch. esp. Urol. 24 (1971) 48

Goldberg, V.: Semennije pusirki (Die Samenblasen). Sowetskaja Enziklopedia, Moscow 101 (1968) 882

Goldberg, V.: Wesikulografia. Sowetskaja Enziklopedia, Moscow 101 (1958) 882

Grayhack, J., J. Wilson, M. Scherbenske: Benign Prostatic Hyperplasia. Bethesda, Maryland. U.S. Government Printing Office, Washington 1975.

Gursel, E., M. Roberts, R. J. Veenema: Regressive Veränderungen des Prostata-Carcinoms nach wiederholter kryochirurgischer Behandlung der Vorsteherdrüse. J. Urol. (Baltimore) 108 (1972) 928

Hansen, R. I.: Prostatakryoresektion. Villadsen & Kristensen, Copenhagen 1973

Harzmann, R., K. H. Bichler u. Mitarb.: Lokale Hochfrequenz-Hyperthermie des Brown-Pearce-Karzinoms des Kaninchens. Urologe A 17 (1978) 130–134

Haschek, H.: Latest developments in cryosurgery. International Congress of Cryosurgery. Verlag der Wiener Medizinischen Akademie, Wien 1972

Haschek, H., H. J. Reuter: Vergleich der Spätergebnisse nach suprapubischer Prostatektomie und transurethraler Elektroresektion (je 1 000 Fälle). Urol. Int. 23 (1968) 454–469

Heise, G.-W., E. Hienzsch, M. Mebel, W. Krebs: Allgemeine und spezielle Urologie, Vol. I. VEB Thieme, Leipzig 1977

Heredia, C. P.: La T.U.R. de la prostata con pressiòn intravesical baja. Rev. Soc. Peruana Urol. 9 (1979) 24

Hösel, M.: Ein neues Resektoskop. Chirurg 26 (1955) 191–192

Hösel, M.: Die endourethrale Prostatektomie und Behandlung des Prostatakarzinoms. Schattauer, Stuttgart 1964

Iglesias, J. J., J. Kamat, J. Seebode: A new resectoscope with continuous irrigation in front of the lens. Scientific exhibit, presented at Annual Meeting of the American Urological Association, Washington D.C. 1972

Iglesias, J. J., E. Perez-Castro, S. Madduri, A. Sporer, J. Seebode: Hydraulic hemostasis in transurethral resection of the prostate using the Iglesias continuous suction resectoscope. Z. Urol. 70 (1977) 3, 306

Iglesias, J. J., U. K. Stams: Das neue Iglesias-Resektoskop. Urologe A 14 (1975) 229–231

Ignatoff, J. M., J. O'Conor Jr.: Complications of transurethral resection of the prostate. Int. Urol. Nephrol. 9 (1977) 33

Jacobellis, U., H. J. Reuter: Irrigazione fisiologica a bassa pressione e drenaggio sovrapubico nella resezione transuretrale. Atti del 47. Congresso Società Italiana di Urologia, Vol. II. (1974) 93–100

Jacobellis, U., A. Tallarigo: Considerazioni su 176 tumori vegetanti della vescica trattati con resezione endoscopica. Atti del 50. Congresso Società Italiana di Urologia, Vol. II. (1977) 181–190

Keller, A., D. Völter: Cryo-Cautery of the prostate. Scan. J. Urol. Nephrol., Suppl. Nr. 48 (1978)

Kiesswetter, H.: Prostatektomie: Methoden, Ergebnisse, Komplikationen. Wien. Med. 120 (1970) 771 ff.

Kölln, C. P., R. H. Flocks: Anatomical factors influencing the technique of transurethral resection for benign prostatic hypertrophy. Endoscopy 3 (1971) 20

Krebs, W.: Fehler und Gefahren bei transurethralen Eingriffen. VEB Thieme, Leipzig 1970

van Leden, H., W. Cahan: Cyrogenics in Surgery. Medical Examination Publishing Co., New York 1971

Leibundgut, B.: Cryosurgery of the prostate. Akt. gerontol. 6 (1976) 167–169

Leroi, R.: Malignomtherapie mit neuen Iscador-Präparaten. Krebsgeschehen, H. 5 (1975)

Lutzeyer, W., S. Lymberopoulos: Kältechirurgie im urologischen Bereich (Forschungsbericht, DFG). Boldt, Boppard 1977

McDonald Jr., J. P.: zit. bei Reuter 1974

Madsen, P. O., K. G. Naber: The importance of the pressure in the prostatic fossa and absorption of irrigating fluid during transurethral resection of the prostate. J. Urol. (Baltimore) 109 (1973) 446–452

Madsen, R. E.: Über die Irrigationsflüssigkeiten bei der transurethralen Prostataresektion. Z. Urol. 58 (1965) 10 f.

Maier-Leibnitz, H.: Zit. n. Lutzeyer

Morera, J.: Reseccion Transurethral. Lopez, Buenos Aires 1977

Naber, K., H. Kuni, H. Sommerkamp, K. H. Bichler: Der quantitative Verlauf der Einschwemmung von Spülflüssigkeit bei der Transurethralen Prostatektomie (TUR) und seine klinische Bedeutung. Urologe A 10 (1971) 261–265

Naber, K., K. Möhring, P. O. Madsen: Zum Problem der Spülflüssigkeitseinschwemmung bei der transurethralen Prostataresektion. Urologe A 12 (1973) 206–209

Nesbit, R. M.: Transurethral Prostatectomy. Thomas, Springfield, Ill. 1943

Perrin, P., R. Barnes, H. Hadley, R. T. Bergmann: Forty years of transurethral prostatic resections. J. Urol. (Baltimore) 116 (1976) 757

Politano, V. J.: Klinische Demonstration, Miami 1973

Politano, V. A., M. P. Small, J. M. Harper, C. M. Lynn: Periurethral teflon injection for urinary incontinence. J. Urol. (Baltimore) 111 (1974) 180–183

Puigvert, A.: Endoscopia urinaria. Editorial ECO, Barcelona 1976

Rand, R., A. Rinfret, H. v. Leden: Cryosurgery. Thomas, Springfield, IL 1968

Rautenberg, W.: Zur Leistungsbreite der transurethralen Elektroresektion beim Prostataadenom. Urologe 2 (1963) 117

Reuter, H. J.: Fermentative Lokalbehandlung der Cystitis necroticans. Visum 1 (1961) 127

Reuter, H. J.: Chirurgische und transurethrale Behandlung von Blasentumoren. Z. Urol. 55 (1962) 523

Reuter, H. J.: Urologische Photo-Film-Fernsehendoskopie. Urologe 2 (1963) 187

Reuter, H. J.: Transurethrale Prostatektomie von Riesenadenomen. Z. Urol. 57 (1964) 363

Reuter, H. J.: Transurethrale Prostatektomie bei Prostatasteinen. Urologia int. (Basel) 20 (1965a) 336

Reuter, H. J.: Urological endophotography and endocinematography. J. Urol. 93 (1965b) 512

Reuter, H. J.: Rektalschild für transurethrale und chirurgische Blasen- und Prostataoperationen. Z. Urol. 58 (1965c) 125

Reuter, H. J.: Die transurethrale Elektroresektion des Ureterostiums. Z. Urol. 59 (1966a) 663–677

Reuter, H. J.: Die Mortalität der Prostataoperationen in ihrer Abhängigkeit von Lebensalter, Operations- und Narkoseverfahren. 7th International Congress of Gerontology, Kongreßband Wien 1966b

Reuter, H. J.: Neue Erfahrungen mit Zytostatica, insbesondere ihrer intraarteriellen Anwendung bei Blasentumoren. Z. Urol. 59 (1966c) 125

Reuter, H. J.: Die transurethrale Elektroresektion des Ureterostiums. Z. Urol. 59 (1966d) 663

Reuter, H. J.: Operative Angiographie als Grundlage urologischer zytostatischer Therapie. Kongreßband der Angiographietagung 1965. Thieme, Stuttgart (1966e) #104

Reuter, H. J.: Neue Gesichtspunkte in der Anwendung der verschiedenen Verfahren der Prostatektomie. Chirurg 38 (1967a) 299

Reuter, H. J.: Ist die blinde Lithotripsie noch zeitgemäß? Z. Urol. 60 (1967b) 247

Reuter, H. J.: Die Kältechirurgie der Prostata. Verh. dtsch. Ges. Urol. 22 (1968a) 350–355

Reuter, H. J.: Elektronisches Überwachungsgerät Hydropur für Katheter und Sonden. Med. Markt. Acta mediotechn. 16 (1968b) 7, 296

Reuter, H. J.: Elektrische Lithotripsie mit Urat.-1. Med. Markt. Acta mediotechn. 16 (1968c) 10, 414

Reuter, H. J.: Endophotographie, Kinematographie und Television der Harnblase auf extraurethralem Weg. Med. Markt 5 (1969a)

Reuter, H. J.: Das Trokarzystoskop – ein neues Endoskop zur diagnostischen und operativen Zystoskopie auf suprapubischem Weg. Endoscopy 1 (1969b) 35–37

Reuter, H. J.: Electric lithotripsy, a new method for transurethral treatment of bladder stones. Endoscopy 1 (1969c) 2, 63

Reuter, H. J.: Erfolg und Mißerfolg der Prostatektomie in Abhängigkeit vom Lebensalter, Operations- und Narkoseverfahren. Mat. med. Nordm. 21 (1969d) 153–172

Reuter, H. J.: Die endoskopische Kältechirurgie von Prostata- und Blasentumoren (Erfahrungen an 300 Fällen). Z. Urol. 63 (1970a) 7, 531

Reuter, H. J.: Urologische Kältechirurgie. Voytjech, Wien 1970b

Reuter, H. J.: Electronic instrument for supervising catheters and probes. J. Urol. 104 (1970c) 916–917

Reuter, H. J.: Cryosurgery in urology. In: Cyrogenic Surgery, hrsg. von H. v. Leeden u. a. Medical Examination Publishing Co., Flushing/N. Y. 1971a

Reuter, H. J.: Endoscopic Cryosurgery. Voytjech, Wien 1971b

Reuter, H. J.: abc für Prostatakranke, 3. Aufl. Thieme, Stuttgart 1971c

Reuter, H. J.: Die permanente TUR unter physiologischem Blasendruck (Niederdruckirrigation und kontinuierliche Wasserableitung). Urologe A 3 (1974a) 114

Reuter, H. J.: Cryosurgery in Urology. Thieme, Stuttgart 1974b

Reuter, H. J.: Urologische Operationslehre. Transurethrale Operationen. In: Allgemeine und spezielle Urologie. Vol. VI, ed by G.-W. Heise, E. Hienzsch, M. Mebel, W. Krebs. VEB Thieme, Leipzig 1977a

Reuter, H. J.: Die Kältechirurgie von Blasentumoren. Verh. dtsch. Ges. Urol. 29 (1977b) 113–117

Reuter, H. J.: Die Bedeutung des regionalen Lymphsystems und seine szintigraphische Diagnostik bei Tumorerkrankungen des kleinen Beckens. Krebsgeschehen 1978, 104–105

Reuter, H. J.: Ärztlicher Rat für Prostatakranke, 4. Aufl. Thieme, Stuttgart 1979

Reuter, H. J., J. Enderle: Die theoretischen und technischen Grundlagen der urologischen Kältechirurgie. Techn. Med. 2 (1971) 52

Reuter, H. J., L. W. Jones: Physiologic low pressure irrigation for transurethral resection: suprapubic trocar drainage. J. Urol. (Baltimore) 111 (1974) 210

Reuter, H. J., W. Krebs: Transurethrale Operationen. In: Urologische Operationslehre, Vol. VI, hrsg. von G. W. Heise, E. Hienzsch. VEB Thieme, Leipzig 1977.

Reuter, H. J., M. A. Reuter: 20 Jahre Prostataoperationen. Z. Urol. u. Nephrol. 73 (1980) 279–290. VEB Thieme, Leipzig

Reuter, H.-J., W. Schuck: Die Nadelbiopsie der Prostata zur zytologischen Karzinomdiagnostik. Erfahrungen an 1 500 Fällen. Z. Urol. H. 11 (1971)

Reuter, M. A., E. Loenicker, H. J. Reuter: Szintigraphische Darstellung der regionalen Lymphknoten der Prostata und Blase mit der Gammakamera. Z. Urol. u. Nephrol. 73 (1979) 185–187

Reuter, M. A., H. J. Reuter: Prevention of irrigant absorption during TURP: continuous low pressure irrigation. Int. Urol. Nephrol. 10 (1978) 293–300

Rilling, S.: Nicht toxische Additivtherapie und diagnostische Verfahren beim Karzinom. Fischer, Frankfurt/M. 1979

Schubert, H.: Technische Entwicklung und Stand der Endophotographie. Medizinalmarkt 7 (1957) 269

Schubert, H.: Die Photo-Endoskopie im Zeichen des Elektronenblitzes. Medizinalmarkt 10 (1961) 413

Sinagowitz, E., M. Reuter, H. Sommerkamp: Erfahrungen mit der Niederdruckirrigation bei der TUR (Trokar-TUR). Vortr. 19. Tg. Südwestdtsch. Ges. Urol., Frankfurt 1978.

Soanes, W. A., M. J. Gonder, S. Shulman: Apparatus and technique for cryosurgery of the prostate. J. Urol. (Baltimore) 96 (1966) 508–511

Steffens, L.: Vergleichende Statistik zur Komplikationsrate bei TUR, Kryotherapie der Prostata und Prostataadenektomie. Z. Urol. 67 (1974) 201–204

Theurer, K.: Multifaktorielle Krebstherapie mit hochmolekularen Organextrakten und tumortropen Antikörperfragmenten Phys. Med. Rehab. 12 (1971) 127

Thiel, U., G. Schwarzer, H. Krebs: Wie gefährlich ist eine transurethrale Elektroresektion der Prostata? Z. Urol. 70 (1977) 797–809

Tramoyeres Celma, A.: Criocirurgia transuretral de la próstata. Editorial Gasri, Madrid 1975

Tramoyeres Celma, A.: Actas del III. Congreso internationale de Criocirurgia 1977. Tipografia Artistica Puertes, Valencia 1978

Whitmore Jr., W. F., B. Hilaris, H. Grabstald.: Retropubic implantation of Iodine 125 in the treatment of prostatic cancer. J. Urol. (Baltimore) 108 (1972) 918–920

Whitehead, E. D.: Current Operative Urology, Harper & Row, Hagerstown 1977

Wolf, R.: 100 Jahre Cystoskop (1879–1979). Eigenverlag, Knittlingen 1979

Weyrauch, H. M.: Surgery of the Prostate, Chap. 13. Saunders, Philadelphia 1959

Recommended Readings*

Aso, Y., Yokoyama, M., Fukutani, K., Kakizoe, T.: New trial for fiberoptic cystourethroscopy: the use of metal sheath. J. Urol. *115*:99–101, 1976.

Crassweller, P. D., Farrow, G. A., Robson, C. J., Russell, J. L., Colapinto, V.: Traumatic rupture of the supramembranous urethra. J. Urol. *118*:770–771, 1977.

Datta, N. S.: Method of performing cystoscopy in patients with problem in positioning on cystoscopic table. Urology *8*:598, 1976.

Dunn, M., Smith, P. J., Abrams, P. H.: Endoscopic examination in children. Br. J. Urol. *50*:586–590, 1978.

Engel, G., Schaeffer, A. J., Grayhack, J. T., Wendel, E. F.: The role of excretory urography and cystoscopy in the evaluation and management of women with recurrent urinary tract infection. J. Urol. *123*:190–191, 1980.

Finney, R. P.: Passing Foley catheters through cystoscope sheath. Urology *10*:56, 1977.

Gonzales, E. T., Jr., Perlmutter, A. D.: In vivo trigonal measurements and their relationship to competence of the ureterovesical junction. J. Urol. *120*:338–340, 1978.

Hanani, Y., Hertz, M., Jonas, P.: Congenital urethral polyp in children. Urology *16*:162–164, 1980.

Iglesias, J. J., Kardasluan, J. F., Lauteri, V. J., Berdini, J. L., Sporer, A., Seebode, J. J.: Iglesias articulated endoscopy teaching attachment. J. Urol. *120*:465–468, 1978.

Iglesias, J. J., Sporer, A., Seebode, J. J.: Iglesias resectoscope with continuous irrigation, suction and low intravesical pressure. Br. J. Urol. *47*:683–686, 1975.

Johnson, D. K., Kroovand, R. L., Perlmutter, A. D.: The changing role of cystoscopy in the pediatric patient. J. Urol. *123*:232–233, 1980.

Johnston, J. H., Koff, S. A., Glassberg, K. I.: The pseudo-obstructed bladder in enuretic children. Br. J. Urol. *50*:505–510, 1978.

Kelami, A.: Use of extra-long urethro-cysto-resectoscope in patients with penile prostheses. Urology *13*:421, 1979.

Kimbrough, H. M., Jr., Crampton, R. S., Gillenwater, J. Y.: Cardiac rhythm in men during cystoscopy. J. Urol. *113*:846–849, 1975.

Koike, R.: A new apparatus with interchangeable lens groups for fluorescence cystoscopy, photography, biopsy and coagulation. J. Urol. *111*:31–33, 1974.

Koyanagi, T., Hisajima, S., Goto, T., Tokunaka, S., Tsuji, I.: Everting ureteroceles: radiographic and endoscopic observation and surgical management. J. Urol. *123*:538–543, 1980.

*Selected from the American and British literature of the past decade by Roland J. Kohen, M.D., F.A.C.S.

Koyanagi, T., Tsuji, I.: Endoscopic management of urethral stricture. Urology *12*:423–426, 1978.

Linker, D. G., Tanagho, E. A.: Complete external sphincterotomy: correlation between endoscopic observation and the anatomic sphincter. J. Urol. *113*:348–352, 1975.

Lockhart, J. L., Reeve, H. R., Krueger, R. P., Glenn, J. F., Henry, H. H. II: Megalourethra. Urology *12*:51–54, 1978.

Loening, S., Fallon, B., Narayana, A., Penich, G. D., Hawtrey, C., Culp, D. A., Bonney, W. W.: Urinary cytology and bladder biopsy in patients with bladder cancer. Urology *11*:591–595, 1978.

Lyon, E. S., Kyker, J. S., Schoenberg, H. W.: Trausurethral ureteroscopy in women: a ready addition to the urological armamentarium. J. Urol. *119*:35–36, 1978.

Maddocks, R. A., Leadbetter, G. W., Jr.: Absence of vesicoureteral reflux after stone basket manipulation. Reflections on iatrogenic reflux. Urology *7*:272–275, 1976.

Marshall, V. F., Seybolt, J. F.: Early detection but delayed appearance of a bladder tumor. J. Urol. *118*:175–176, 1977.

Moore, T.: Vesicoureteric reflux following endoscopic extraction of lower ureteric calculi. Br. J. Urol. *51*:357–358, 1979.

Noe, H. N., Dale, G. A.: Evaluation of children with meatal stenosis. J. Urol. *114*:455–456, 1975.

O'Dea, M. J., Malek, R. S.: Foreign body in bladder and perivesicular inflammation masquerading as pelvic lipomatosis. J. Urol. *116*:669–670, 1976.

Page, B. H., Levison, V. B., Curwen, M. P.: The site of recurrence of non-infiltrating bladder tumors. Br. J. Urol. *50*:237–242, 1978.

Rajendran, L. J., Rao, M. S., Bapna, B. C., Dutta, T. K., Reddy, M. J., Subudhi, C. L., Rao, K. M., Vaidyanathan, S.: Peripelvic extravasation and formation of perinephric urinoma after cystoscopy. Urology *16*:199–201, 1980.

Roberts, J. A.: Renal cystoscopy. Urology *8*:537–540, 1976.

Romero, R. E., Hicks, T. H., Galindo, G. H., Drach, G. W.: Evaluation of importance of cystoscopy in staging gynecologic carcinomas. J. Urol. *121*:64–65, 1979.

Silber, L. M., Ratnathicam, W., Addonizio, J. C.: Indirect-direct cystoscopy. Urology *15*:405, 1980.

Sommer, J. T., Stephens, F. D.: Dorsal urethral diverticulum of the fossa navicularis: symptoms, diagnosis and treatment. J. Urol. *124*:94–97, 1980.

Vondermark, J. S., Brannen, G. E., Wettlaufer, J. N., Modarelli, R. O.: Suprapubic endoscopic vesical neck suspension. J. Urol. *122*:165–167, 1979.

Walther, P. C., Kaplan, G. W.: Cystoscopy in children: indications for its use in common urologic problems. J. Urol. *122*:717–720, 1979.

Wise, G. J., Jensen, A.: Bivalve endoscopic sheath for direct vision insertion of urethral catheter. Urology *16*:519, 1980.

Index

(Page numbers in *italic* type refer to illustrations.)